国家卫生健康委员会"十三五"规划教材

全国高等职业教育教材

供医学检验技术专业用

医学检验技术英语

第 2 版

U0207978

主 编 张 刚

副主编 金月玲 王太重

编 者（按姓氏笔画排序）

王 敏（河南医学高等专科学校）　　张 瑞（襄阳职业技术学院）

王太重（右江民族医学院）　　　　张 燕（长治医学院）

刘 微（吉林医药学院）　　　　　张 鑫（大庆医学高等专科学校）

刘 鎏（黑龙江护理高等专科学校）　张丹丹（昆明卫生职业学院）

关 庆（哈尔滨医科大学大庆校区）　陈松建（河南医学高等专科学校）

孙秀萍（楚雄医药高等专科学校）　　金月玲（上海健康医学院）

李 晶（福建卫生职业技术学院）　　胡 南（南阳医学高等专科学校）

李 霞（黄冈职业技术学院）　　　　洪 会（安徽卫生健康职业学院）

李立胜（江苏护理职业学院）　　　　唐玉莲（右江民族医学院）

吴 怡（沈阳医学院）　　　　　　彭丽桦（四川护理职业学院）

吴思士（安徽医学高等专科学校）　　韩利伟（鹤壁职业技术学院）

张 刚（河南医学高等专科学校）　　裴聪聪（皖北卫生职业学院）

人民卫生出版社

·北 京·

图书在版编目（CIP）数据

医学检验技术英语/张刚主编. —2 版. —北京：
人民卫生出版社，2021.2（2024.7 重印）
ISBN 978-7-117-31267-7

Ⅰ.①医… Ⅱ.①张… Ⅲ.①医学检验–英语–高等
学校–教材 Ⅳ.①R446

中国版本图书馆 CIP 数据核字（2021）第 028499 号

人卫智网	www.ipmph.com	医学教育、学术、考试、健康， 购书智慧智能综合服务平台
人卫官网	www.pmph.com	人卫官方资讯发布平台

医学检验技术英语
Yixue Jianyanjishu Yingyu
第 2 版

主　　编：张　刚
出版发行：人民卫生出版社（中继线 010-59780011）
地　　址：北京市朝阳区潘家园南里 19 号
邮　　编：100021
E - mail：pmph @ pmph.com
购书热线：010-59787592　010-59787584　010-65264830
印　　刷：北京华联印刷有限公司
经　　销：新华书店
开　　本：850×1168　1/16　印张：13　插页：8
字　　数：411 千字
版　　次：2015 年 2 月第 1 版　2021 年 2 月第 2 版
印　　次：2024 年 7 月第 2 次印刷
标准书号：ISBN 978-7-117-31267-7
定　　价：45.00 元
打击盗版举报电话：010-59787491　E-mail：WQ @ pmph.com
质量问题联系电话：010-59787234　E-mail：zhiliang @ pmph.com

为了深入贯彻落实党的二十大精神,落实全国教育大会和《国家职业教育改革实施方案》新要求,更好地服务医学检验人才培养,人民卫生出版社在教育部、国家卫生健康委员会的领导和全国卫生职业教育教学指导委员会的支持下,成立了第二届全国高等职业教育医学检验技术专业教育教材建设评审委员会,启动了第五轮全国高等职业教育医学检验技术专业规划教材的修订工作。

全国高等职业教育医学检验技术专业规划教材自1997年第一轮出版以来,已历经多次修订,在使用中不断提升和完善,已经发展成为职业教育医学检验技术专业影响最大、使用最广、广为认可的经典教材。本次修订是在2015年出版的第四轮25种教材(含配套教材6种)基础上,经过认真细致的调研与论证,坚持传承与创新,全面贯彻专业教学标准,加强立体化建设,以求突出职业教育教材实用性,体现医学检验专业特色:

1. **坚持编写精品教材** 本轮修订得到了全国上百所学校、医院的响应和支持,300多位教学和临床专家参与了编写工作,保证了教材编写的权威性和代表性,坚持"三基、五性、三特定"编写原则,内容紧贴临床检验岗位实际、精益求精,力争打造职业教育精品教材。

2. **紧密对接教学标准** 修订工作紧密对接高等职业教育医学检验技术专业教学标准,明确培养需求,以岗位为导向,以就业为目标,以技能为核心,以服务为宗旨,注重整体优化,增加了《医学检验技术导论》,着力打造完善的医学检验教材体系。

3. **全面反映知识更新** 新版教材增加了医学检验技术专业新知识、新技术,强化检验操作技能的培养,体现医学检验发展和临床检验工作岗位需求,适应职业教育需求,推进教材的升级和创新。

4. **积极推进融合创新** 版式设计体现教材内容与线上数字教学内容融合对接,为学习理解、巩固知识提供了全新的途径与独特的体验,让学习方式多样化、学习内容形象化、学习过程人性化、学习体验真实化。

本轮规划教材共25种(含配套教材5种),均为国家卫生健康委员会"十三五"规划教材。

教材目录

序号	教材名称	版次	主编	配套教材
1	临床检验基础	第5版	张纪云　龚道元	√
2	微生物学检验	第5版	李剑平　吴正吉	√
3	免疫学检验	第5版	林逢春　孙中文	√
4	寄生虫学检验	第5版	汪晓静	
5	生物化学检验	第5版	刘观昌　侯振江	√
6	血液学检验	第5版	黄斌伦　杨晓斌	√
7	输血检验技术	第2版	张家忠　陶　玲	
8	临床检验仪器	第3版	吴佳学　彭裕红	
9	临床实验室管理	第2版	李　艳　廖　璞	
10	医学检验技术导论	第1版	李敏霞　胡　野	
11	正常人体结构与机能	第2版	苏莉芬　刘伏祥	
12	临床医学概论	第3版	薛宏伟　高健群	
13	病理学与检验技术	第2版	徐云生　张　忠	
14	分子生物学检验技术	第2版	王志刚	
15	无机化学	第2版	王美玲　赵桂欣	
16	分析化学	第2版	闫冬良　周建庆	
17	有机化学	第2版	曹晓群　张　威	
18	生物化学	第2版	范　明　徐　敏	
19	医学统计学	第2版	李新林	
20	医学检验技术英语	第2版	张　刚	

第二届全国高等职业教育医学检验技术专业教育教材建设评审委员会名单

主任委员

胡 野 张纪云 杨 晋

秘 书 长

金月玲 黄斌伦 窦天舒

委 员（按姓氏笔画排序）

王海河 王翠玲 刘观昌 刘家秀 孙中文 李 晖
李好蓉 李剑平 李敏霞 杨 拓 杨大干 吴 茅
张家忠 陈 菁 陈芳梅 林逢春 郑文芝 赵红霞
胡雪琴 侯振江 夏金华 高 义 曹德明 龚道元

秘 书

许贵强

数字内容编者名单

主　编　张　刚

副主编　金月玲　王太重

编　者（按姓氏笔画排序）

王　敏（河南医学高等专科学校）　　　　张　燕（长治医学院）

王太重（右江民族医学院）　　　　　　　张　鑫（大庆医学高等专科学校）

刘　微（吉林医药学院）　　　　　　　　张丹丹（昆明卫生职业学院）

刘　鎏（黑龙江护理高等专科学校）　　　陈松建（河南医学高等专科学校）

关　庆（哈尔滨医科大学大庆校区）　　　罗秀秀（右江民族医学院）

孙秀萍（楚雄医药高等专科学校）　　　　罗艳红（右江民族医学院）

李　晶（福建卫生职业技术学院）　　　　金月玲（上海健康医学院）

李　霞（黄冈职业技术学院）　　　　　　胡　南（南阳医学高等专科学校）

李北林（右江民族医学院附属医院）　　　洪　会（安徽卫生健康职业学院）

李立胜（江苏护理职业学院）　　　　　　郭子维（右江民族医学院）

吴　怡（沈阳医学院）　　　　　　　　　唐玉莲（右江民族医学院）

吴思士（安徽医学高等专科学校）　　　　彭丽桦（四川护理职业学院）

邹佳峻（右江民族医学院）　　　　　　　韩利伟（鹤壁职业技术学院）

张　刚（河南医学高等专科学校）　　　　裴聪聪（皖北卫生职业学院）

张　瑞（襄阳职业技术学院）　　　　　　潘广琴（右江民族医学院）

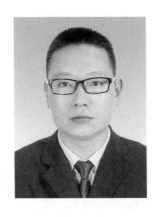

张刚,副教授,硕士,英语专业八级,英语翻译三级,河南医学高等专科学校外语教研室主任,全国职场英语考试一级培训师,全国国际商务英语考试一级培训师,全国国际商务英语考试一级口语考官。从事大学英语教学与研究工作近20年,执教大学英语精读、大学英语听力、医学英语及护理英语等课程。2015—2016年参加中国援非医疗队工作,担任英语翻译,荣获"河南省援外医疗工作先进个人"。主编教材3部,参编教材5部。主持课题6项,参与课题10余项,其中获教育部职业院校外语类专业教学指导委员会教学成果一等奖1项,河南省卫健委科研成果一等奖2项、二等奖2项,河南省社科联科研成果一等奖2项、二等奖3项。发表学术论文20余篇。

寄语:

医学检验为临床诊断、治疗疾病、预后判断等提供科学的实验室证据,是现代医学不可或缺的重要组成部分。医学检验技术英语对正确使用进口检验仪器设备和试剂、保证医学检验质量起到关键性作用。因此,掌握医学检验技术英语已经成为医学检验专业必备的职业技能。希望同学们潜心学习,掌握技能,精检细验,不断探索,在就业、升学、出国深造、修炼成为检验达人的路上为自己插上梦想的翅膀!

　　我国卫生健康事业和高等职业教育的快速发展,不仅要求医学检验工作者具备扎实的专业知识与技能,还需要具备一定的专业英语知识。本教材正是为了培养和提高医学检验技术专业学生及临床检验工作者具备阅读和理解专业英文文献的能力而编写。

　　本教材的编写团队由从事检验医学与英语教育及临床检验一线工作的专家、教授组成,以医学与英语专业博士、硕士和海归学者为主。根据党的二十大精神进教材要求和高等职业教育医学检验技术专业培养目标要求,本教材遵循"三基、五性、三特定"原则,结合医院检验科日常工作,从大量英文原始资料中精心挑选既贴近医学检验工作岗位,又方便医学检验技术专业学生及临床检验工作者学习的内容进行编写。本教材围绕医学检验专业用语选定词汇与短语并标注了美式音标,以便于学习者进行英语口语学习与交流;同时,为了培养和提高学习者对医学检验技术专业英文文献的阅读理解能力,教材结合章节内容设置了思考题、填空题和翻译题,并在附录部分附有填空题和翻译题的参考答案。

　　本教材共五章,四十七课,分别从医学检验学、实验室基本技能、临床检验技术、病理学检验技术、拓展阅读五个方面,对医学检验技术专业知识与技能进行系统地归纳和整理,围绕检验医学特定主题展开,内容相对独立,有利于教师在教学过程中根据需要选择教学内容。教材章节内容主要包括学习目标、课文导学、课文文本、生词短语、课文注释和课后练习六个部分。为了向学习者提供更优质的服务,本教材在纸质内容的基础上提供了数字内容,具体包括自学要点 PPT、正文教学 PPT、课文音频、课文翻译、单词微课和扫一扫与练一练等。

　　本教材适用于高等职业院校医学检验技术专业学生学习,还可作为临床检验工作者、临床医护人员与生物技术实验工作人员的参考书籍。

　　本教材在编写过程中参考并引用了大量英文原始资料,未能一一注明,在此向英文资料作者表示诚挚感谢!本教材的编写工作得到了全体编者所在单位领导和家人的大力支持,谨致谢忱。

　　由于水平有限,不足之处,敬请斧正。

教学大纲(参考)

张　刚

2023 年 10 月

Contents
目　录

Leading In

Medical laboratory science is a subject, which provides the basis for the prevention, diagnosis and treatment of diseases by conducting clinical tests on in vitro specimens from human body in terms of microbiology, immunology, biochemistry, hematology, cytology and molecular biology. Through the study of this chapter, you will have a basic understanding of the history, category and classification of clinical laboratory medicine, which mainly includes basic clinical laboratory medicine, clinical hematology, clinical biochemistry, clinical immunology, clinical microbiology and clinical molecular biology; you will also know about their laboratory technology, related application and development tendency, and understand how clinical testing is carried out. Furthermore, this chapter will help you establish an overall understanding of clinical laboratory medicine, which will provide the foundation for your following in-depth study.

Lesson 1   Laboratory Medicine
检验医学

Learning Objectives

After studying this lesson, students are expected to be able to

1. master the definition of clinical laboratory medicine;

2. be familiar with the general work flow of Clinical Laboratory;

3. know about the prospects of clinical laboratory medicine, the classification of medical laboratories, the constituents and functions of professional laboratories.

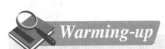 **Warming-up**

1. What is clinical laboratory medicine?

2. What is the function of Clinical Laboratory?

3. Do you know the professional laboratories in Clinical Laboratory?

Text A Clinical Laboratory Medicine
临床检验医学

As the developing trend of medical laboratory science (MLS), clinical laboratory medicine (CLM) becomes a branch of medicine. It is a science that combines clinical medicine with modern laboratory technologies, and provides an important basis for the diagnosis, management, prevention, treatment and health assessment of human diseases by conducting a series of tests on specimens from the human body and issuing test results through the clinical laboratories (either the Clinical Laboratory or laboratories in a hospital, or the independent medical laboratories).

As a bridge connecting basic medicine and clinical medicine, CLM is a comprehensively applied multidisciplinary and interdisciplinary subject based on laboratory medicine. It consists of clinical biochemistry, clinical immunology, clinical microbiology, parasitology, hematology, osology and transfusion science, etc. It is an important part of medical and health work and medical research, involving chemistry, physics, biology, biochemistry, biophysics, optics, statistics, artificial intelligence, immunology, microbiology, physiology, pathology, cytology, genetics, molecular biology and many other natural disciplines.

CLM can be generally divided into two subfields, anatomic pathology and clinical pathology, each of which can be further divided into a number of subjects. The former includes histopathology, cytopathology, electron microscopy and some relevant subjects such as anatomy, physiology, histology, pathology, pathophysiology; while the latter usually includes the following subjects: clinical microbiology, clinical chemistry, hematology, immunohematology, genetics and reproduction biology.

CLM is playing an increasingly prominent role in modern medicine. Correspondingly, clinical laboratory testing is crucial for quality medical care. Firstly, more than 70% medical decisions provided by health care personnel are based on clinical laboratory tests. Secondly, clinical laboratory tests can tailor patients care to meet individual needs and improve the quality of care. Thirdly, clinical laboratory tests can save time, costs and lives by enabling early detection and prevention of disease. Fourthly, clinical laboratory tests can provide patients with prevention, accurate diagnosis, early treatment, less invasive care, faster recovery, less disability, fewer relapses, slower disease progression, fewer complications.

In recent decades, CLM keeps pursuing high theory, high technology and high level. With the breakthrough and application of new technology in molecular biology, material science, information science and computer science, the continuous integration and innovation with other disciplines, and the development of laboratory automation, point-of-care testing (POCT) and molecular diagnostics, CLM can better serve the patients in evaluation of disease risk stratification, diagnosis of diseases, monitoring of disease, assessment of curative effect and prognosis. Thus, the function of current hospital can be well upgraded from pure treatment to prevention, health care, treatment and rehabilitation to adapt to modern medical mode.

Text B Clinical Laboratory
检验科

A medical testing laboratory refers to the medical institution with an independent legal representative where clinical tests on the specimens from humans body are performedin terms of clinical hematology and osology, clinical chemistry, clinical immunology, clinical microbiology, clinical cellular and molecular genetics and clinical pathology, and clinical test reports are issued, for the purpose of providing the relevant information for the diagnosis, management, prevention and treatment of human diseases, and for the assessment of health.

In many countries, there are two main types of laboratories for processing the majority of medical specimens. Hospital laboratories are attached to a hospital, where most of clinical decisions are based on laboratory testing, and perform tests on patients. Private (or community) laboratories receive samples from general practitioners, insurance companies, clinical research sites and other health clinics for analysis.

Clinical Laboratory is mainly responsible for the daily examinations of various human specimens from the wards, the Outpatient Department, the Emergency Department, all physical examinations and scientific researches.

In accordance with *Basic Standards for Medical Test Laboratory* issued by the National Health and Family Planning Commission (NHFPC) on July 20, 2016, Clinical Laboratory generally involves the following five professional laboratories: Clinical Hematology and Body Fluids Laboratory, Clinical Chemistry Laboratory, Clinical Immunology Laboratory, Clinical Microbiology Laboratory, and Clinical Cellular and Molecular Genetics Laboratory.

Clinical Hematology and Body Fluids Laboratory can carry out routine testing items for basic clinical tests, such as clinical blood cell number and morphological analysis, clinical hemorrhage and thrombosis analysis, clinical urine analysis, clinical stool analysis, clinical semen analysis, clinical cell number, and morphological analysis of other body fluids.

Clinical Chemistry Laboratory functions as a place for routine tests of clinical chemistry, such as liver function test, renal function test, glucose metabolism test, blood lipid test, electrolyte detection, related protein detection, related enzyme detection, and therapeutic drug monitoring.

Clinical Immunology Laboratory can do routine clinical immunization testing items, including pathogenic markers detection of infectious diseases, tumor markers detection, thyroid function detection, hormone detection, cardiac markers detection, autoimmune disease related detection, and related inflammatory factors detection.

Clinical Microbiology Laboratory is for routine clinical microbial testing items, including the cultivation, isolation and identification of various pathogenic microorganisms, and drug sensitivity testing.

Clinical Cellular and Molecular Genetics Laboratory carries out routine testing items for clinical gene amplification, including viral nucleic acid quantification of infectious diseases and detection of pathogen nucleic acids, diseases (such as tumors, genetic diseases) related gene detection, and drug-related gene detection.

New Words

specimen /ˈspesɪmən/ *n.* 样品,样本,标本

biochemistry /ˌbaɪoʊˈkemɪstri/ *n.* 生物化学

immunology /ˌɪmjuˈnɑːlədʒi/ *n.* [免疫] 免疫学

microbiology /ˌmaɪkroʊbaɪˈɑːlədʒi/ *n.* 微生物学

parasitology /ˌpærəsaɪˈtɑlədʒi/ *n.* 寄生虫学

hematology /ˌhiməˈtɑlədʒi/ *n.* [基医] 血液学

osology /oʊˈsɑlədʒɪ/ *n.* 体液学

transfusion /trænsˈfjuːʒn/ *n.* [临床] 输血,输液

physiology /ˌfɪziˈɑːlədʒi/ *n.* 生理学

pathology /pəˈθɑːlədʒi/ *n.* 病理(学)

cytology /saɪˈtɑːlədʒi/ *n.* 细胞学

genetics /dʒəˈnetɪks/ *n.* 遗传学(genetic 遗传的,基因的)

molecular /məˈlekjələr/ *adj.* 分子的,由分子组成的

anatomic /ˌænəˈtɑmɪk/ *adj.* 组织的,解剖(学)的(等于 anatomical)

histopathology /ˌhistəʊpəˈθɔlədʒi/ *n.* 组织病理学

cytopathology /ˌsaitəʊpəˈθɔlədʒi/ *n.* [病理] 细胞病理学

microscopy /maɪˈkrɑːskəpi/ *n.* 显微镜学

pathophysiology /ˌpæθoˌfɪziˈɑlədʒi/ *n.* 病理生理学

immunohematology /ˌɪmjənoˌhiməˈtalədʒi/ n. 免疫血液学

diagnostics /ˌdaɪəɡˈnɑstɪks/ n. 诊断学（用作单数）

prognosis /prɑːɡˈnoʊsɪs/ n. ［医］预后，预知（复数 prognoses）

rehabilitation /ˌriːəˌbɪlɪˈteɪʃn/ n. 复原，康复

fluid /ˈfluɪd/ n. 液体

morphological /ˌmɔːrfəˈlɑːdʒɪkl/ adj. 形态学的

hemorrhage /ˈhɛmərɪdʒ/ n. ［病理］出血（等于 haemorrhage）

thrombosis /θrɑːmˈboʊsɪs/ n. ［病理］血栓形成，血栓症（复数 thromboses）

semen /ˈsiːmən/ n. ［生理］精液，精子

electrolyte /ɪˈlɛktrəlaɪt/ n. 电解液，电解质

protein /ˈproʊtiːn/ n. 蛋白质，朊

therapeutic /ˌθerəˈpjuːtɪk/ adj. 治疗的，治疗学的

pathogenic /ˌpæθəˈdʒenɪk/ adj. 致病的，病原的，发病的（等于 pathogenetic）

infectious /ɪnˈfekʃəs/ adj. 传染的，传染性的

thyroid /ˈθaɪrɔɪd/ n. 甲状腺

autoimmune /ˌɔːtoʊɪˈmjuːn/ adj. 自身免疫的

inflammatory /ɪnˈflæmətɔːri/ adj. 炎症性的

microorganism /ˌmaɪkroʊˈɔːrɡənɪzəm/ n. ［微］微生物

sensitivity /ˈsensəˈtɪvəti/ n. 敏感，敏感度，敏感性

pathogen /ˈpæθədʒən/ n. ［基医］病原体，病原菌，致病菌

Phrases and Expressions

Clinical Hematology and Body Fluids Laboratory	临床血液与体液检验室
Clinical Chemistry Laboratory	临床化学检验室
Clinical Immunology Laboratory	临床免疫检验室
Clinical Microbiology Laboratory	临床微生物检验室
Clinical Cellular and Molecular Genetics Laboratory	临床细胞分子遗传学检验室
clinical blood cell number and morphological analysis	临床血细胞数量与形态分析检测
clinical hemorrhage and thrombosis analysis	临床出血与血栓分析检测
viral nucleic acid quantification of infectious diseases	感染性疾病病毒核酸定量
detection of pathogen nucleic acids	病原体核酸检测

Notes

1. It is a science that combines clinical medicine with modern laboratory technologies, and provides an important basis for the diagnosis, management, prevention and treatment or health assessment of human diseases by conducting a series of tests on specimens from the human body and issuing test results through the clinical laboratories (either the Clinical Laboratory or laboratories in a hospital, or the independent medical laboratories).

临床检验医学是一门将临床医学和现代实验室技术相结合，由临床实验室（既可以是医院的检验科或实验室，也可以是独立的检验所）对来自人体的标本进行一系列检验工作并出具检验结果，从而为人类疾病的诊断、管理、预防和治疗或健康评估提供重要依据的一门科学。

2. As a bridge connecting basic medicine and clinical medicine, CLM is a comprehensively applied multi-disciplinary and interdisciplinary subject based on laboratory medicine.

作为基础医学与临床医学之间的桥梁学科，临床检验医学是一门以检验医学为基础，多学科相互渗透、交叉配合的综合性应用学科。

3. CLM can be generally divided into two subfields, anatomic pathology and clinical pathology, each of

which can be further divided into a number of subjects.

临床检验医学一般分成两部分,解剖病理学和临床病理学。这两部分进一步被分为许多单元。

4. CLM is playing an increasingly prominent role in modern medicine. Correspondingly, clinical laboratory testing is crucial for quality health care.

临床检验医学在现代医学中发挥着越来越突出的作用。相应地,临床实验室检验在提供优质医疗服务中起着至关重要的作用。

5. With the breakthrough and application of new technologies in molecular biology, material science, information science and computer science, the continuous integration and innovation with other disciplines, and the development of laboratory automation, point-of-care testing (POCT) and molecular diagnostics, CLM can better serve the patients in evaluation of disease risk stratification, diagnosis of diseases, monitoring of disease, assessment of curative effect and prognosis. Thus, the function of hospital can be well upgraded from pure treatment to prevention, health care, treatment and rehabilitation to adapt to modern medical mode.

随着分子生物学、材料科学、信息科学、计算机技术新成果和新技术的应用及其与其他学科的不断融合和创新,以及实验室全自动化、即时检验(POCT)、分子诊断学技术的发展,检验医学能更好地在疾病危险性分层评价、疾病诊断、病情监测、疗效判断和预后评价中为病人服务,从而使医院由单纯的治疗向预防、保健、治疗和康复四大功能转型升级,以适应现代医学模式。

6. A medical testing laboratory refers to the medical institution with an independent legal representative where clinical tests on the specimens from humans body are performed in terms of clinical hematology and osology, clinical chemistry, clinical immunology, clinical microbiology, clinical cellular and molecular genetics and clinical pathology, and clinical test reports are issued, for the purpose of providing the relevant information for the diagnosis, management, prevention and treatment of human diseases, and for the assessment of health.

医学检验实验室指以提供人类疾病诊断、管理、预防和治疗或健康评估的相关信息为目的,对来自人体的标本进行临床检验,包括临床血液与体液检验、临床化学检验、临床免疫检验、临床微生物检验、临床细胞分子遗传学检验和临床病理检查等,并出具检验结果,具有独立法人资质的医疗机构。

7. Clinical Laboratory is mainly responsible for the daily examinations of various human specimens from the wards, the Outpatient Department, the Emergency Department, all physical examinations and scientific researches.

检验科主要承担来自病房、门诊、急诊、各类体检及科学研究的各种人体标本的日常检验检测工作。

8. In accordance with *Basic Standards for Medical Test Laboratory* issued by the National Health and Family Planning Commission (NHFPC) on July 20, 2016, Clinical Laboratory generally involves the following five professional laboratories: Clinical Hematology and Body Fluids Laboratory, Clinical Chemistry Laboratory, Clinical Immunology Laboratory, Clinical Microbiology Laboratory, and Clinical Cellular and Molecular Genetics Laboratory.

依据国家卫生和计划生育委员会 2016 年 7 月 20 日颁发的《医学检验实验室基本标准》,检验科一般设有临床血液与体液检验室、临床化学检验室、临床免疫检验室、临床微生物检验室和临床细胞分子遗传学检验室等 5 个专业实验室。

9. Clinical Microbiology Laboratory is for routine clinical microbial testing items, including the cultivation, isolation and identification of various pathogenic microorganisms, and drug sensitivity testing.

临床微生物检验室可以进行临床微生物的常规项目检测,包括:各种(型)病原微生物的培养、分离与鉴定和药物敏感性检测等。

10. Clinical Cellular and Molecular Genetics Laboratory carries out routine testing items for clinical gene amplification, including viral nucleic acid quantification of infectious diseases and detection of pathogen nu-

cleic acids, diseases (such as tumors, genetic diseases) related gene detection, and drug-related gene detection.

临床细胞分子遗传学实验室可以开展临床基因扩增等常规项目检测,具体包括:感染性疾病的病毒核酸定量及病原体核酸检测、疾病(如肿瘤、遗传性疾病)相关基因检测和药物相关基因检测等。

Exercises

Ⅰ. Fill in the blanks according to the texts.

1. CLM is a comprehensive applied multi-disciplinary and interdisciplinary subject based on _____ ____. (Text A)

2. CLM can be generally divided into two subfields, anatomic pathology and _____. (Text A)

3. More than 70% medical decisions made by health care providers are based on _____. (Text A)

4. A medical testing laboratory aims to provide the relevant information for the diagnosis, management, prevention and treatment of human diseases, and for the _____ of health. (Text B)

5. Clinical Laboratory is mainly responsible for the daily examinations of various human specimens from the wards, the Outpatient Department, the _____, all physical examinations and scientific researches. (Text B)

Ⅱ. Translate the following into Chinese.

In many countries, there are two main types of laboratories for processing the majority of medical specimens. Hospital laboratories are attached to a hospital, where most of clinical decisions are based on laboratory testing, and perform tests on patients. Private (or community) laboratories receive samples from general practitioners, insurance companies, clinical research sites and other health clinics for analysis.

Lesson 2 Basic Clinical Laboratory Medicine
临床检验基础

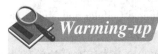 *Learning Objectives*

After studying this lesson, students are expected to be able to

1. master the ways of blood routine examination;

2. be familiar with the changes in the number of abnormal blood cells;

3. know about the procedures of specimen (blood, urine and stool) collection.

Warming-up

1. What is basic clinical laboratory medicine mainly about?

2. What is the Complete Blood Count?

3. What is the fecal occult blood test used for?

Text A Basic Clinical Laboratory Medicine
临床基础检验学

Basic clinical laboratory medicine is a branch of health science, which involves the clinical testing and analysis of the samples of tissues, blood and other body fluids from patients by using a wide variety of instruments, microscopes, computers, chemicals or other methods.

Basic clinical examinations are mainly undertaken in the Clinical Hematology and Body Fluids Laboratory in most Chinese hospitals. Basic clinical examination can obtain information about diagnosing, monitoring and treating diseases, most of which is helpful for doctors to diagnose and treat diseases. An estimated 60% of all diagnostic medical decisions are based on the results produced by basic clinical laboratory testing.

Basic clinical laboratory medicine is typically concerned with the following three aspects:

1. Study blood samples by identifying the number of cells, the cell morphology, blood type, and compatibility with other blood types;

2. Analyze body fluids, such as blood, urine, cerebrospinal fluid, serous effusion, joint effusion, semen, prostatic fluid, vaginal discharge, sputum and amniotic fluid, and record normal or abnormal findings;

3. Operate automated laboratory equipment computerized instruments capable of performing a number of clinical tests, such as microscopes and cell counters.

Basic clinical laboratory medicine has shifted from a manual, "hands-on" process providing a simple test menu to an instrument-centric, high-volume clinical engine inside the modern healthcare enterprise. Laboratory automation began in the 1950s, and its history includes the evolution of laboratory instruments, the growth of the laboratory information (management) systems (LIS or LIMS), and development of pre-analytic and post-analytic automation. Automation has been popular for clinical medical laboratory scientists as a result of the pressure of producing quicker results, improving patient care and minimizing costs. Laboratory automation is designed to maximize efficiency and minimize errors by integrating mechanical, electronic, and informatics tools to perform an ever expanding variety of laboratory tasks. Following the installation of automation error reduction rates exceed 70%, while staff time per specimen collection is reduced by over 10%.

Text B　Basic Clinical Laboratory Techniques
临床基础检验技术

Basic clinical laboratory techniques perform tests to analyze blood, urine, feces and other body fluids, providing crucial information for detecting, diagnosing, treating and monitoring diseases.

Complete Blood Count（CBC）

CBC, also called full blood count (FBC), is a test that evaluates the cells that circulate in blood. Blood consists of three types of cells suspended in fluid called plasma: white blood cells (WBCs), red blood cells (RBCs) and platelets (PLTs). A CBC is typically performed using an automated instrument that measures various parameters including counts of the cells. A standard CBC includes the following:

1. White Blood Cells

There are five different types of WBCs (i. e., neutrophils, monocytes, lymphocytes, eosinophils and basophils), with which the body can maintain a healthy state and to fight infections and other injuries. These numbers may temporarily shift higher or lower depending on what is going on in the body.

2. Red Blood Cells

Red blood cells are produced in the bone marrow and released into the bloodstream as they mature. They contain hemoglobin, a protein that transports oxygen throughout the body.

3. Platelets

Platelets, also called thrombocytes, are special cell fragments that play an important role in normal blood clotting. A person who does not have enough platelets may be at an increased risk of excessive bleeding and bruising. An excess of platelets can cause excessive clotting, or excessive bleeding if the platelets are not functioning properly.

Clinical Urine Tests

Clinical urine tests are various tests for diagnostic purposes. The target parameters that can be measured or quantified in urinalysis, including naked eye examination of color and odor tests, as well as analysis of many substances, and other properties, such as urine specific gravity.

1. Rapid urine test

A rapid urine test is the quickest way to test urine. This involves dipping a test strip with small square colored fields on it into the urine sample for a few seconds. Depending on the concentration of the particular substance you are testing, the fields on the test strip change color. Then the resulting colors of the fields are compared with a color table.

2. Urinalysis

Urinalysis is often part of a routine examination and is frequently performed when people are admitted to a hospital and before surgery. It can also be used to check abnormal results from a rapid urine test. Urinalysis can also test creatinine, bacteria, urinary casts, crystal, epithelial cells, etc.

Stool Test

A stool test analysis includes microscopic examination, chemical tests, and microbiological tests. The stool may be examined for occult blood, fat, meat fibers, bile, white blood cells, sugars and bacteria.

1. Visual examination

The patient and / or health care worker is able to make some important observations. The stool will be checked for color, consistency, amount, shape, odor, and the presence of mucus.

2. Fecal occult blood test

It can be used to diagnose many conditions that cause bleeding in the gastrointestinal system, including colorectal cancer and stomach cancer. Cancers and precancerous lesions that are ulcerated also may shed blood into the stool, which can be identified by a hemoglobin assay.

3. Microbiological test

Parasitic diseases such as ascariasis, hookworm, strongyloidiasis and whipworm can be diagnosed by examining stools under a microscope for the presence of worm larvae or eggs. Some bacterial diseases can be detected with a stool culture. Viruses such as rotavirus can also be found in stools.

New Words

cerebrospinal /ˌsɛrəbroˈspaɪnl/ *adj.* ［解剖］脑脊髓的

prostatic /ˈprɔsteitik/ *adj.* 前列腺的

vaginal /vəˈdʒaɪnl/ *adj.* ［解剖］阴道的

sputum /ˈspjuːtəm/ *n.* ［生理］痰,唾液

feces /ˈfiːsiːz/ *n.* 排泄物,粪便,渣滓

neutrophil /ˈnjuːtrəfil/ *n.* 中性粒细胞

lymphocyte /ˈlɪmfəsaɪt/ *n.* ［免疫］淋巴细胞,淋巴球

basophil /ˈbeisəfil/ *n.* 嗜碱性粒细胞

eosinophil /ˌiəˈsɪnəfɪl/ *n.* 嗜酸性粒细胞

monocyte /ˈmɑːnəsaɪt/ *n.* ［基医］单核细胞

marrow /ˈmærou/ *n.* 髓,骨髓,精华,活力

hemoglobin /ˌhɛmoˈglobɪn/ *n.* ［生化］血红蛋白(等于 haemoglobin)

assay /əˈseɪ/ *n.* 化验,试验

thrombocyte /ˈθrɑmbəˌsaɪt/ *n.* ［组织］血小板,凝血细胞

clotting /ˈklɔtiŋ/ *n.* 凝血,结块

urinalysis /ˌjʊrəˈnæləsɪs/ *n.* 尿液分析

strip /strɪp/ *n.* 条,长条

odor /ˈoʊdər/ *n.* 气味

crystal /ˈkrɪstl/ *n.* 晶体

epithelial /ˌɛpɪˈθiliəl/ *adj.* ［生物］上皮的

stool /stuːl/ *n.* 粪便

fecal /ˈfiːkl/ *adj.* 排泄物的

parasitic /ˌpærəˈsɪtɪk/ *adj.* 寄生的(等于 parasitical)

larvae /ˈlɑːrvi/ *n.* 幼虫,幼体(larva 的复数)

rotavirus /ˌrotəˈvaɪrəs/ *n.* 轮状病毒

Phrases and Expressions

fecal occult blood test	粪便隐血检验
complete blood count（CBC）/ full blood count（FBC）	全血细胞计数
urinary casts	尿管型
naked eye（unaided eye）	肉眼

Notes

1. Basic clinical laboratory medicine is a branch of health science, which involves the clinical testing and analysis of the samples of tissues, blood and other body fluids from patients by using a wide variety of instruments, microscopes, computers, chemicals or other methods.

临床基础检验学是卫生科学的一个分支,涉及使用各种仪器、显微镜、计算机、化学物品或其他方法对来自病人的组织、血液和其他体液等标本进行临床检验和分析。

2. Blood consists of three types of cells suspended in fluid called plasma: white blood cells（WBCs）, red blood cells（RBCs）and platelets（PLTs）.

血液由悬浮在血浆中的 3 种类型的细胞组成:白细胞(WBCs)、红细胞(RBCs)和血小板(PLTs)。

3. Platelets, also called thrombocytes, are special cell fragments that play an important role in normal blood clotting. A person who does not have enough platelets may be at an increased risk of excessive bleeding and bruising.

血小板,又名血栓细胞,是在正常血液凝固中起重要作用的特殊细胞碎片。没有足够血小板的人可能会增加出血和瘀伤的风险。

4. A stool test analysis includes microscopic examination, chemical tests, and microbiological tests. The stool may be examined for occult blood, fat, meat fibers, bile, white blood cells, sugars and bacteria.

粪便检测分析包括显微镜检查、化学检测和微生物检测,可以检查粪便中潜血、脂肪小滴、肌肉纤维、胆汁、白细胞、糖和细菌。

5. It can be used to diagnose many conditions that cause bleeding in the gastrointestinal system, including colorectal cancer and stomach cancer. Cancers and precancerous lesions that are ulcerated also may shed blood into the stool, which can be identified by a hemoglobin assay.

它(粪便隐血检验)可用于诊断导致胃肠系统出血的许多疾病,包括结肠直肠癌、胃癌等。癌症和溃疡性癌前病变也可使血液进入粪便,可通过血红蛋白测定法鉴定。

Exercises

Ⅰ. Fill in the blanks according to the texts.

1. Basic clinical laboratory medicine has shifted from a manual, "hands-on" process providing a simple test menu to an instrument-centric, _____ clinical engine inside the modern healthcare enterprise. (Text A)

2. Basic Clinical Laboratory Techniques perform tests to analyze blood, _____, feces and other body fluids. (Text B)

3. An excess of platelets can cause excessive clotting, or excessive bleeding if the platelets are not functioning properly, excessive_____. (Text B)

4. Cancers and precancerous lesions that are ulcerated also may shed blood into the stool, which can be identified by a_____ assay. (Text B)

5. _____ diseases such as ascariasis, hookworm, strongyloidiasis and whipworm can be diagnosed by examining stools under a microscope for the presence of worm larvae or eggs. (Text B)

Ⅱ. Translate the following into Chinese.

Red blood cells, also called erythrocytes, are produced in the bone marrow and released into the bloodstream as they mature. They contain hemoglobin, a protein that transports oxygen throughout the body.

Lesson 3 Clinical Laboratory Hematology
临床血液学检验

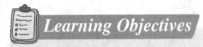

Learning Objectives

After studying this lesson, students are expected to be able to

1. master some key words, phrases and the concept of clinical hematology;
2. be familiar with the methods of hematological examination;
3. know about the relationship between clinical hematology and hematological testing;
4. understand the main idea of the whole texts.

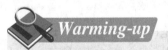

Warming-up

1. What is the relationship between hematology and hematological diseases?
2. What is the purpose of hematological examination?

Text A Clinical Hematology
临床血液学

Hematology is an independent branch of medical science, which mainly deals with blood and hematopoietic tissues. Human blood is composed of blood cells and plasma, accounting for approximately 35%-45% and 55%-65% respectively. Blood cells include red blood cells, white blood cells and platelets, which are called the formed elements of blood. Plasma is the liquid elements, and mainly composed of water (about 90%), plasma protein (about 7%), glucose, amino acid, inorganic salt and other elements (about 7%), which plays an important role in the normal physiological function of the human body.

The main function of blood is to transport nutrients and oxygen to all the tissues and organs throughout the human body, and to excrete the metabolic wastes from the body. At the same time, blood (white blood cells) has the immune-defense function, which can protest the body from bacteria, viruses, fungi, parasites and other foreign matter's invasion. In addition, blood (platelets) also owns the blood clotting function, when the human body bleeds, it plays the role of coagulation and hemostasis.

Red blood cells contain hemoglobin (Hb), which makes blood appear red. It is also the component that transports oxygen to organs, systems, tissues and cells to sustain life. Anemia is caused by an insufficient amount of red blood cells or hemoglobin. There are five types of WBCs (leukocytes): neutrophils (polymorphonuclear leukocytes, PMNLs), monocytes, lymphocytes, eosinophils and basophils. Each has a specific function to protect the body from infection. For example, neutrophil mainly responds to bacterial infection, while lymphocytes react to the virus infection. Therefore, any increase in lymphocytes and neutrophils may indicate invasive microorganisms. White blood cells, especially immature ones, are produced too much from the bone marrow then released into the peripheral blood system, which is known as leukemia.

According to the different research contents and categories, hematology can be divided into multiple sub-disciplines, including blood cell morphology, blood cell physiology, blood biochemistry, blood immunology, genetic hematology and hemorheology. In recent years, with the development of basic medical science and experimental technology, the research content and scope of hematology have been continuously deepened and extended, and many new fields of hematology research have emerged, such as blood cell biology and blood molecular biology.

Clinical hematology is a comprehensive discipline closely integrated with basic theory and clinical practice. Clinical hematology focuses on the pathogenesis, clinical manifestations, diagnosis and treatment of various blood diseases (e. g., leukemia, aplastic anemia, hemophilia and deep vein thrombosis). In addition, hematological abnormalities caused by other clinical diseases (such as liver diseases, kidney diseases, coronary heart disease, diabetes, cerebrovascular diseases, respiratory diseases, infectious diseases, immune diseases, obstetrical diseases, malignant tumors, genetic diseases, as well as surgical operations, severe trauma and drug treatment) are also studied.

Text B   Laboratory Techniques in Hematology
血液学检验技术

With the hematological theory as the basis, hematopathy as the research object, immunological, molecular and biological, chemical and physical techniques as the means and methods, laboratory techniques in hematology aims to analyze and study the pathological changes of hematopoietic organs and blood, so as to provide the experimental basis for the diagnosis, treatment and prognosis of clinical diseases.

Providing a wide variety of information, complete blood count (CBC) is the most commonly used testing method in the clinical laboratories. Most clinical laboratories, large or small, are equipped with automated instruments for CBC. Automated hemocytometer has been available in the past 30 years, and newer and more sophisticated technology has provided it with more features and expanded functions. Besides performing red blood cells, white blood cells and platelet counts, measuring hemoglobin and calculating hematocrit, the hemocytometer also distinguished each white blood cell according to the size, karyoplasm and cytoplasmic characteristics.

Flow cytometry is one of the newest technological innovations in the clinical hematology laboratory. A flow cytometer can not only count cells but also help differentiate cell types according to how cells scatter a laser light beam. Using a panel of fluorescent-labeled antibodies, a patient's lymphocytes can be divided into two major types: B lymphocytes and T lymphocytes. Then they further move on to a specific stage of development. This is essential for the accurate identification of different types of leukemia and for the provision of appropriate treatment for patients.

In recent years, with the rapid development of molecular biology technology, nucleic acid molecular hybridization, polymerase chain reaction, gene chip and proteomics technology have been widely applied in hematological examination. The laboratory prevention, diagnosis and treatment of diseases have risen from the original cell level to molecular and molecular group level. The newly-discovered molecular markers, such as blood cell CD molecules, fusion genes and small molecule non-encoded RNA, provide higher laboratory indexes of specificity and sensitivity for accurate diagnosis and division of malignant hematopathy such as leukemia and lymphoma. The development of hematologic tumors molecular biology has promoted the development of blood cell chromosome testing techniques. Developed in the 1980s, fluorescence in situ hybridization (FISH) has played an important role in the cytogenetical diagnosis of leukemia and detection of minimal residual leukemia.

New Words

hematopoietic /ˌhɛmətopɔɪˈitɪk/ *adj.* 造血的，生血的

plasma /ˈplæzmə/ *n.* ［生理］血浆

leukemia /luˈkimɪə/ *n.* ［内科］［肿瘤］白血病

carbohydrate /ˌkɑːrboʊˈhaɪdreɪt/ *n.* ［有化］碳水化合物，糖类

metabolic /ˌmetəˈbɑːlɪk/ *adj.* 变化的，新陈代谢的

anemia /əˈnimiə/ *n.* 贫血

leukocyte /ˈlʊkəˌsaɪt/ *n.* 白细胞（等于 leucocyte）

hemophilia /ˌhɛməˈfɪlɪr/ *n.* ［内科］血友病（等于 haemophilia）

diabetes /ˌdaɪəˈbiːtiːz/ *n.* 糖尿病

respiratory /ˈrespərətɔːri/ *adj.* 呼吸的

surgical /ˈsɜːrdʒɪkl/ *adj.* 外科的

hybridization /ˌhaɪbrɪdəˈzeɪʃn/ *n.* ［化学］杂交，杂化，反应

micronutrient /ˌmaɪkroˈnjʊtrɪənt/ *n.* ［生化］微量营养素

Phrases and Expressions

hematopoietic tissue	造血组织
polymerase chain reaction	聚合酶链反应
flow cytometry	流式细胞术

Notes

1. Hematology is an independent branch of medical science, which mainly deals with blood and hematopoietic tissues.

血液学是医学的一个独立分支，主要研究对象是血液和造血组织。

2. Human blood is composed of blood cells and plasma, accounting for approximately 35%-45% and 55%-65% respectively. Blood cells include red blood cells, white blood cells and platelets, which are called the formed elements of blood.

人体血液由血细胞和血浆两部分组成，分别占 35%～45% 和 55%～65%。血细胞包括红细胞、白细胞和血小板，是血液中的有形成分。

3. Plasma is the liquid elements, and mainly composed of water (about 90%), plasma protein (about 7%), glucose, amino acid, inorganic salt and other elements (about 7%), which plays an important role in the normal physiological function of the human body.

血浆是血液中的液态成分，主要由水组成（约占 90%），还含有血浆蛋白（约占 7%）、葡萄糖、氨基酸、无机盐等其他成分（约占 7%），这些成分在人体的正常生理功能当中发挥了重要的作用。

4. Clinical hematology is a comprehensive discipline closely integrated with basic theory and clinical practice. Clinical hematology focuses on the pathogenesis, clinical manifestations, diagnosis and treatment of various blood diseases (e. g. , leukemia, aplastic anemia, hemophilia and deep vein thrombosis).

临床血液学是一门与基础理论与临床实践紧密结合的综合性学科。临床血液学重点研究各种血液疾病（如白血病、再生障碍性贫血、血友病、深静脉血栓）的发病机制、临床表现、诊断和治疗。

5. With the hematological theory as the basis, hematopathy as the research object, immunological, molecular and biological, chemical and physical techniques as the means and methods, laboratory techniques in hematology aims to analyze and study the pathological changes of hematopoietic organs and blood, so as to provide the experimental basis for the diagnosis, treatment and prognosis of clinical diseases.

血液学检验技术是以血液学的理论为基础，以临床血液病为研究对象，以免疫学、分子生物学、化学、物理技术为手段和方法，来分析和研究造血器官和血液的病理变化，从而为临床疾病的诊断、治疗和预后判断提供实验依据。

6. Providing a wide variety of information, complete blood count (CBC) is the most commonly used testing method in the clinical laboratories. Most clinical laboratories, large or small, are equipped with automated instruments for CBC.

由于提供的信息丰富多样,全血细胞计数(CBC)是临床实验室中最常用的检测方法。在大多数临床实验室,无论大小,全血细胞计数都是使用自动化仪器进行的。

7. The newly-discovered molecular markers, such as blood cell CD molecules, fusion genes and small molecule non-encoded RNA, provide higher laboratory indexes of specificity and sensitivity for accurate diagnosis and division of malignant hematopathy, such as leukemia and lymphoma.

新发现的分子标志物,如血细胞 CD 分子、融合基因和小分子非编码 RNA 等,为白血病及淋巴瘤等恶性血液病的精确诊断与分型提供了更高特异性和灵敏度的实验室指标。

Exercises

Ⅰ. Fill in the blanks according to the texts.

1. Human blood is composed of blood cells and _____. (Text A)

2. WBCs include neutrophils, lymphocytes, monocytes, eosinophils, and _____. (Text A)

3. _____ is caused by a lack of red blood cells or hemoglobin. (Text A)

4. Immature leukocytes are produced too much from the bone marrow then released into the peripheral system, which is called _____. (Text A)

5. A patient's lymphocytes can be divided into two major types: _____ and T lymphocytes. (Text B)

Ⅱ. Translate the following into Chinese.

The main function of blood is to transport nutrients and oxygen to all the tissues and organs throughout the human body, and to excrete the metabolic wastes from the body. At the same time, blood (white blood cells) has the immune-defense function, which can help the body against bacteria, viruses, fungi, parasites and other foreign matter's invasion. In addition, blood (platelets) also owns the blood clotting function, when the human body bleeds, it can play the role of coagulation and hemostasis.

Lesson 4 Clinical Laboratory Biochemistry
临床生物化学检验

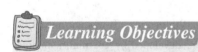 **Learning Objectives**

After studying this lesson, students are expected to be able to

1. master some key words, phrases and the testing indexes in the biochemical laboratory;

2. be familiar with common technologies used in biochemical testing;

3. know about the types of specimen in the biochemical laboratory;

4. understand the main idea of the whole texts.

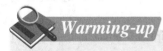 **Warming-up**

1. What are the biochemical components in the blood?

2. Why do we have to empty stomach when we have a health examination?

3. What are the diagnostic criteria for diabetes?

Text A　Clinical Biochemistry
临床生物化学

The clinical biochemistry laboratory is one of the main laboratories in a hospital. In a biochemistry laboratory, clinical laboratory staff examine the biochemical components of body fluids. The humoral specimens in this department include plasma, serum, urine, cerebrospinal fluid (CSF), peritoneal fluid, pericardial fluid, synovial fluid and other specimens. The function of the clinical biochemistry laboratory is to help the trial applicants provide interpretation of a patient's results so as to aid their diagnosis, treatment or further treatment.

Common clinical chemistry examinations are divided into basic metabolic panel (BMP) and comprehensive metabolic panel (CMP). The former is one of the most common laboratory tests ordered by health care workers. It provides critical information that can be used to assess, monitor and screen problems that patients may need to solve.

The latter is a set of 14 or more blood tests, which is served as an initial and extensive screening tool for medical staff. It is an important and comprehensive examination of kidney function, liver function, electrolyte and humoral balance. It is conceivable that CMP provides an important benchmark for a patient's basic physiology, so it is often formulated as a regular part of an annual physical examination. It is also used to monitor the status of patients with chronic diseases, such as diabetes.

Laboratory medical data influence approximately 70% of clinical decisions, especially in biochemical laboratories, and therefore require high quality analytical services. Fortunately, laboratory medical experts have successfully improved the quality of laboratory tests in recent years. The internal quality control (IQC) and external quality assessment (EQA) are implemented. The international standards (e. g., ISO 15189) are being widely adopted.

When introducing new methods and analyzers into clinical laboratories, we should also ensure that their performance meets the specified quality standards. The conventional performance indicators are as follows: analytical sensitivity, specificity, detection limit, measurement range and linearity. This is the premise to ensure that the test results are accurate.

Text B　Laboratory Techniques in Biochemistry
生物化学检验技术

As we all know, initially artificial biochemical tests began in the late 19th century. It was not until 1957 that automated instruments were put into use. The first automated analyzer, developed by Tektronix, dominated the market at an early stage.

There are many technologies that have been applied in the field of biochemistry tests, such as electrophoresis technology, absorption spectrum analysis technology, emission spectrum analysis technology, centrifugal technology, scattering spectral analysis technology, electrochemical analysis and so on. They are frequently used in the highly complex and automated instruments. With these instruments we can provide general practitioners with a relatively accurate result.

Examinations of organ and tissue diseases often include examination of liver function, kidney function, myocardial marker, pancreas disease, endocrine disease, bone disease, etc.

The liver function examination includes total protein, albumin, total bilirubin, direct bilirubin, ALT (alanine transaminase) and AST (aspartate transaminase), etc. They reflect the synthesis, biotransformation and damage status of liver cells. Although ALT is widely distributed, a significant increase in their activity in the plasma usually indicates liver damage. Therefore, ALT is often used to identify liver damage caused by inflammation or necrosis.

The renal function test includes the test of creatinine, uric acid and urea, etc. The results reflect the filtration, secretion and reabsorption functions of kidney. The medium of the experiment is serum or plasma, not urine. The principal use of uric acid measurements is in the diagnosis and treatment of gout. Hyperuricaemia is usually present in gout, but not always. In gout treatment, the monitoring of uric acid is essential.

The detection of cardiac markers includes the test of creatine kinase and troponin. The increase of concentration indicates that the heart cells are damaged to some extent.

The detection of metabolites usually includes tests of blood glucose, blood lipids, electrolytes and plasma proteins. Serum glucose level is measured to diagnose and monitor diabetes. High and low concentrations of blood sugar are all associated with glucose metabolism disorders. The patient should receive the appropriate interventions. Glucose is a dedicated energy source for erythrocytes. Therefore, the whole blood glucose decreases at the rate of 0.4 mmol/(L·h) in vitro at room temperature, unless there are glycolysis inhibitors, which will decrease if refrigerated. For this reason, specimens that measure blood sugar are usually collected in test tubes containing fluoride (as a glycolysis inhibitor) and citric acid salts, EDTA (Ethylene Diamine Tetraacetic Acid) or oxalate (as anticoagulants). Blood lipid includes cholesterol, triglycerides, etc. Abnormal blood lipid levels represent the possibility of atherosclerosis. When subjects are asked to test for blood glucose or lipids, they needed to have an empty stomach and not eat for at least eight hours.

New Words

component /kəmˈpoʊnənt/ n. 组成部分，成分，组件，元件

humoral /ˈhjʊmərəl/ adj. 体液的

performance /pərˈfɔːrməns/ n. 性能，绩效，表演，执行，表现

specificity /ˌspesɪˈfɪsəti/ n. ［免疫］特异性，特征，专一性

electrophoresis /ɪˌlɛktrofəˈrisɪs/ n. ［化学］电泳

spectrum /ˈspektrəm/ n. 光谱，频谱

myocardial /ˌmaɪəˈkɑrdɪəl/ n. 心肌衰弱

pancreas /ˈpæŋkrɪəs/ n. ［解剖］胰腺

endocrine /ˈendəkrɪn/ adj. 内分泌（腺）的 n. 内分泌，内分泌腺，内分泌物

bilirubin /ˌbɪlɪˈruːbɪn/ n. ［生化］胆红素

biotransformation /ˌbaɪoˌtrænsfɚˈmeʃən/ n. ［环境］生物转化

creatinine /kriˈætənin/ n. ［生化］肌氨酸酐，肌酸酐

urea /jʊˈriːə/ n. ［肥料］尿素

secretion /sɪˈkriːʃn/ n. 分泌（物）

reabsorption /ˌriːəbˈsɔːpʃən/ n. 再吸收

troponin /ˈtroʊpənɪn/ n. ［生化］肌钙蛋白

dedicated /ˈdedɪˌkeɪtɪd/ adj. 专用的，专注的

fluoride /ˈflɔːraɪd/ n. 氟化物

Phrases and Expressions

basic metabolic panel（BMP）	基础代谢功能检查试验组合
comprehensive metabolic panel（CMP）	代谢功能全套试验
internal quality control（IQC）	室内质量控制
external quality assessment（EQA）	室间质量评价
detection limit	检测范围（极限）
measurement range	测量范围
ALT（alanine transaminase）	谷丙转氨酶
AST（aspartate transaminase）	谷草转氨酶
EDTA（Ethylene Diamine Tetraacetic Acid）	乙二胺四乙酸

Notes

1. The humoral specimens in this department include plasma, serum, urine, cerebrospinal fluid (CSF), peritoneal fluid, pericardial fluid, synovial fluid and other specimens.

本科室的标本包括血浆、血清、尿液、脑脊液、腹膜液、心包液、滑膜液以及其他标本。

2. The latter is a set of 14 or more blood tests, which is served as an initial and extensive screening tool for medical staff. It is an important and comprehensive examination of kidney function, liver function, electrolyte and humoral balance.

后者(代谢功能全套试验)作为医务人员初步和全面筛查工具,是一个由 14 个或更多的血液测试组成的组套。它对肾功能、肝功能、电解质和体液平衡的状态进行了一个重要的综合检查。

3. When introducing new methods and analyzers into clinical laboratories, we should also ensure that their performance meets the specified quality standards. The conventional performance indicators are as follows: analytical sensitivity, specificity, detection limit, measurement range and linearity.

在将新方法和分析仪引入临床实验室时,我们还应确保其性能符合规定的质量标准。常规的性能指标如下:分析灵敏度、特异性、检出限、测量范围和线性范围。

4. There are many technologies that have been applied in the field of biochemistry tests, such as electrophoresis technology, absorption spectrum analysis technology, emission spectrum analysis technology, centrifugal technology, scattering spectral analysis technology, electrochemical analysis and so on.

有很多技术被应用在生物化学检测领域,如电泳技术、吸收光谱分析技术、发射光谱分析技术、离心技术、散射光谱分析技术和电化学分析等。

5. Examinations of organ and tissue diseases often include examination of liver function, kidney function, myocardial marker, pancreas disease, endocrine disease, bone disease, etc.

器官和组织疾病的检查通常包括肝功能、肾功能、心肌标记物、胰腺疾病、内分泌疾病、骨骼疾病的检测等。

6. The renal function test includes the test of creatinine, uric acid and urea, etc. The results reflect the filtration, secretion and reabsorption functions of kidney.

肾功能测试包括肌酐、尿酸、尿素等的测定,结果集代表了肾脏滤过、分泌和重吸收功能。

7. Glucose is a dedicated energy source for erythrocytes. Therefore, the whole blood glucose decreases at the rate of 0.4 mmol/(L·h) in vitro at room temperature, unless there are glycolysis inhibitors, which will decrease if refrigerated. For this reason, specimens that measure blood sugar are usually collected in test tubes containing fluoride (as a glycolysis inhibitor) and citric acid salts, EDTA (Ethylene Diamine Tetraacetic Acid) or oxalate (as anticoagulants).

葡萄糖是红细胞的专用能量来源,因此,体外全血中的葡萄糖在室温下以 0.4mmol/(L·h)的速率下降,除非存在糖酵解抑制剂,如果冷藏则会降低。正因如此,血糖测量通常被收集到含有氟化物(作为糖酵解抑制剂)和柠檬酸盐、乙二胺四乙酸或草酸盐(作为抗凝血剂)的试管中。

Exercises

Ⅰ. Fill in the blanks according to the texts.

1. In a biochemistry laboratory, clinical laboratory staff examine the biochemical components of _____ _____. (Text A)

2. Common clinical chemistry examinations are divided into_____ and comprehensive metabolic panel (CMP). (Text A)

3. When introducing new methods and analyzers into clinical laboratories, we should also ensure that their performance_____ the specified quality standards. (Text A)

4. The_____ examination includes total protein, albumin, total bilirubin, direct bilirubin, ALT (alanine transaminase) and AST (aspartate transaminase), etc. (Text B)

5. _____ is often used to identify liver damage caused by inflammation or necrosis. (Text B)

II. Translate the following into Chinese.

The liver function examination includes total protein, albumin, total bilirubin, direct bilirubin, ALT (alanine transaminase) and AST (aspartate transaminase), etc. They reflect the synthesis, biotransformation and damage status of liver cells. Although ALT is widely distributed, a significant increase in their activity in the plasma usually indicates liver damage. Therefore, ALT is often used to identify liver damage caused by inflammation or necrosis.

Lesson 5 Clinical Laboratory Immunology
临床免疫学检验

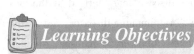
Learning Objectives

After studying this lesson, students are expected to be able to

1. master some key words and the concept of clinical immunology;
2. be familiar with the major developing direction of clinical immunology;
3. know about the structure of the immune system;
4. understand the main idea of the whole texts.

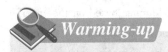
Warming-up

1. What diseases do you know correlated with the immune system?
2. Why should we get vaccinated?
3. At present, why can't humans control the diseases such as AIDS and Ebola hemorrhagic fever well?

Text A Clinical Immunology
临床免疫学

Clinical immunology is a general term for multiple subdisciplines, which combines the basic immunological theory, clinical medical diseases and immunological techniques to study the immunopathological mechanism, diagnosis and differential diagnosis, therapeutic effect evaluation, and prognosis of diseases, including immunopathology, infection immunology, transplantation immunology and tumor immunology.

The major developing direction of clinical immunology is to apply the theoretical results of basic immunological researches to the diagnosis and treatment of clinical diseases, explore the relationship between new immunological phenomena and clinical diseases, and further promote the developments of clinical immunology and related disciplines, so as to make an important contribution to human life and health.

The core of immunology is to study the structure and function of the immune system. The immune system is composed of immune organs, immune cells and immune molecules. The immune response is divided into the innate immune response and the acquired (or adaptive) immune response, the latter of which is further divided into the humoral immune response and the cellular immune response. Clinical immunology is to study the diseases caused by the immune system disorders, including multipleorgnfilure, dysfunction, and the malignant growth of cellular elements of the immune system. It also involves the diseases of other systems, and the immune responses play a role in the pathological and clinical features of these diseases.

The humoral (antibody) immune response is defined as the interaction between antibodies (immunoglob-

17

ulin) and antigens. Antibodies are special proteins that are secreted by plasma cells which differentiated from B lymphocytes when stimulated by an antigen. In human body, there are five types of antibody, known as IgA, IgD, IgE, IgG and IgM. They are all named with a prefix "Ig" that stands for immunoglobulin (another name of antibody) and differ in the biological properties, functional locations and abilities to deal with different antigens. An antigen is defined as a substance that induces the production of antibodies. Therefore, antigens are the "source" of antibodies. The specificity of antibodies and antigen responses has made it an excellent tool for detecting substances by various diagnostic techniques.

Diseases caused by the immune system disorders fall into two categories: immunodeficiency diseases and autoimmune diseases. Immunodeficiency diseases, that is, a partial loss or insufficiency of the immune system, result in the immune dysfunction. AIDS is a kind of immunodeficiency disease characterized by the lack of $CD4^+$ ("helper") T cells and macrophages, which are destroyed by HIV. Autoimmune diseases, are a kind of disease that the immune system attacks its own host's body (e. g. , systemic lupus erythematosus, rheumatoid arthritis, Hashimoto's disease and myasthenia gravis). Other diseases caused by the immune system include a variety of hypersensitivities, in which the immune system reacts inappropriately to harmless substances (e. g. , asthma and other allergies) or reacts too strongly.

Text B　Laboratory Techniques in Immunology
免疫学检验技术

Laboratory techniques in immunology is a subject that studies the immunological technology and its application in the medical testing field. The emergence of various immunological techniques based on the specific binding reactions between antigens and antibodies, allows us to detect the presence or quantity of the corresponding antigens or antibodies in clinical specimens, which can be used for the diagnosis and treatment of diseases.

The development of laboratory techniques in immunology, can be divided into three basic phages: classic immunological laboratory technology, modern immunological laboratory technology and automatic immunological laboratory technology. Classic immunological laboratory technology mainly refer to agglutination, precipitation reaction and complement fixation test. At present, agglutination (for Widal test) and precipitation reaction are still commonly used in the clinical practice. The marker immunological examination belongs to the modern immunological laboratory technology, mainly including fluoroimmunoassay, radioimmunoassay, enzyme immunoassay and chemiluminescence immunoassay. Since the 1990s, the development of the immunoassay reagents and antibodies of gene engineering has broadened the development path of immunology technology.

Based on different application purposes, immunological laboratory technology can be divided into screening tests, diagnostic tests and validation tests. Enzyme-linked immunosorbent assay (ELISA), chemiluminescence immunoassay and other screening tests are the screening tests because of low positive predictive value, which are used for clinical asymptomatic examination, such as Hepatitis C virus and HIV. The diagnostic tests for diseases with specific clinical symptoms, belong to the diagnostic tests because of high positive predictive value. Immunoblotting are usually used in the validation tests, such as the validation test for HIV.

There are a variety of immunological laboratory techniques. In the clinical practice, the most common techniques are immunoturbidimetry, marker immunolabeling technique (enzyme marker, radionuclide marker, fluorescein marker, illuminant marker, etc.) and immunoagglutination test. Different techniques are used for different markers or measurement cases. For example, immunoturbidimetry with relatively-low sensitivity is usually used for the detection of immunoglobulins and complements with high levels in the body. The immunolabeling techniques with high sensitivity are mostly used for the detection of low-level substances, such as hormones, antigens of pathogens, markers of antibodies and tumor. In certain situations, immunofluorescence technique has unique application value, such as for the autoantibody detection and rapid diagnosis of pathogen infection. As a point-of-care test, gold or selenium immunolabeling technique is widely used in emergency medicine, blood transfusion medicine and individual self-examination.

New Words

immunopathology /ˌɪmjʊnəʊpəˈθɒlədʒɪ/ *n.* 免疫病理学

acquired /əˈkwaɪrd/ *adj.* [医] 后天的, 已获得的

antibody /ˈæntɪbɒːdɪ/ *n.* [免疫] 抗体

antigen /ˈæntɪdʒən/ *n.* [免疫] 抗原

isotype /ˈaɪsəʊtaɪp/ *n.* 同型抗原

autoimmunity /ˌɔːtəʊɪˈmjuːnətɪ/ *n.* [免疫] 自身免疫(性)

hypersensitivity /ˌhaɪpərˌsensəˈtɪvətɪ/ *n.* 过敏症

allergy /ˈælərdʒɪ/ *n.* 过敏反应, 过敏症, 反感, 厌恶

detect /dɪˈtekt/ *vt.* 检测, 探测, 察觉, 发现

agglutination /əˌɡluːtənˈeʃən/ *n.* 凝集(反应), 胶合

complement /ˈkɑmpləmənt/ *n.* 补体, 补充物

fluoroimmunoassay /ˈfluərəˌɪˈmjənoˈæse/ *n.* 荧光免疫技术

radioimmunoassay /ˈrediˌɔɪmjənoˈæse/ *n.* 放射免疫检定法

immunoassay /ˌɪmjənoˈæse/ *n.* 免疫分析, 免疫测定

chemiluminescence /ˌkɛməˌlʊməˈnɛsəns/ *n.* 化学发光, 化合光

immunosorbent /ˌɪmjunəʊˈsɔːbənt/ *adj.* [生化] 免疫吸附的 *n.* 免疫吸附剂

immunoblot /ˈɪmjʊnoʊblɒt/ *n.* 免疫印迹

radionuclide /ˈrediɔˈnjʊˌklaɪd/ *n.* [核] 放射性核素

fluorescein /ˈfluɔˈrɛsiɪn/ *n.* [试剂] 荧光素, 荧光黄

immunoturbidimetry /ˌɪmjənoˌtɔːbiˈdimitri/ *n.* 免疫比浊

immunoglobulin /ˌɪmjənoˈɡlɑbjələn/ *n.* [免疫] [生化] 免疫球蛋白, 免疫血球素

immunofluorescence /ˈɪmjunəʊˌfluəˈresns/ *n.* [免疫] 免疫荧光, 免疫荧光法

autoantibody /ˌɔtoˈæntɪˌbɑdi/ *n.* [免疫] 自身抗体, 自体抗原

selenium /səˈliːniəm/ *n.* [化学] 硒

Phrases and Expressions

acquired (or adaptive) immune response	获得性(或适应性)免疫应答
AIDS (acquired immune deficiency syndrome)	艾滋病(获得性免疫缺陷综合征)
Hashimoto's disease	慢性甲状腺炎, 桥本病
myasthenia gravis	重症肌无力
Widal test	肥达试验
precipitation reaction	沉淀反应
complement fixation test	补体结合实验
enzyme-linked immunosorbent assay (ELISA)	酶联免疫吸附测定
human immunodeficiency virus (HIV)	人类免疫缺陷病毒
immunoagglutination test	免疫凝集试验
immunolabeling techniques	免疫标记技术

Notes

1. Clinical immunology is a general term for multiple subdisciplines, which combines the basic immunological theory, clinical medical diseases and immunological techniques to study the immunopathological mechanism, diagnosis and differential diagnosis, therapeutic effect evaluation, and prognosis of diseases, including

immunopathology, infection immunology, transplantation immunology and tumor immunology.

临床免疫学是将免疫学基础理论、临床医学疾病与免疫学技术相结合,用于研究疾病的免疫病理机制、诊断与鉴别诊断、评价治疗效果和判断预后的多个分支学科的总称,包括免疫病理学、感染免疫学、移植免疫学和肿瘤免疫学。

2. The major developing direction of clinical immunology is to apply the theoretical results of basic immunological researches to the diagnosis and treatment of clinical diseases, explore the relationship between new immunological phenomena and clinical diseases, and further promote the developments of clinical immunology and related disciplines, so as to make an important contribution to human life and health.

临床免疫学的主要发展方向是将基础免疫学研究所取得的理论成果应用于临床疾病的诊治,探讨新的免疫现象与临床疾病的关系,进一步推动临床免疫学与相关学科的发展,从而为人类的生命健康做出重要贡献。

3. Clinical immunology is to study the diseases caused by the immune system disorders, including multipleorgnfilure, dysfunction, and the malignant growth of cellular elements of the immune system. It also involves the diseases of other systems, and the immune responses play a role in the pathological and clinical features of these diseases.

临床免疫学研究免疫系统紊乱引起的疾病,包括功能衰竭、功能异常以及免疫系统中细胞成分的恶性生长。它还涉及其他系统的疾病,免疫反应在这些疾病的病理和临床特征中发挥作用。

4. An antigen is defined as a substance that induces the production of antibodies. Therefore, antigens are the "source" of antibodies. The specificity of antibodies and antigen responses has made it an excellent tool for detecting substances by various diagnostic techniques.

抗原被定义为能诱导产生抗体的物质。因此,抗原是产生抗体的"来源"。抗体和抗原反应的特异性,成为各种诊断技术检测物质的极好工具。

5. The development of laboratory techniques in immunology, can be divided into three basic phages: classic immunological laboratory technology, modern immunological laboratory technology and automatic immunological laboratory technology.

免疫学检验技术的发展,可大致分为经典免疫检验技术、现代免疫检验技术和自动化免疫检验技术 3 个基本阶段。

6. Based on different application purposes, immunological laboratory technology can be divided into screening tests, diagnostic tests and validation tests.

根据应用目的不同,免疫学检验技术可分为筛查试验、诊断试验和确认试验。

7. There are a variety of immunological laboratory techniques. In the clinical practice, the most common techniques are immunoturbidimetry, marker immunolabeling technique (enzyme marker, radionuclide marker, fluorescein marker, illuminant marker, etc.) and immunoagglutination test.

免疫学检验技术多种多样。在临床实践中,最常见的有免疫比浊、标记免疫技术(酶标记、放射性核素标记、荧光素标记、发光物标记等)和免疫凝集试验。

Exercises

Ⅰ. Fill in the blanks according to the texts.

1. Clinical immunology includes _____, infection immunology, transplantation immunology and tumor immunology. (Text A)

2. The immune system consists of immune organs, immune cells and immune _____. (Text A)

3. In human body, there are five types of _____, known as IgA, IgD, IgE, IgG and IgM. (Text A)

4. Classic immunological laboratory techniques are mainly _____, precipitation reaction and complement fixation test. (Text B)

5. As a point-of-care test, gold or selenium standard _____ technique is widely used in emer-

gency medicine, blood transfusion medicine and individual self examination. (Text B)

Ⅱ. Translate the following into Chinese.

Laboratory techniques in immunology is a subject that studies the immunological technology and its application in the medical testing field. The emergence of various immunological techniques based on the specific binding reactions between antigens and antibodies, allows us to detect the presence or quantity of the corresponding antigens or antibodies in clinical specimens, which can be used for the diagnosis and treatment of diseases.

Lesson 6   Clinical Laboratory Microbiology
临床微生物学检验

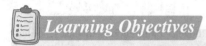

After studying this lesson, students are expected to be able to

1. master the techniques of Gram staining;
2. be familiar with the bacterial culture techniques;
3. know about the principle of antibiotic susceptibility testing;
4. use the Gram staining to study bacterial cell morphology properly.

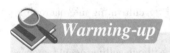

1. What are the main types of microbial culture media?
2. What is the antibiotic susceptibility testing?
3. What is the principle of Gram staining?

Text A   Clinical Microbiology
临床微生物学

Clinical microbiology, as a major branch of medical microbiology, is a medicine-related subject that deals with the prevention, diagnosis and treatment of infectious diseases. There are three kinds of microorganisms causing infectious disease, i. e., bacteria, fungi and viruses, and clinical microbiology is the study of the three pathogens which are of great medical importance to humans.

Clinical microbiology mainly studies the characteristics, the transmission methods, the infection and growth mechanisms of pathogens. Clinical microbiology concentrates on the etiological diagnosis and drug sensitivity of clinical specimens to detect the presence of infectious diseases. The diagnosis of infections may involve clinical specimens isolated from humans, animals or foods, as well as the samples collected from the environment.

The research of clinical microbiology includes molecular and cellular biology of pathogenic bacteria, pathogenesis, clinical manifestations of infectious diseases, epidemiology, diagnosis and treatment, which is beneficial for disease treatment. Clinical microbiologists often serve as the consultants for physicians, provide the identification of pathogens and suggestion for treatment options. In addition, they take on the tasks of recognizing the potential health risks, monitoring the evolution of potentially virulent or drug-fast strains of microbes, and assisting the health care in the community. They can also assist in preventing or controlling epidemics and the outbreaks of diseases.

In the past, culture-based laboratory techniques on microorganisms have been the identification standard for the clinical microbiology laboratory. Recently, a real-time quantitative PCR that can simultaneously detect multiple nucleic acid target sequences has been proved to be of high sensitivity and specificity in the detection of clinical microorganisms, which is superior in testing performance to the traditional culture methods and routine PCR methods.

Text B Laboratory Techniques in Microbiology
微生物学检验技术

Clinical laboratory microbiology offers diagnostic testing and consultative services for infectious diseases caused by bacteria, mycobacteria, fungi, and viruses. In addition, it performs antimicrobial and antifungal susceptibility testing, to direct anti-infective therapy.

Microbial culture

Microbiological culture is the primary method used for isolating pathogens of infectious diseases. Selective medium or identification of the growth of medium microorganism is to test if the specific pathogen exists in tissue or fluid samples. The three main types of media used for testing are listed as follows:

1. Solid media: A solid surface is combined with the mixture of nutrients, salts and agar at a concentration of 1.5%-2.0%. A single microbe on an agar plate can then grow into colonies containing thousands of cells. Solid medium can be used for isolating bacteria or for determining the colony characteristics of the isolate.

2. Semisolid media: They are prepared with agar at concentrations of 0.5% or less. They have some properties of solids, and some properties of liquids. Semisolid media are useful for cultivating microaerophilic bacteria or for determination of bacterial motility.

3. Liquid media: These media contains specific amounts of nutrients but without gelling agents such as gelatin or agar. Microorganisms can grow in liquid medium. Broth medium serves various purposes (e. g., enrichment and fermentation studies) and other different tests (e. g., sugar fermentation test and MR-VR broth test).

Gram staining

Gram staining, also called Gram's staining method, is a method of staining used to distinguish bacterial species. According to Gram's staining method, bacteria is classified into two large groups (Gram-positive and Gram-negative) based on the physical characteristics of cell wall. The name came from the Danish bacteriologist Hans Christian Gram, who first invented and used this technique. Gram staining is always used as the first step to preliminarily identify bacterial organisms. The process involves four steps:

1. Make a slide of bacteria sample to be stained. Then fasten the sample to the slide by carefully passing the slide with a small piece of sample on it through alcohol lamp flame three times;

2. Add the primary stain (crystal violet) to the sample or slide and incubate for 1 minute. Rinse slide with a gentle stream of water to remove unbound crystal violet. Add Gram's iodine for 1 minute. Wash the slide with gentle water again.

3. Rinse sample or slide with acetone or alcohol for 30 seconds and rinse with a gentle stream of water.

4. Add the secondary stain safranin to the slide and incubate for 1 minute. Add a drop of immersion oil on the stained sample and observe under the oil immersion objective.

Antibiotic Susceptibility Testing

Antibiotic susceptibility testing (AST) examines the susceptibility of bacteria to different antibiotic agents. AST is usually carried out to determine which antibiotic will be most successful in treating a bacterial infection in vivo. There are two possible ways to get an antibiogram.

1. A semi-quantitative way based on diffusion (Kirby-Bauer method): small discs containing different antibiotics are laid in different zones of the culture on an agar plate. The antibiotic will diffuse in the area sur-

rounding each tablet, and a disc of bacterial lysis will become visible. Since the concentration of the antibiotic was the highest at the centre, and the lowest at the edge of this zone, the diameter is suggestive for the minimum inhibitory concentration (MIC).

2. A quantitative way based on dilution: A dilution series of antibiotics is established. The last vial in which no bacteria grow contains the antibiotic at the MIC.

New Words

bacteria /bæk'tɪrɪə/ *n.* ［微］细菌

fungi /'fʌndʒaɪ/ *n.* 真菌(fungus 的复数)

virus /'vaɪrəs/ *n.* 病毒

epidemiology /ˌepɪˌdiːmi'ɑːlədʒi/ *n.* 流行病学,传染病学

physician /fɪ'zɪʃn/ *n.* 医师,内科医师

virulent /'vɪrələnt/ *adj.* 剧毒的

mycobacteria /ˌmaikəubæk'tiəriə/ *n.* ［微］分枝杆菌

agar /'eɪɡɑːr/ *n.* 琼脂

motility /məʊ'tɪlətɪ/ *n.* 运动性

fermentation /f3ːmen'teɪʃ(ə)n/ *n.* 发酵

safranin /'sæfrənɪn/ *n.* 盐基性红色染料

antibiotic /ˌæntibaɪ'ɑːtɪk/ *n.* 抗生素 *adj.* 抗菌的

lysis /'laɪsɪs/ *n.* (生物)溶胞,溶菌,溶解,分解

Phrases and Expressions

Gram staining	革兰氏染色
crystal violet	结晶紫(试剂)
immersion oil	镜油
antibiotic susceptibility testing (AST)	抗生素药物敏感性试验
minimum inhibitory concentration (MIC)	最小抑菌浓度,最低抑菌浓度

Notes

1. Clinical microbiology, as a major branch of medical microbiology, is a medicine-related subject that deals with the prevention, diagnosis and treatment of infectious diseases.

临床微生物学,作为医学微生物学的一大分支,是研究传染性疾病预防、诊断和治疗的一门与医学相关的学科。

2. The research of clinical microbiology includes molecular and cellular biology of pathogenic bacteria, pathogenesis, clinical manifestations of infectious diseases, epidemiology, diagnosis and treatment, which is beneficial for disease treatment.

临床微生物学的研究包括致病菌分子和细胞生物学、发病机制,感染性疾病的临床表现、流行病学、诊断和治疗,这些信息有助于疾病的治疗。

3. Microbiological culture is the primary method used for isolating pathogens of infectious diseases. Selective medium or identification of the growth of medium microorganism is to test if the specific pathogen exists in tissue or fluid samples.

微生物培养是在实验室中分离感染性疾病病原体的主要方法,通过选择性培养基或鉴别培养基中微生物的生长情况,来判定待检测组织或体液样品中是否存在特定病原体。

4. Gram staining, also called Gram's staining method, is a method of staining used to distinguish bacterial species. According to Gram's staining method, bacteria is classified into two large groups (Gram-positive and Gram-negative) based on the physical characteristics of cell wall.

革兰氏染色,也称为革兰氏染色法,是一种用于鉴别细菌的染色方法。根据细胞壁的物理特性,革兰氏染色将细菌分为两大种类(革兰氏阳性菌和革兰氏阴性菌)。

5. Antibiotic susceptibility testing (AST) examines the susceptibility of bacteria to different antibiotic agents. AST is usually carried out to determine which antibiotic will be most successful in treating a bacterial infection in vivo.

抗生素药物敏感性试验(AST)是细菌对不同抗生素的敏感性实验。AST 也通常被用来确定哪种抗生素在体内治疗细菌感染方面会取得最佳效果。

6. The antibiotic will diffuse in the area surrounding each tablet, and a disc of bacterial lysis will become visible.

抗生素将在每个药片周围的区域扩散,就可观察到细菌抑菌圈。

7. A dilution series of antibiotics is established. The last vial in which no bacteria grow contains the antibiotic at the MIC.

建立抗生素系列稀释梯度,没有细菌生长的最后一个小瓶含有的抗生素浓度为最小抑菌浓度。

Exercises

Ⅰ. Fill in the blanks according to the texts.

1. There are three kinds of microorganisms causing infectious disease: bacteria, fungi and _____. (Text A)

2. _____ culture is the primary method used for isolating pathogens of infectious diseases. (Text B)

3. Semisolid media are useful for the cultivation of microaerophilic bacteria or for determination of bacterial_____. (Text B)

4. A semi-quantitative way based on_____ (Kirby-Bauer method): small discs containing different antibiotics are laid in different zones of the culture on an agar plate. (Text B)

5. Since the concentration of the antibiotic was the highest at the centre, and the _____ at the edge of this zone, the diameter is suggestive for the minimum inhibitory concentration (MIC). (Text B)

Ⅱ. Translate the following into Chinese.

Gram staining, also called Gram's staining method, is a method of staining used to distinguish bacterial species. According to Gram's staining method, bacteria is classified into two large groups (Gram-positive and Gram-negative) based on the physical characteristics of cell wall. The name came from the Danish bacteriologist Hans Christian Gram, who first invented and used this technique. Gram staining is always used as the first step to preliminarily identify bacterial organisms.

Lesson 7 Clinical Laboratory Molecular Biology
临床分子生物学检验

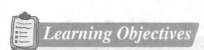

Learning Objectives

After studying this lesson, students are expected to be able to

1. master the main tasks and aims of clinical laboratory molecular biology;

2. be familiar with the core techniques, including amplification technique, molecular hybridization technique and sequencing technique;

3. know about the clinical application prospects of laboratory techniques in molecular biology.

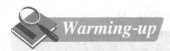

Warming-up

1. How do we predict the risk of breast cancer?
2. What is the technology applied in noninvasive prenatal screening?

Text A   Clinical Molecular Biology
临床分子生物学

In 1940, Pauling found a E6V mutation in hemoglobin, i. e., the valine replacement of the glutamic acid, to be the cause of disease for sickle cell anemia. In 1959, Jerome identified the first chromosomal disorder-trisomy 21 syndrome (Down's syndrome). Since then, scientists began to understand the nature of diseases-genetic variation or defects, which ushered in an era of molecular clinical medicine. In accordance with the central dogma, clinical molecular biology studies association between structures and functions of human disease-related biomolecules as well as the occurrence and development of diseases at genome, transcriptome, proteome and metabolome levels. It addresses two major issues: to elucidate the molecular mechanism of occurrence and development of diseases and to provide effective measures for the diagnosis, treatment and prevention of diseases. The clinical molecular biology has a broad spectrum of application:

Molecular diagnosis of infectious diseases

As genomes of various pathogenic microorganisms have been "decoded", molecular biological technology allows for not only a definite diagnosis of microbial infection, but also typing and drug resistance test of infectious pathogens. At present, molecular diagnosis has been applied to widespread infectious diseases, such as viral hepatitis, AIDS, influenza and tuberculosis.

Molecular diagnosis of genetic diseases

Diseases caused by abnormality of genetic material (gene or chromosome) are called genetic diseases. All genetic diseases are related to the mutations of one or more genes. By analyzing alterations of DNA, RNA, protein and metabolite from patients, occurrence and development relevant biomarkers (e. g., genotype, genetic mutation and karyotype) of specific genetic diseases could be revealed. Molecular biological technology is often used in prenatal diagnosis. Before the birth of a fetus, certain genetic diseases of the fetus can be predicted by analyzing some pathogenic genes.

Molecular diagnosis of tumors

Tumorigenesis-relative gene includes oncogene and suppressor. Activation of oncogene and inactivation of suppressor are important mechanisms of tumorigenesis. Through detection of structures, copy numbers and expression products of these genes, early diagnosis, treatment and prognosis analysis of tumor disease would be greatly improved in clinical practice. For example, the risk of breast cancer can be predicted by detection of the mutations of HER2 and ER genes.

Molecular diagnosis in pharmacogenetics

Pharmacogenetics means that the effect of a drug in a specific patient's body depends on his genes. The metabolic differences of the same drug in different individuals lead to different drug effects. Molecular biological detection of pharmacogenetics will help provide an accurate drug treatment regimen for clinical practice. For example, doctors can determine the metabolic capacity of patients to warfarin and adopt an appropriate therapeutic dose by detecting the mutations of CYP2C9 and VKORC1.

Text B   Laboratory Techniques in Molecular Biology
分子生物学检验技术

Laboratory techniques in molecular biology are defined as a disease-oriented new generation techniques which targets biomolecular markers. It focuses mostly on nucleic acids. By analyzing alterations of structures and expressions of relevant genes, these techniques provide accurate information for the diagnosis, treatment and prediction of disease. There are mainly three core techniques: amplification technique, molecular hybridization technique and sequencing technique.

Amplification technique

Polymerase chain reaction (PCR) technique invented by Mullis brings about the way of DNA amplification in vitro. It is capable of detecting trace amounts of genes and has been widely applied in clinical diagnosis, forensic identification and archaeology. Clinically, the real-time fluorescent quantitative PCR (RT-PCR) developed on the basis of PCR technology has achieved a breakthrough in molecular biological analysis from qualitatively to quantitatively and used for nucleic acid quantification and analysis of mRNA expression level.

Molecular hybridization technique

Molecular hybridization refers to the process of two single-stranded nucleic acids (DNA or RNA) with heterogenous sequences to form a heteroduplex complying with the principle of complementary base pairing. The most commonly used molecular hybridization techniques included the in-situ hybridization (ISH) and chip techniques. ISH is often used for chromosome abnormality detection, gene mutation analysis and gene diagnosis of leukemia. Chip technology is often used in drug screening, gene typing and SNP detection.

Sequencing technique

The first-generation sequencing technique, the dideoxy chain termination method, was invented by Sanger et al. It is accurate in reading sequence and suitable for sequencing repetitive regions of the genome, while the disadvantage is that it detects only one sequence each time. It is mainly applied in detection of gene mutations.

The second-generation sequencing technique, principally, slices the sequence into small segments, which would further go through PCR amplification with simultaneous sequencing. Bases are detected by capturing newly synthesized end labels and millions of sequences can be concurrently detected by this method. The second-generation sequencing technology has been applied in non-invasive prenatal screening. The method is not only safe but also highly accurate to determine whether the fetus has genetic diseases by detecting the free DNA of the fetus in the plasma of pregnant women.

The third-generation sequencing technique, also called single-molecule sequencing technique, abandoned PCR enrichment while cast separate sequencing on every single sequence. It can be used in whole genome sequencing, transcriptome sequencing, miRNA sequencing and DNA methylation analysis, etc.

Detection methods of clinical molecular biology have been undergoing rapid developments, from qualitative detection to quantitative detection, low throughput to high throughput sequencing, and manual operation to automation.

New Words

mutation /mjuˈteʃən/ *n.* 突变

biomolecule /ˌbaɪəʊˈmɒlɪkjuːl/ *n.* 生物分子

genome /ˈdʒiːnoʊm/ *n.* 基因组,染色体组

transcriptome /trænskˈrɪptɒm/ *n.* 转录组

proteome /ˈprəʊtɪəʊm/ *n.* 蛋白质组

metabolome /metæboʊˈlɒm/ *n.* 代谢组

influenza /ˌɪnfluˈɛnzə/ *n.* [内科] 流行性感冒(简写 flu),家畜流行性感冒

tuberculosis /tuːbɜːrkjəˈloʊsɪs/ *n.* 肺结核

chromosome /ˈkroʊməsoʊm/ *n.* [遗] [细胞] [染料] 染色体

biomarker /ˈbaɪɒmɑːkər/ *n.* 生物标志物

genotype /ˈdʒenətaɪp/ *n.* 基因型,遗传型

karyotype /ˈkærɪəˌtaɪp/ n. 核型

tumorigenesis /ˌtʊmərəˈdʒɛnɪsɪs/ n. 肿瘤发生

oncogene /ˈɑŋkəˌdʒin/ n. ［遗］［肿瘤］致癌基因

pharmacogenetics /ˌfɑrməkodʒəˈnɛtɪks/ n. 遗传药理学

warfarin /ˈwɔːrfərɪn/ n. 华法林

amplification /ˌæmplɪfɪˈkeɪʃn/ n. ［电子］扩增

sequencing /ˈsiːkwənsɪŋ/ n. ［计］排序，测序

archaeology /ˌɑːrkɪˈɑːlədʒi/ n. 考古学

heteroduplex /ˌhetərəʊˈdjuːpleks/ adj. 异源双链核酸分子的

dideoxy /ˈdɪdiːˌɒksɪ/ n. 双脱氧法

simultaneous /ˌsaɪmlˈteɪnɪəs/ adj. 同时的，联立的，同时发生的

fetus /ˈfiːtəs/ n. 胎儿

methylation /ˌmeθɪˈleɪʃən/ n. ［有化］甲基化，甲基化作用

throughput /ˈθruːpʊt/ n. 生产量，生产能力，通量，吞吐量

Phrases and Expressions

sickle cell anemia	镰状细胞贫血
Trisomy 21 syndrome（Down's syndrome）	21 三体综合征（唐氏综合征）
central dogma	中心法则
drug resistance test	耐药性检测
genetic disease	遗传病
in-situ hybridization	原位杂交
the first-generation sequencing technique	第一代测序技术
non-invasive prenatal screening	无创产前筛查

Notes

1. In accordance with the central dogma, clinical molecular biology studies association between structures and functions of human disease-related biomolecules as well as the occurrence and development of diseases at genome, transcriptome, proteome and metabolome levels.

临床分子生物学遵循生物体的中心法则，从基因组、转录组、蛋白质组、代谢物组等水平研究人类疾病相关的生物分子的结构、功能与疾病发生发展之间的关系。

2. As genomes of various pathogenic microorganisms have been "decoded", Molecular biological technology allows for not only a definite diagnosis of microbial infection, but also typing and drug resistance test of infectious pathogens. At present, molecular diagnosis has been applied to many widespread infectious diseases, such as viral hepatitis, AIDS, influenza and tuberculosis.

随着多种病原微生物的基因组被"破译"，分子生物学技术不仅可以对微生物感染作出确诊，还可以对感染性病原体进行分型和耐药性检测。目前，分子诊断已经应用于很多传播广泛的传染性疾病，如病毒性肝炎、艾滋病、流感和结核病等。

3. All genetic diseases are related to the mutations of one or more genes. By analyzing alterations of DNA, RNA, protein and metabolite from patients, occurrence and development relevant biomarkers (e. g., genotype, genetic mutation and karyotype) of specific genetic diseases could be revealed.

遗传性疾病的分子诊断是通过分析病人体内遗传物质的结构或表达水平的变化，揭示与该遗传病发生发展相关的生物标志物（如基因型、基因突变和染色体核型）。

4. Tumorigenesis-relative gene includes oncogene and suppressor. Activation of oncogene and inactivation of suppressor are important mechanisms of tumorigenesis.

与肿瘤发生相关的基因有癌基因和抑癌基因，癌基因的激活与抑癌基因的失活是引发肿瘤的重

要机制。

5. The metabolic differences of the same drug in different individuals lead to different drug effects. Molecular biological detection of pharmacogenetics will help provide an accurate drug treatment regimen for clinical practice.

同种药物在不同个体存在代谢差异,导致药效不同。药物遗传学的分子生物学检测为临床提供准确的药物治疗方案。

6. Clinically, real-time fluorescent quantitative PCR (RT-PCR) developed on the basis of PCR technology has achieved a breakthrough in molecular biological analysis from qualitatively to quantitatively and used for nucleic acid quantification and analysis of mRNA expression level.

临床上,以 PCR 技术为基础发展起来的实时荧光定量 PCR,实现了分子生物学检验从定性到定量的突破,用于核酸定量和 mRNA 表达水平分析。

7. Molecular hybridization refers to the process of two single-stranded nucleic acids (DNA or RNA) with heterogenous sequences to form a heteroduplex complying with the principle of complementary base pairing.

分子杂交是指异源序列的两条核酸单链(DNA 或 RNA),按照碱基互补配对原则形成异质双链的过程。

8. The first-generation sequencing technique, the dideoxy chain termination method, was invented by Sanger et al. It is accurate in reading sequence and suitable for sequencing repetitive regions of the genome, while the disadvantage is that it detects only one sequence each time.

第一代测序技术,双脱氧链末端终止法,是由 Sanger 等人发明的。这种方法的优点是读取序列准确,适合重复序列测序,缺点是每次只能检测单一序列。

9. The second-generation sequencing technique, principally, slices the sequence into small segments, which would further go through PCR amplification with simultaneous sequencing. Bases are detected by capturing newly synthesized end labels and millions of sequences can be concurrently detected by this method.

第二代测序技术是将待测序列剪切成小片段,在利用 PCR 富集序列的同时进行测序,通过捕捉新合成的末端标记来确定碱基,这种方法可以同时检测几百万条序列。

10. The third-generation sequencing technique, also called single-molecule sequencing technique, abandoned PCR enrichment while cast separate sequencing on every single sequence.

第三代测序技术也称单分子测序技术,这种方法不需要进行 PCR 富集,实现了对每一条序列的单独测序。

Exercises

Ⅰ. Fill in the blanks according to the texts.

1. Tumorigenesis-relative gene includes oncogene and suppressor. _____ of oncogene and inactivation of suppressor are important mechanisms of tumorigenesis. (Text A)

2. Diseases caused by abnormality of genetic material (gene or chromosome) are called _____. (Text A)

3. Clinically, real-time fluorescent quantitative PCR (RT-PCR) developed on the basis of the PCR technology has achieved a breakthrough in molecular biological analysis from qualitatively to _____ and used for nucleic acid quantification and analysis of mRNA expression level. (Text B)

4. The most commonly used molecular hybridization techniques included the in-situ hybridization (ISH) and _____. (Text B)

5. The method is not only safe but also highly accurate to determine whether the fetus has genetic diseases by detecting the free _____ of the fetus in the plasma of pregnant women. (Text B)

Ⅱ. Translate the following into Chinese.

The first-generation sequencing technique, the dideoxy chain termination method, was invented by Sanger et al. It is accurate in reading sequence and suitable for sequencing repetitive regions of the genome, while the disadvantage is that it detects only one sequence each time.

笔记

Chapter II　Basic Skills in the Laboratory
实验室基本技能

Leading In

Through the study of this chapter, you will learn the basic skills, related medical knowledge and terms involved in the clinical laboratory. You will have the ability to identify the types of laboratory biohazards and occupational exposure risks in the laboratory, have the concept of aseptic techniques and understand the uses of clinical reagents, standard solutions and in vitro diagnostic reagents. Moreover, you will be able to know the process flow of clinical specimens and the basic principles and uses of experimental instruments, know about the significance of medical equipment calibration and test validity, and largely understand the benefits of External Quality Assessment.

Lesson 1　Laboratory Safety—Everyone is Responsible
实验安全人人有责

Learning Objectives

After studying this lesson, students are expected to be able to

1. master some medical words and terms about biological hazards;
2. be familiar with the types ofbiological hazards in the clinical laboratory;
3. know about the risks of occupational exposure.

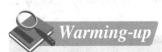

1. What do biological hazards include?
2. What do Level 1 and Level 4 stand for?
3. What is occupational exposure?

Text A　Laboratory Hazards
实验危害

In some laboratories, the conditions are no more dangerous than in any other room. In many labs, however, hazards are present. Laboratory hazards are as varied as the subjects of study in laboratories, and might include extreme temperatures; lasers, strong magnetic fields or high voltage; flammable; explosive; or radioactive materials; poisons; infectious agents. Biological hazards primarily refer to biological substances that pose a threat to the health of humans. This can include medical waste or samples of a microorganism, virus or toxin (from a biological source) that can impact human health. It can also include substances harmful to animals. The United States' Centers for Disease Control and Prevention (CDC) categorizes various diseases in levels of biohazard. Level 1 is minimum risk and Level 4 is extreme risk. Laboratories and other facilities are categorized as BSL (Biosafety Level) 1-4 or as P1 through P4 for short (Pathogen or Protection Level).

In the laboratories where dangerous conditions might exist, safety precautions are important. The Occupational Safety and Health Administration (OSHA) in the United States have tailored a standard for occupational exposure to hazardous chemicals in laboratories, due to the unique characteristics of the laboratory workplace. This standard is often referred to as the "Laboratory Standard". Under this standard, a laboratory is required to produce a Chemical Hygiene Plan (CHP) which addresses the specific hazards found in its location, and its approach to them.

A clinical laboratory means a workplace where diagnostic or other screening procedures are performed on blood or other potentially infectious materials. In any laboratory where work involves the use of and / or exposure to human blood, certain other body fluids, or unfixed human tissue, there is the danger of exposure to bloodborne pathogens, the disease-causing microorganisms that may be found in such materials. Working with any of these materials in a laboratory setting usually requires that workers be enrolled in the Bloodborne Pathogens Program. The Bloodborne Pathogens Program requires each department or laboratory to develop an Exposure Control Plan documents how the risk of exposure will be reduced or eliminated. These rules must be followed at all times.

Text B　Occupational Exposure
职业暴露

Occupational exposure means reasonably anticipated skin, eye, mucous membrane, or parenteral contact with blood or other potentially infectious materials that may result from the performance of an employee's duties. Bacteria, viruses and other microorganisms have the potential to cause illness in a number of exposure situations if the proper precautions and procedures are not in place. Universal precautions shall be observed to prevent contact with blood or other potentially infectious materials. Under circumstances in which differentiation between body fluid types is difficult or impossible, all body fluids shall be considered potentially infectious materials.

Needleless system is a device that does not use needles for: (1) the collection of body fluids or withdrawal of body fluids after initial venous or arterial access is established; (2) the administration of medication or fluids; (3) any other procedure involving the potential for occupational exposure to bloodborne pathogens due to percutaneous injuries from contaminated sharps.

Other potentially infectious materials include: (1) the following human body fluids, i. e., semen, vaginal discharge, cerebrospinal fluid, synovial fluid, pleural fluid, pericardial fluid, peritoneal fluid, amniotic fluid, saliva in dental procedures, any body fluid that is visibly contaminated with blood, and all body fluids in situations where it is difficult or impossible to differentiate between body fluids; (2) any unfixed tissue or organ (other than intact skin) from a human (living or dead); (3) cell or tissue cultures and organ cultures with human immunodeficiency virus (HIV), culture medium or other solutions with HIV or hepatitis B virus (HBV), and blood, organs, or other tissues from experimental animals infected with HIV or HBV.

New Words
flammable /ˈflæməbl/ *adj.* 易燃的,可燃的
explosive /ɪkˈsploʊsɪv/ *adj.* 爆炸(性)的
radioactive /ˌreɪdioʊˈæktɪv/ *adj.* [核] 放射性的

tailor /ˈteɪlər/ v. 量身定制，使合适，使适应

address /əˈdres/ v. 演说，从事，提出

borne /bɔːrn/ v. 忍受，负荷

enroll /ɪnˈroʊl/ v. 参加，登记

anticipated /ænˈtɪsəˌpetɪd/ adj. 预期的，期望的

mucous /ˈmjuːkəs/ adj. 黏液的

membrane /ˈmembreɪn/ n. 膜，薄膜

parenteral /pəˈrentərəl/ adj. 肠胃外的

precaution /prɪˈkɔːʃn/ n. 预防（措施），警惕

differentiation /ˌdɪfəˌrenʃiˈeɪʃn/ n. ［生物］变异，分化，区别

device /dɪˈvaɪs/ n. 设备，仪器

venous /ˈviːnəs/ adj. 静脉的

arterial /ɑːrˈtɪriəl/ adj. ［解剖］动脉的，干线的

access /ˈækses/ n. 通道，进入，机会 v. 接近，使用，访问

administration /ədˌmɪnɪˈstreɪʃn/ n. 管理，行政

medication /ˌmedɪˈkeɪʃn/ n. 药物治疗，药物

percutaneous /ˌpɜːrkjuːˈteɪniəs/ adj. 通过皮肤的

contaminate /kənˈtæmɪneɪt/ vt. 污染，弄脏

amniotic /ˌæmnɪˈotɪk/ adj. ［昆］羊膜的

saliva /səˈlaɪvə/ n. 唾液

immunodeficiency /ˌɪˌmjuːnoʊdɪˈfɪʃnsi/ n. ［免疫］免疫缺陷

hepatitis /ˌhepəˈtaɪtɪs/ n. 肝炎

Phrases and Expressions

infectious agent	传染性试剂，传染因子
biological hazard	生物危害
centers for disease control and prevention（CDC）	疾病预防控制中心
Occupational Safety and Health Administration（OSHA）	职业安全与健康管理局
occupational exposure	职业暴露
Chemical Hygiene Plan（CHP）	化学卫生计划
blood borne pathogen	经血液传播的病原体
disease-causing microorganism	致病微生物
hepatitis B virus（HBV）	乙型肝炎病毒

Notes

1. In some laboratories, the conditions are no more dangerous than in any other room.

部分实验室的状况如同普通房间一样，不存在危险。

2. Biological hazards, refer to biological substances that pose a threat to the health of living organisms, primarily that of humans.

生物危害，是指对生物体的健康，主要是人的健康构成威胁的生物物质。

3. Under this standard, a laboratory is required to produce a Chemical Hygiene Plan（CHP）which addresses the specific hazards found in its location, and its approach to them.

在这个标准下，实验室需要制订一个化学卫生计划（CHP），强调本实验室区域内以及实验室附近的特殊危害，并提出针对危害的预防措施。

4. Clinical laboratory means a workplace where diagnostic or other screening procedures are performed on

blood or other potentially infectious materials.

临床实验室是对血液或其他具有潜在传染性生物材料进行诊断分析或其他筛选检验的实验室。

5. In any laboratory where work involves the use of and / or exposure to human blood, certain other body fluids, or unfixed human tissue, there is the danger of exposure to bloodborne pathogens, the disease-causing microorganisms that may be found in such material.

凡是涉及应用和/或暴露于人血液、某些其他体液,或未固定的人体组织进行工作的实验室,都具有暴露于血源性病原体的危险,致病性微生物可能存在于以上这些生物材料中。

6. The Bloodborne Pathogens Program requires each department or laboratory to develop an Exposure Control Plan that documents how the risk of exposure will be reduced or eliminated.

血源性病原体程序要求各部门或实验室进一步制订暴露控制计划,将如何减少或消除暴露的风险形成文件。

7. Under circumstances in which differentiation between body fluid types is difficult or impossible, all body fluids shall be considered potentially infectious materials.

在难以或不可能区分体液类型的条件下,所有体液应该被视为潜在的传染性材料。

8. Needleless system is a device that does not use needles for: (1) the collection of bodily fluids or withdrawal of body fluids after initial venous or arterial access is established; (2) the administration of medication or fluids; (3) any other procedure involving the potential for occupational exposure to bloodborne pathogens due to percutaneous injuries from contaminated sharps.

无针系统是在以下情况下不使用针的设施:(1)建立静脉或动脉通路收集体液或抽出体液时;(2)向体内输入治疗药物或液体时;(3)通过任何其他污染锐器损伤皮肤而导致的职业暴露风险时。

Exercises

Ⅰ. Fill in the blanks according to the texts.

1. In some laboratories, the conditions are no more _____ than in any other room. (Text A)

2. The Occupational Safety and Health Administration (OSHA) in the United States, have tailored a standard for _____ exposure to hazardous chemicals in laboratories, due to the unique characteristics of the laboratory workplace. (Text A)

3. In any laboratory where work involves the use of and / or exposure to human blood, certain other body fluids, or unfixed human tissue, there is the danger of exposure to bloodborne _____, the disease-causing microorganisms that may be found in such material. (Text A)

4. Occupational exposure means reasonably anticipated skin, eye, mucous membrane, or parenteral contact with blood or other potentially _____ materials that may result from the performance of an employee's duties. (Text B)

5. Under circumstances _____ differentiation between body fluid types is difficult or impossible, all body fluids shall be considered potentially infectious materials. (Text B)

Ⅱ. Translate the following into Chinese.

Bacteria, viruses and other microorganisms have the potential to cause illness in a number of exposure situations if the proper precautions and procedures are not in place. Universal precautions shall be observed to prevent contact with blood or other potentially infectious materials.

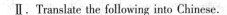

Lesson 2　Asepsis
无菌术

Learning Objectives

After studying this lesson, students are expected to be able to
1. master some key words and phrases;
2. be familiar with the differences between sterilization and disinfection;
3. know about the aseptic techniques;
4. choose appropriate aseptic techniques for different items.

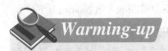

1. What is asepsis?
2. Can you tell the common aseptic techniques?

Text A　Brief Introduction to Asepsis
无菌术简介

Asepsis is a basic operational procedure in clinical medicine, and it is particularly important for surgery. A variety of microorganisms are prevalent in human body and surrounding environment. In the process of surgery, puncture, intubation, injection and dressing change, a series of strict measures must be taken to prevent microorganisms from entering human wounds or tissues, otherwise infection could occur. Asepsis includes a series of preventive measures aiming at killing microorganisms and interdicting infection pathways.

Asepsis mainly includes sterilization and disinfection, and there are some differences between them. Firstly, sterilization refers to killing all living microorganisms, including spores, while disinfection means killing pathogenic microorganisms and other harmful microorganisms, not all microorganisms. The goal of disinfection is only that the site and the article reach the level of harmlessness, while the aim of sterilization is that no living bacteria exist. Secondly, the techniques of sterilization and disinfection are different. The techniques of sterilization are more demanding and more difficult to operate than those of disinfection. For sterilization, only the physical technique or the chemical disinfectants that can kill the most resistant microorganisms (bacterial spores) could medical staff select, while the physical technique, the chemical disinfectants or the biological disinfectants which just have some sterilization effect still could be selected. Thirdly, the items which they are appropriate for are different. The items used in the surgical area or wound are usually treated according to the sterilization requirements, which means physical technique (e. g. , high temperature) or chemical technique (e. g. , glutaraldehyde) are used to eliminate all microorganisms on the related items completely, while some special surgical instruments, the arm of the operator, the skin of the patient and the air in the operating room are treated according to the standard of disinfection, which means just removing harmful microorganisms.

Asepsis involves various techniques of sterilization and disinfection and the related operation rules as well as the management system are very important. In the process Skf medical operation, medical staff shall follow a set of operating procedures to keep sterile articles and sterile areas from contamination and prevent pathogenic microorganisms from invading the human body. All medical personnel must consciously observe and strictly enforce these rules and regulations to ensure the implementation of aseptic procedures.

With the development of our country, many hospitals have updated their instruments and equipment in recent years, which has greatly improved the appearance of asepsis. The establishment of laminar flow operating room, the extensive use of ethylene oxide and plasma gas sterilization, as well as the preparation of disposable medical materials and other series of measures have significantly improved the effect of sterilization and disinfection. What's more, they play an excellent role in safeguarding various surgical clinical works.

Text B   Aseptic Techniques
无菌操作

Sterilization mainly consists of the following techniques: high-pressure steam sterilization, chemical gas sterilization, boiling, liquid immersion, dry heat sterilization and ionizing radiation.

High-pressure steam sterilization which is the most widely used sterilization technique in hospitals can be divided into two types: downdraft and pre-vacuum. There are many styles of the downdraft sterilizer, including portable, horizontal and vertical, but their basic structure and principle of action are the same. As the steam enters the human sterile room, accumulation as well as pressure increases and the indoor temperature also rises. When high-pressure steam reaches certain temperature and lasts for certain time, it can kill all microorganisms, including bacteria spores that have a strong resistance.

Many hospitals now use more advanced pre-vacuum steam sterilizers, the principle of which is that the air in sterilizer is blotted up to make its assuming vacuum state, then central gas supplier sends the steam to the person sterilization room directly. Through this can medical staff assure the steam in sterilization room is distributed equably and the time that the whole sterilization process takes could be reduced.

Chemical gas sterilization is applicable to sterilization of medical materials that are not resistant to high temperature or humidity, such as electronic instruments, optical instruments, endoscopes and their special instruments, cardiac catheters, catheters and other rubber products. At present, ethylene oxide gas sterilization, argon peroxide plasma sterilization and formaldehyde steam sterilization are prevalent. The emissions of residual ethylene oxide and formaldehyde gas cannot adopt natural volatilization, so special emission system should be set.

The boiling technique is suitable for metal instruments, glass products and rubber items. Common bacteria can be killed in boiling water for 15-20 minutes, while killing bacterial spores takes at least 1 hour. This technique is easy to use and proves effective. In order to save time and guarantee sterilization quality, a pressure cooker can be used in plateau area. The steam pressure in the pressure cooker can reach 127.5 kPa, and the highest temperature in the pot is about 124℃, so the sterilization effect can be achieved in 10 minutes with the pressure cooker.

The liquid infusion technique is appropriate for sharp surgical instruments, endoscopy, etc. 2% neutral glutaraldehyde is mostly used as the infusion in clinical practice currently, and the sterilization effect can be achieved in 30 minutes. Other kinds of immersion solution used for disinfection include 10% formaldehyde, 70% ethanol, 1:1 000 benzalkonium bromides and 1:1 000 chlorhexidine.

Dry heat sterilization applies to the articles that are resistant to heat but moisture, such as glass, powder and oil. The whole process of sterilization takes at least 2 hours when the dry heat temperature is heated to 160℃, 170℃ takes 1 hour, 180℃ takes 30 minutes.

Ionizing radiation technique is suitable for industrial sterilization and mainly used in sterile medical consumables (such as disposable syringes, silk threads) and some drugs. For example, the radiation of ^{60}Co and the electronic radiation produced by accelerator are usually used for sterilization.

New Words

asepsis /æˈsɛpsɪs/ n. 无菌,无菌(操作)

puncture /ˈpʌŋktʃər/ v. 刺穿,戳破,揭穿 n. 穿刺,刺痕

intubation /ˌɪntjuˈbeɪʃən/ n. [临床]插管,插管法

sterilization /ˌsterələˈzeɪʃn/ n. [医][食品]杀菌,使不孕,无用状态

disinfection /ˌdɪsɪnˈfekʃn/ n. 消毒,杀菌

disinfectant /ˌdɪsɪnˈfektənt/ n. 消毒剂 adj. 消毒的

contamination /kənˌtæmɪˈneɪʃn/ n. 污染,玷污,污染物

laminar /ˈlæmɪnə/ adj. 层状的,薄片状的,板状的

immersion /ɪˈmɜːrʒn/ n. 沉浸,陷入,专心

autoclave /ˈɔːtoʊkleɪv/ n. 高压灭菌器,高压锅 v. 用高压锅烹饪

downdraft /ˈdaʊndræft/ n. 下坡,向下之气流或风

horizontal /ˌhɔːrɪˈzɑːntl/ adj. 水平的,地平线的

vertical /ˈvɜːtɪkl/ adj. 垂直的,直立的;[解剖]头顶的,顶点的

accumulation /əˌkjuːmjəˈleɪʃn/ n. 积聚,累积,堆积物

endoscope /ˈendəskoʊp/ n. [临床]内镜

cardiac /ˈkɑːrdiæk/ n. 强心剂,强胃剂 adj. 心脏的,心脏病的

catheter /ˈkæθətər/ n. [医]导管,导尿管,尿液管

residual /rɪˈzɪdʒuəl/ n. 剩余,残渣 adj. 剩余的,残留的

radiation /ˌreɪdiˈeɪʃn/ n. 辐射,放射物

Phrases and Expressions

high-pressure steam sterilization	高压蒸汽灭菌
chemical gas sterilization	化学气体灭菌
liquid immersion	液浸灭菌
dry heat sterilization	干热灭菌
ionizing radiation	电离辐射灭菌
autoclave sterilization	高压灭菌器消毒

Notes

1. The items used in the surgical area or wound are usually treated according to the sterilization requirements, which means physical technique (e.g., high temperature) or chemical technique (e.g., glutaraldehyde) are used to eliminate all microorganisms on the related items completely, while some special surgical instruments, the arm of the operator, the skin of the patient and the air in the operating room are treated according to the standard of disinfection, which means just removing harmful microorganisms.

手术区或伤口使用的物品通常按照灭菌要求进行处理,即使用物理技术(如高温等)或化学技术(如戊二醛等)彻底清除相关物品上的所有微生物;而一些特殊的手术器械,操作人员的手臂、病人的皮肤和手术室的空气都是按照消毒的标准来处理的,也就是去除有害的微生物。

2. Many hospitals now use more advanced pre-vacuum steam sterilizers, the principle of which is that the air in sterilizer is blotted up to make its assume vacuum state, then central gas supplier sends the steam to the person sterilization room directly.

现在很多医院都在使用更先进的预真空蒸汽灭菌器,其原理是灭菌器内的空气被吸干,使其处于真空状态,然后中央燃气供应商将蒸汽直接送到消毒室。

3. The liquid infusion technique is appropriate for sharp surgical instruments, endoscopy, etc. 2% neutral glutaraldehyde is mostly used as the infusion in clinical practice currently, and the sterilization effect can be achieved in 30 minutes. Other kinds of immersion solution used for disinfection include 10% formalde-

hyde，70% ethanol，1∶1 000 benzalkonium bromides and 1∶1 000 chlorhexidine.

液体浸泡技术适用于尖锐的手术器械、内镜等。目前临床主要采用2%中性戊二醛输注，灭菌效果可在30min内完成。其他用于消毒的浸泡液包括10%甲醛、70%乙醇、1∶1 000苯扎溴铵和1∶1 000氯己定。

Exercises

Ⅰ. Fill in the blanks according to the texts.

1. A variety of _____ are prevalent in human body and surrounding environment.（Text A）

2. All medical personnel must consciously observe and strictly enforce these rules and regulations to ensure the_____ of aseptic procedures.（Text A）

3. _____ steam sterilization which is the most widely used sterilization technique in hospitals can be divided into two types.（Text B）

4. Chemical gas sterilization is applicable to sterilization of medical materials that are not _____ to high temperature or humidity.（Text B）

5. In order to save time and guarantee sterilization quality，a pressure cooker can be used in _____ area.（Text B）

Ⅱ. Translate the following into Chinese.

Many hospitals now use more advanced pre-vacuum steam sterilizers，the principle of which is that the air in sterilizer is blotted up to make its assuming vacuum state，then central gas supplier sends the steam to the person sterilization room directly.

Lesson 3　Laboratory Purified Water and Solution Concentration
化验用纯水与溶液浓度

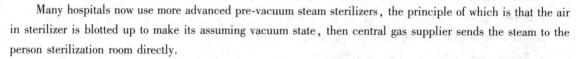
Learning Objectives

After studying this lesson，students are expected to be able to

1. master the definition and technical standards of purified water；

2. be familiar with the concentration of a solute in chemistry；

3. know about why the highest grades of ultra-pure water should not be stored in glass or plastic containers.

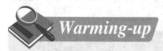
Warming-up

1. What is the color，state and taste of water？

2. Can tap water be used directly in the chemical experiments？

3. How do we express the solution concentration？

Text A　Purified Water
纯化水

Water（H_2O）is the most abundant compound on the earth，covering about 70% of the earth's surface. It is essential for all life on Earth. Water usually makes up 55%-78% of the human body.

In nature, it exists in liquid, solid, and gaseous states. At room temperature, it is a tasteless and odorless liquid, nearly colorless with a hint of blue. Water is a good solvent due to its polarity. Many substances dissolve in water. Substances that will mix well and dissolve in water (e. g. , salts) are known as hydrophilic ("water-loving") substances, while those that do not mix well with water (e. g. , fats and oils), are known as hydrophobic ("water-fearing") substances. In general, ionic and polar substances such as acids, alcohols and salts are relatively in water, and non-polar substances such as fats and oils are not.

Purified water is water from any source that is physically processed to remove impurities. Purified water is suitable for laboratory testing. Technical standards on water quality have been established by a number of professional organizations, including the U. S. National Committee for Clinical Laboratory Standards (NCCLS) which is now named Clinical and Laboratory Standards Institute (CLSI). The International Standardization Organization (ISO) 3696 (1987) and NCCLS (1988) classify purified water into Grade 1-3 or Types Ⅰ-Ⅲ depending upon the level of purity. Regardless of which organization's water quality norm is used, even Type Ⅰ water may require further purification depending upon the specific laboratory application. For example, water used to analyze trace metals may require elimination of trace metals to a standard beyond that of the Type Ⅰ water norm. Water for microbiology experiments needs to be completely sterile, which is usually accomplished by autoclaving. Water that is being used for molecular-biology experiments needs to be deoxyribonuclease (DNase) or ribonuclease (RNase)-free, which requires special additional treatment or functional testing.

The highest grades of ultra-pure water should not be stored in glass or plastic containers because these container materials leach (release) contaminants at very low concentration. Storage vessels made of silica are used for less demanding applications and vessels of ultra-pure tin are used for the highest purity applications.

Text B Solution and Concentration
溶液与浓度

An aqueous solution is a solution in which the solvent is water. As water is an excellent solvent and is also naturally abundant, it is a ubiquitous solvent in chemistry. The ability of a substance to dissolve in water is determined by whether the substance can match or exceed the strong attractive forces that water molecules generate between themselves. If the substance lacks the ability to dissolve in water the molecules form a precipitate. Aqueous solutions that conduct electric current efficiently contain strong electrolytes, while ones that conduct poorly are considered to have weak electrolytes. Those strong electrolytes are substances that are completely ionized in water, whereas the weak electrolytes exhibit only a small degree of ionization in water. Nonelectrolytes are substances that dissolve in water, but which maintain their molecular integrity (do not dissociate into ions). Examples include sugar, urea and glycerol.

The concentration of a solute is very important in studying chemical reactions. In chemistry, concentration is defined as the abundance of a constituent divided by the total volume of a mixture. Concentration may be expressed in a number of ways. For example:

(1) molar concentration equals the number of moles of a specified component per unit volume of the system in which it is contained. It is also called molarity, amount-of-substance concentration, amount concentration, substance concentration, or simply concentration. The SI-unit is mol/m^3. However, more commonly the unit mol/L is used. A solution of concentration 1 mol/L is also denoted as "1 molar" (1 M).

$$1 \text{ mol/L} = 1 \text{ mol/dm}^3 = 1 \text{ M} = 1000 \text{ mol/m}^3.$$

The molarity of a solution is the number of moles of solute per liter of solution. e. g. , a solution of glucose in water containing 180. 16 grams (1 mole) of glucose per liter of solution is referred to as one molar (1 M).

(2) number concentration equals the number of specified particles or molecular entities per unit volume of the system in which it is contained. It is expressed in m^{-3}. Note: The concentration of a solute in solution

may sometimes be expressed in more convenient units, especially in a percentage, e. g., (for solids) as the mass of solute in grams per 100 milliliters of solution (abbr.: %, w/v), or (for liquids) as the number of volumes of solute per 100 volumes of solution (abbr.: %, v/v).

020303

New Words

gaseous /ˈgæsɪəs/ *adj.* 气体的,气体状态的
odorless /ˈodəlɪs/ *adj.* 无气味的,无臭的
solvent /ˈsɑːlvənt/ *n.* 溶剂
polarity /pəˈlærəti/ *n.* [物] 极性,两极,对立
dissolve /dɪˈzɑːlv/ *v.* 溶解,分解
impurities /ɪmˈpjʊrətiz/ *n.* 杂质(impurity 的复数)
deoxyribonuclease (DNase) /diˌoksiˌraɪboˈnʊkliˌes/ *n.* [生化] 脱氧核糖核酸酶
ribonuclease (RNase) /ˌraɪboˈnjʊklɪez/ *n.* [生化] 核糖核酸酶
soluble /ˈsɑːljəbl/ *adj.* [化学] 可溶解的
hydrophilic /ˌhaɪdrəˈfɪlɪk/ *adj.* [化学] 亲水的(等于 hydrophilous)
hydrophobic /ˌhaɪdrəˈfoʊbɪk/ *adj.* 疏水的
ionic /aɪˈɑːnɪk/ *adj.* 离子的
analyze /ˈænəlaɪz/ *v.* 分析
elimination /ɪˌlɪmɪˈneɪʃn/ *n.* 排除,除去
sterile /ˈsterəl/ *adj.* 无菌的,不生育的
autoclaving /ˌɔːtəuˈkleiviŋ/ *n.* [医] 高压灭菌法,高压蒸气养护
silica /ˈsɪlɪkə/ *n.* 二氧化硅,[材] 硅土
ultra /ˈʌltrə/ *adj.* 过激的
leach /liːtʃ/ *v.* 浸出
release /rɪˈliːs/ *v.* 释放,发射 *n.* 释放,发布
contaminant /kənˈtæmɪnənt/ *n.* 污染物
concentration /ˌkɑːnsnˈtreɪʃn/ *n.* 浓度,浓缩
aqueous /ˈeɪkwɪəs/ *adj.* 水的,水般的
nonelectrolyte /ˌnɔnɪˈlektrəlaɪt/ *n.* 非电解质
precipitate /prɪˈsɪpɪteɪt/ *n.* 沉淀物
ubiquitous /juːˈbɪkwɪtəs/ *adj.* 普遍存在的
dissociate /dɪˈsoʊʃieɪt/ *v.* 离解,分离
constituent /kənˈstɪtʃuənt/ *n.* 成分
molarity /məʊˈlærɪtɪ/ *n.* [化学] 摩尔浓度

Phrases and Expressions

make up	组成,构成,占据
due to ...	由于……,因为……
ultra-pure water	超纯净水
refer to ... as ...	把……称作……
National Committee for Clinical Laboratory Standards (NCCLS)	美国临床实验室标准化委员会
Clinical and Laboratory Standards Institute (CLSI)	美国临床与实验室标准化研究所
International Standardization Organization (ISO)	国际标准化组织

Notes

笔记

1. In general, ionic and polar substances such as acids, alcohols and salts are relatively in water, and

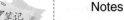

non-polar substances such as fats and oils are not.

一般而言,离子与极性物质诸如酸类、醇类和盐类相对溶于水,非极性物质如脂肪和油类不溶于水。

2. Regardless of which organization's water quality norm is used, even Type Ⅰ water may require further purification depending upon the specific laboratory application.

不管使用哪个组织的正常水质标准,即使Ⅰ类水体也可能要根据特殊实验室应用要求进行进一步的纯化。

3. Water for microbiology experiments needs to be completely sterile, which is usually accomplished by autoclaving. Water that is being used for molecular-biology experiments needs to be deoxyribonuclease (DNase) or ribonuclease (RNase)-free, which requires special additional treatment or functional testing.

微生物实验用水需要完全无菌,通常采用高压蒸汽灭菌法达到无菌要求。分子生物学实验用水则要求无脱氧核糖核酸酶(DNase)和无核糖核酸酶(RNase),需要用额外的处理方法或功能测试。

4. The ability of a substance to dissolve in water is determined by whether the substance can match or exceed the strong attractive forces that water molecules generate between themselves.

物质溶解于水的能力,取决于该物质与水分子的作用力是否超过或者与水分子之间的吸引力相当。

5. The concentration of a solute in solution may sometimes be expressed in more convenient units, especially in a percentage, e. g. , (for solids) as the mass of solute in grams per 100 millilitres of solution (abbr. : %, w/v), or (for liquids) as the number of volumes of solute per 100 volumes of solution (abbr. : %, v/v).

溶液中溶质的浓度,有时采用更方便的单位表示,尤其是用百分比。例如,(对于固体溶质)以每100毫升溶液中溶解的溶质克数表示(缩写:%,w/v),或(对于液体溶质)以每100体积溶液中所含溶质的体积数表示(缩写:%,v/v)。

Exercises

Ⅰ. Fill in the blanks according to the texts.

1. Water (H₂O) is the most abundant _____ on Earth's surface, covering about 70%. (Text A)

2. Water is a good _____ due to its polarity. (Text A)

3. Purified water is water from any source that is physically _____ to remove impurities. (Text A)

4. The ability of a substance to _____ in water is determined by whether the substance can match or exceed the strong attractive forces that water molecules generate between themselves. (Text B)

5. In chemistry, _____ is defined as the abundance of a constituent divided by the total volume of a mixture. (Text B)

Ⅱ. Translate the following into Chinese.

Technical standards on water quality have been established by a number of professional organizations, including the U. S. National Committee for Clinical Laboratory Standards (NCCLS) which is now Clinical and Laboratory Standards Institute (CLSI). The International Standardization Organization (ISO) 3696 (1987) and NCCLS (1988) classify purified water into Grade 1-3 or Types Ⅰ-Ⅲ depending upon the level of purity.

Lesson 4 Chemical and Diagnostic Reagents
化学试剂与诊断试剂

 Learning Objectives

After studying this lesson, students are expected to be able to

1. master the definition of chemical reagents and IVD reagents;
2. be familiar with a standard solution and the primary standards;
3. know about the uses of chemical reagents, a standard solution and IVD reagents;
4. properly use the diagnostic reagents in the clinical laboratory.

Warming-up

1. Can you tell any kinds of diagnostic reagents?
2. Do you know any purity standards for reagents?
3. What are the main types of in vitro diagnostic products?

Text A Chemical Reagents
化学试剂

Reagents are substances or compounds that are added to a system in order to bring about a chemical reaction or are added to see if a reaction occurs. Solvents and catalysts, although involved in the reaction, are usually not referred to as reactants. Some reagents are just a single element. However, most processes require reagents made of chemical compounds.

Reagent-grade describes chemical substances of sufficient purity for use in chemical analysis, chemical reactions or physical testing. Purity standards for reagents are set by organizations such as American Society for Testing and Materials (ASTM) International. For instance, reagent-quality water must have very low levels of impurities like sodium and chloride ions, and bacteria, as well as a very high electrical resistivity.

Commercial chemicals are available at several levels of purity. Chemicals labeled "technical" or "commercial" are usually quite impure. The grade "USP" indicates only that the chemical meets the requirements of the United States Pharmacopeia. The term "CP" only means that the chemical is purer than "technical." Chemicals designated "reagent grade" or "analyzed reagent" are specially purified materials which usually have been analyzed to establish the levels of impurities. American Chemical Society has established specifications and tests for purity for some chemicals. Materials which meet these specifications are labeled "Meets ACS Specifications".

A standard solution is a solution containing a precisely known concentration of an element or a substance i. e., a known weight of solute is dissolved to make a specific volume. The concentrations of standard solutions are normally expressed in units of moles per liter (mol/L). Standard solutions are used to determine the concentrations of other substances, such as solutions in titrations. In analytical chemistry, Standard solution is prepared using a standard substance, such as a primary standard. A primary standard is typically a reagent which can be weighed easily, and which is so pure that its weight truly represents the number of moles of substance contained. Primary standards are used to calibrate other standards referred to as working standards.

Text B　In Vitro Diagnostic Reagents
体外诊断试剂

Living organisms are extremely complex functional systems. This extraordinary complexity of living organisms is a great barrier to the identification of individual components and the exploration of their basic biological functions. In vitro diagnostic (IVD) tests are medical devices intended to perform diagnoses from assays in a test tube, or more generally in a controlled environment outside a living organism. Colloquially, these experiments are commonly referred to as "test tube experiments".

In vitro diagnostic products (IVDs) are those reagents, instruments, and systems intended for use in the diagnosis of diseases or other conditions, including a determination of the state of health, in order to cure, mitigate, treat, or prevent disease or its sequelae. Such products are intended for use in the collection, preparation, and examination of specimens taken from the human body. ISO 23640 (2011) is applicable to the stability evaluation of in vitro diagnostic medical devices, including reagents, calibrators, control materials, diluents, buffers and reagent kits, hereinafter called IVD reagents.

Developing rapidly, the IVD reagents plays a more and more important role in medical practices, such as physical examination, disease diagnoses, curative effect evaluation, prognosis, and so on. Many manufacturers manufacture diagnostic kits that can be used in all clinical chemistry laboratories on a variety of automated clinical analysers. The quality and diagnostic value of IVDs becomes the focus point of medical agency and the public. So, for the safety of people's health, we need to strengthen the management of IVDs market access to make sure that only the IVDs with high quality can be approved to the market.

Assuring the performance characteristics of IVDs is a major objective of product evaluations. This includes using sets of well-planned and controlled trials in order to (1) analyze product performance characteristics; (2) validate design specifications; (3) assess product safety. Performance parameters, like sensitivity, specificity, precision, robustness, are assessed in order to assure that the product design consistently meets performance specifications upon manufacturing.

New Words

reagent /riˈeɪdʒənt/ n. ［试剂］试剂,反应物

reactant /rɪˈæktənt/ n. ［化学］反应物,反应剂

catalyst /ˈkætəlɪst/ n. ［物化］催化剂,刺激因素

ion /ˈaɪən/ n. 离子

pharmacopeia /ˈfɑrməkəˈpiə/ n. 药典,处方汇编

titration /tɪˈtreɪʃn/ n. ［分化］滴定,滴定法

calibrate /ˈkælɪbreɪt/ v. 校准

sufficient /səˈfɪʃnt/ adj. 足够的,充足的

designated /ˈdɛzɪɡˌnetɪd/ adj. 指定的,特定的

mitigate /ˈmɪtɪɡeɪt/ v. 使缓和,使减轻

sequelae /sɪˈkwili/ n. 后遗症(sequela 的复数)

diluent /ˈdɪljʊənt/ n. 稀释液

curative /ˈkjʊrətɪv/ adj. 有疗效的

approve /əˈpruːv/ v. 批准,核准,赞成

validate /ˈvælɪdeɪt/ v. 证实,验证

identification /aɪˌdentɪfɪˈkeʃn/ n. 鉴别,识别

diagnoses /ˌdaɪəɡˈnəusiːz/ n. 诊断,调查分析,评价(diagnosis 的复数形式)

colloquially /kəˈloʊkwɪəlɪ/ adv. 口语地,用通俗语

buffer /ˈbʌfər/ n. 缓冲器 v. 缓冲

hereinafter /ˌhɪrɪnˈæftər/ *adv.* 以下,在下文中

consistently /kənˈsɪstəntli/ *adv.* 一贯地,坚持地

parameter /pəˈræmɪtər/ *n.* 参数,系数,参量

robustness /rouˈbʌstnəs/ *n.* [计] 稳健性

evaluation /ɪˌvæljuˈeɪʃn/ *n.* 评价;[审计] 评估,估价,求值

calibrator /ˈkæliˌbreɪtə/ *n.* [仪] 校准器,口径测量器(等于 calibrater)

kit /kɪt/ *n.* 试剂盒,成套用品

Phrases and Expressions

American Society for Testing and Materials(ASTM)	美国试验与材料学会
for instance	例如
reagent-quality	试剂质量
electrical resistivity	电阻系数
American Chemical Society(ACS)	美国化学学会
Association of Caribbean States(ACS)	加勒比国家联盟
United States Patent(USP)	美国专利
primary standard	基准物质
in vitro	在(活)体外,在试管内
performance characteristics	运行特性

Notes

1. Reagents are substances or compounds that are added to a system in order to bring about a chemical reaction or are added to see if a reaction occurs.

如果某种物质或者化合物加入一个体系中后,能引发化学反应或是能用于判断是否存在反应,那么它们就被称之为试剂。

2. Reagent-grade describes chemical substances of sufficient purity for use in chemical analysis, chemical reactions or physical testing.

试剂级别描述化学物质用于化学分析、化学反应或物理试验的足够纯度。

3. A standard solution is a solution containing a precisely known concentration of an element or a substance i. e. , a known weight of solute is dissolved to make a specific volume.

标准溶液是指精确知道所含成分或物质浓度的溶液,也就是说,已知质量的溶质溶解在特定体积的溶液中。

4. A primary standard is typically a reagent which can be weighed easily, and which is so pure that its weight truly represents the number of moles of substance contained.

基准物质通常是一种易于称重的试剂,它的高纯度使得其重量能真实地代表所含物质的摩尔数。

5. So, for the safety of people's health, we need to strengthen the management of IVDs market access to make sure that only the IVDs with high quality can be approved to the market.

因此,为了人民的健康安全,我们需要加强管理 IVDs 的市场准入,确保只有高质量的 IVDs 被批准进入市场。

6. Performance parameters, like sensitivity, specificity, precision, robustness, are assessed in order to assure that the product design consistently meets performance specifications upon manufacturing.

对敏感性、特异性、精密度和稳定性等性能进行参数评估,以确保产品设计始终符合生产制造的技术指标。

Exercises

Ⅰ. Fill in the blanks according to the texts.

1. _____ describes chemical substances of sufficient purity for use in chemical analysis, chemical reactions or physical testing. (Text A)

2. A _____ solution is a solution containing a precisely known concentration of an element or a substance i. e. , a known weight of solute is dissolved to make a specific volume. (Text A)

3. The concentrations of standard solutions are normally expressed in units of _____ per liter (mol/L). (Text A)

4. In vitro _____ products (IVDs) are those reagents, instruments, and systems intended for use in the diagnosis of diseases or other conditions, including a determination of the state of health, in order to cure, mitigate, treat, or prevent disease or its sequelae. (Text B)

5. In vitro diagnostic (IVD) tests are medical devices intended to perform diagnoses from assays in a test tube, or more generally in a _____ environment outside a living organism. (Text B)

Ⅱ. Translate the following into Chinese.

Standard solutions are used to determine the concentrations of other substances, such as solutions in titrations. In analytical chemistry, Standard solution is prepared using a standard substance, such as a primary standard. A primary standard is typically a reagent which can be weighed easily, and which is so pure that its weight truly represents the number of moles of substance contained. Primary standards are used to calibrate other standards referred to as working standards.

Lesson 4 Scan and Practice

Lesson 5 PPT

Lesson 5   Work Flow for Clinical Specimen Collection
临床标本采集流程

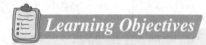
Learning Objectives

After studying this lesson, students are expected to be able to

1. master the work flow of specimen processing and the venipuncture procedure;

2. be familiar with the most commonly collected samples and the fingerstick procedure;

3. know about the function of clinical specimen collection, the three kinds of blood sampling and the heel stick procedure;

4. process the most commonly collected samples and collect blood by venipuncture or fingerstick sampling in the right way.

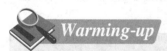
Warming-up

1. What are the most commonly collected samples from clinical cases?

2. What are the three kinds of blood sampling for blood test?

Text A   Specimen Processing and Work Flow
标本处理与工作流程

020501

The information gleaned from any of the specimens collected will only be as good as the techniques used in collecting, handling, and processing these specimens. It goes without saying that the ultimate usefulness of these samples will depend upon the clinician's ability to interpret the results and use them for developing a medical management program.

Use universal precautions when handling specimens containing blood or other potentially infectious mate-

笔记

rial. Work areas contaminated with blood or serum must be disinfected immediately with 10% bleach (hypochlorite at 0.5% final concentration) or other approved disinfectants. Specimens must be handled in a safe manner and according to applicable legal requirements or guidance. Many tests require that the patient be prepared in some specific way to ensure useful results. The best analytical techniques provide results that are only as meaningful as the quality of the specimen that has been submitted for analysis.

The most commonly collected samples from clinical cases include blood, urine, feces, cerebral spinal fluid (CSF), synovial fluid, semen, sputum and swabs. Sample processing will usually start with a set of samples and a request form. Specimen collection is a critical initial step in laboratory diagnosis. Meaningful laboratory results require careful attention to the specimen source, the method of collection, and the timing, storage, transport and handling of the collected specimens. In addition, a completed request form with relevant history, if appropriate, is essential for optimal and efficient laboratory workup of the collected specimens.

Typically, a set of vacutainer tubes containing blood, or any other specimen, will arrive to the laboratory in a small plastic bag, along with the form. The form and the specimens are given a laboratory number. The specimens will usually all receive the same number, often as a sticker that can be placed on the tubes and form. This label has a barcode that can be scanned by automated analyzers and test requests uploaded from the LIS (laboratory information system). Entry of requests onto a laboratory management system involves typing, or scanning (where barcodes are used) in the laboratory number, and entering the patient identification, as well as any tests requested. This allows laboratory machines, computers and staff to know what tests are pending, and also gives a place (such as a hospital department, doctor or other customer) for results to go.

For biochemistry samples, blood is usually centrifuged and serum is separated. If the serum needs to go on more than one machine, it can be divided into separate tubes. Many specimens end up in one or more sophisticated automated analyzers, that process a fraction of the sample and return one or more "results". Some laboratories use robotic sample handlers (laboratory automation) to optimize the work flow and reduce contamination risk and sample handling of the staff.

Text B Methods of Venous Blood Sampling
静脉采血方法

Blood analysis is one of the most important diagnostic tools available to clinicians within healthcare. Blood sampling for any blood test includes arterial blood sampling, such as radial artery puncture, and venous blood sampling, also called venipuncture, and capillary blood sampling, such as blood sampling by finger sticks or a heel stick.

There are many ways in which blood can be drawn from a vein. The best method varies with the age of the patient, equipment available and tests required. Blood is most commonly obtained from the median cubital vein, which lies within the cubital fossa anterior to the elbow. This vein lies close to the surface of the skin, and there is not a large nerve supply. Minute quantities of blood may be taken by finger sticks sampling or by means of an earlobe stick and collected from infants by means of a heel stick or from scalp veins with a winged infusion needle. In medicine, venipuncture, also known as venepuncture or venipuncture, is one of the most routinely performed invasive procedures. Venipuncture is performed by medical laboratory scientists, medical practitioners, phlebotomists, dialysis technicians and other nursing staff.

Venipuncture procedure

Arrange the following supplies on the table next to the drawing chair: safety needle and vacutainer sleeve, tubes, tourniquet, gloves, alcohol swab, bandage, cotton or gauze, and tape. A sharps container should always be within reach. Tubes should be arranged by order of draw: Red Top, Blue Top, Serum-separating tubes(SST), Green Top, Lavender Top, Yellow Top, and Gray Top. Ask the patient say their name to confirm the paperwork.

After putting on gloves, inspect the patient's arms to determine where a sample can be collected. Apply the tourniquet and clean the site with the alcohol swab. After the site has dried, insert the needle into the vein and fill each tube. Remove the tourniquet before removing the needle. The vacutainer tube should be removed from the needle before removing the needle from the vein. The tubes that contain additive must be inverted 8-10 times immediately after drawing. After the needle has been removed, apply direct pressure with a cotton ball or gauze on the insertion site. The bleeding should stop in 5 minutes and the puncture can then be bandaged.

Fingerstick Procedure

The best locations for finger sticks are the 3rd (middle) and 4th (ring) fingers of the non-dominant hand. Avoid sampling from tip and sides of the finger. Also, avoid puncturing a finger that is cold or cyanotic, swollen, scarred, or covered with a rash.

Massage the finger toward the selected site prior to the puncture. Clean the skin with antiseptic.

Using a sterile safety lancet, make a skin puncture just off the center of the finger pad. The lancet should enter the finger perpendicularly otherwise the blood may run along finger pad ridges.

Wipe away the first drop of blood, which tends to contain excess tissue fluid.

Collect drops of blood into the collection tube or device by gentle pressure on the finger. Avoid excessive pressure lest you may squeeze tissue fluid into the drop of blood.

Place a small gauze pad over the puncture site for a few minutes to stop the bleeding.

Heel Stick Procedure

Careful handling of the child is important when a blood sample is being obtained for testing. The recommended location for blood collection on a newborn baby or infant is the heel.

Prewarming the infant's heel (42℃ for 3-5 minutes) is important to obtain capillary blood gas samples and warming also greatly increases the flow of blood for collection of other specimens. However, do not use too high a temperature warmer, because baby's skin is thin and susceptible to thermal injury.

Hold the baby's foot firmly to avoid sudden movement. An assistant may be required to do that.

Clean the skin.

Use a sterile blood safety lancet and puncture the side of the heel in the appropriate regions.

Wipe away the first drop of blood.

Newborns do not often bleed immediately; a gentle pressure is required to produce the drop of the blood. Do not use excessive pressure otherwise the blood may become diluted with tissue fluid.

Fill the required tube or capillary as needed.

After it is done, elevate the heel, place a piece of clean, dry cotton on the puncture site, and hold it in place until the bleeding has stopped.

New Words

glean /gliːn/ *v.* 收集

bleach /bliːtʃ/ *n.* 漂白剂

hypochlorite /ˌhaɪpəˈklɔːraɪt/ *n.* ［无化］次氯酸盐，低氧化氯

workup /ˈwɜːrkʌp/ *n.* 病情检查

vacutainer /ˈvækjʊteɪnə/ *n.* 真空采血管

analyzer /ˈænəˌlaɪzɚ/ *n.* ［计］分析仪，分析者

centrifuge /ˈsentrɪfjuːdʒ/ *v.* 用离心机分离

sophisticated /səˈfɪstɪkeɪtɪd/ *adj.* 精密的

optimize /ˈɑːptɪmaɪz/ *v.* 使最优化，使完善

capillary /ˈkæpəleri/ n. 毛细管,毛细血管 adj. 毛细管的,毛状的

fingerstick /ˈfɪŋgəstik/ n. 手指穿刺,指刺

dialysis /daiˈæləsis/ n. [医][分化]透析,渗析(复数 dialyses)

supplies /səpˈlaɪz/ n.（复数）物资,医疗设备和用品

tourniquet /ˈtɔːrnəkət/ n. [外科]止血带,压脉器,压血带

gauze /gɔz/ n. 纱布

additive /ˈædətɪv/ n. 添加物,添加剂

antiseptic /ˌæntiˈseptɪk/ n. 抗菌剂

lancet /ˈlænsɪt/ n. [外科]柳叶刀

perpendicular /ˌpɜːrpənˈdɪkjələr/ adj. 垂直的

susceptible /səˈseptəbl/ adj. 易受影响的,易受感染的

thermal /ˈθəːrml/ adj. 热的

dilute /daiˈluːt/ vt. 稀释

elevate /ˈelɪveɪt/ vt. 提升,举起

Phrases and Expressions

work flow	工作流程
it goes without saying that	不用说,不言而喻
laboratory information system（LIS）	实验室信息系统
laboratory management system	实验室管理系统
radial artery puncture	桡动脉穿刺
median cubital vein	肘正中静脉
winged infusion needle	有翼输液针
invasive procedures	创伤性操作,侵入性医疗作业
a sharps container	锐器容器
order of draw	采血顺序

Notes

1. The information gleaned from any of the specimens collected will only be as good as the techniques used in collecting, handling, and processing these specimens.

从收集的标本获取的信息将取决于收集、整理和处理这些标本所使用技术的水平。

2. Use universal precautions when handling specimens containing blood or other potentially infectious material. Work areas contaminated with blood or serum must be disinfected immediately with 10% bleach (hypochlorite at 0.5% final concentration) or other approved disinfectants.

在处理含有血液或其他潜在感染性物质的标本时,采取通用预防措施。被血液或血清污染的工作区域必须立即用10%的漂白剂(最终浓度为0.5%的次氯酸盐)或批准的其他消毒剂消毒。

3. The best analytical techniques provide results that are only as meaningful as the quality of the specimen that has been submitted for analysis.

最好的分析技术提供的结果与被提交分析的标本质量一样有意义。

4. Meaningful laboratory results require careful attention to the specimen source, the method of collection, and the timing, storage, transport and handling of the collected specimens.

获取有意义的实验室检查结果要求十分注意标本来源、收集方法,以及收集标本的时间、储藏、运输和处理。

5. In addition, a completed request form with relevant history, if appropriate, is essential for optimal and efficient laboratory workup of the collected specimens.

此外,如果可能的话,一份具有相关病史的完整申请表,对于实现所收集标本的最佳和有效的实验室诊断检查是至关重要的。

6. Entry of requests onto a laboratory management system involves typing, or scanning (where barcodes are used) in the laboratory number, and entering the patient identification, as well as any tests requested.

请求登录实验室管理系统要求打印或扫描(使用条形码的地方)实验室编号、输入病人身份信息,以及其他任何要求化验的项目。

7. This allows laboratory machines, computers and staff to know what tests are pending, and also gives a place (such as a hospital department, doctor or other customer) for results to go.

这就使得实验室仪器、计算机和工作人员知道正在请求什么检验项目,也给出了检验结果的去处(比如医院科室、医生或者其他客户)。

8. Some laboratories use robotic sample handlers (laboratory automation) to optimize the work flow and reduce contamination risk and sample handling of the staff.

一些实验室使用自动化的标本处理机(实验室自动化)使工作流程最优化,并减少标本的污染风险和工作人员的标本处理程序。

9. Tubes should be arranged by order of draw: Red Top, Blue Top, Serum-separating tubes (SST), Green Top, Lavender Top, Yellow Top, and Gray Top. Ask the patient say their name to confirm the paperwork.

试管应按照采血顺序排列:红头试管、蓝头试管、血清分离试管(SST)、绿头试管、紫头试管、黄头试管和灰头试管。要让病人说出姓名以确认书写内容。

10. Remove the tourniquet before removing the needle. The vacutainer tube should be removed from the needle before removing the needle from the vein.

在拔针之前去除止血带。将针从静脉血管拔出之前应将真空采血管从针上去除。

Exercises

Ⅰ. Fill in the blanks according to the texts.

1. The most commonly collected samples from clinical cases include blood, _____, feces, cerebral spinal fluid (CSF), synovial fluid, semen, sputum and swabs. (Text A)

2. Meaningful laboratory results require careful attention to the specimen source, the method of collection, and the timing, storage, _____ and handling of the collected specimens. (Text A)

3. Blood sampling for any blood test includes arterial blood sampling, such as radial artery puncture, and venous blood sampling, also called_____, and capillary blood sampling, such as blood sampling by finger sticks or a heel stick. (Text B)

4. Minute quantities of blood may be taken by finger sticks sampling or by means of an earlobe stick and collected from infants by means of_____ or from scalp veins with a winged infusion needle. (Text B)

5. Arrange the following supplies on the table next to the drawing chair: safety needle and vacutainer sleeve, tubes, _____, gloves, alcohol swab, bandage, cotton or gauze, and tape. (Text B)

Ⅱ. Translate the following into Chinese.

Arrange the following supplies on the table next to the drawing chair: safety needle and vacutainer sleeve, tubes, tourniquet, gloves, alcohol swab, bandage, cotton or gauze, and tape. A sharps container should always be within reach. Tubes should be arranged by order of draw: Red Top, Blue Top, Serum-separating tubes (SST), Green Top, Lavender Top, Yellow Top, and Gray Top. Ask the patient say their name to confirm the paperwork.

Lesson 6   Collection of Blood Plasma and Serum
血浆和血清采集

 Learning Objectives

After studying this lesson, students are expected to be able to

1. master the differences between serum and plasma;
2. be familiar with several common anticoagulants and their applications;
3. know about the components of serum and plasma;
4. understand the main idea of the whole texts.

 Warming-up

1. Why does a hospital have a lot of colored vacuum tubes? What are they used for?
2. What should we pay attention to in the clinical laboratory?
3. Why does bleeding stop automatically after the skin damage?

Text A   Blood Plasma Collection
血浆采集

Blood plasma is a yellowish colored liquid and composed of blood that normally holds the blood cells in suspension, for which we call it extracellular matrix. It makes up about 55% of the body's total blood volume. It is mostly water (up to 95% by volume), and contains dissolved proteins (6%-8%) (i. e., serum albumins, globulins, and fibrinogen), glucose, clotting factors, electrolytes (Na^+, Ca^{2+}, Mg^{2+}, HCO_3^-, Cl^-, K^+, etc.), hormones, carbon dioxide, oxygen and so on .

The main functions of plasma are to transport nutrients, waste material, to provide an appropriate environment for different blood cells, to stop the blood from coagulating in the blood vessels, to prevent blood from losing immediately after injury by the blood coagulation material and anticoagulant material, and to prevent the body from infecting by containing antibodies and so on.

Plasma can also be used to treat diseases, and fresh frozen plasma is on the WHO Model List of Essential Medicines, which is the most important medications needed in a basic health system. It is critical importance in the treatment of many types of traumas which lead to blood loss, and is therefore kept stocked universally in all medical facilities, such as trauma centers, hospitals, ambulances, blood bank, operating room.

Now how to separate plasma from blood? We collect whole blood into a commercially available anticoagulant-treated tube. Blood plasma is separated from the blood by centrifuging the tube . The blood cells fall to the bottom of the tube and the blood plasma which a light yellow liquid is then poured or drawn off. Nowadays, the vacuum tubes are disposable blood collection tube made of plastic with vacuum system to facilitate the predetermined draw volume of blood. The vacuum tubes which have different color for different uses are specially used to collect venous blood. For example, the vacuum tubes EDTA-treated (lavender cap) can be used for complete blood count; citrate-treated (light blue cap) can be used for the detection of coagulation function; citrate-treated (black cap) can be used for the detection of erythrocyte sedimentation rate; heparinized tubes (green cap) are indicated for some other applications, such as the detection of some emergency biochemical and routine biochemical items.

Blood plasma samples should be maintained at 2-8℃ while handling. If the plasma is not analyzed immediately, the plasma should be apportioned into clean pipes, stored, and transported at −20℃ or lower. It is important to avoid freeze-thaw cycles. Samples which are hemolyzed, icteric, or lipemic can invalidate certain tests. Therefore, we should pay attention to these factors that affect the test results when accepting specimens to ensure that we accept qualified specimens, and so as to ensure the authenticity and reliability of the results.

Text B   Serum Collection
血清采集

Serum is also a yellowish colored liquid. It is the liquid fraction of whole blood that is collected after the blood clotting. Serum do not contain fibrinogen, although some clotting factors remained. It includes all the electrolytes, antibodies, hormones, and any exogenous substances (e. g., drugs and microorganisms).

The serum of convalescent patients who successfully recover (or already recovered) from an infectious disease be used as a biological medicine in the treatment of other people with that same disease, because the antibodies which generated by the successful recovery are potent fighters of the pathogen. Such convalescent serum (antiserum) is a form of immunotherapy. In the clinical Laboratory, Serum is used in numerous diagnostic tests, as well as blood typing. Measurements of serum concentrations has proved usefully in many fields. Test results can be used to prevent, diagnose and treat diseases.

Now how do we separate serum from blood? If commercial the vacuum tubes are used, the researcher can use the tubes which with red cap contain no additives. After collection of the whole blood, allow the blood to clot by leaving it undisturbed at room temperature. It usually takes 15-30 minutes. Separate the clot by the centrifugal force of 1000-2000 xg for 10 minutes in a centrifuge. We can use this serum for biochemistry, immunology and serology tests in medical inspection.

We can also use the vacuum tubes with yellow cap. These tubes contain spray coated silicon and micronized silica particles to accelerate clotting. It also contains an inert separator gel on the base of the tube for serum separation. Gently invert the tube 8-10 times and after coagulation, centrifuge at 2000-3000 rpm for 10 minutes at room temperature. The specific gravity make the barrier gel move upward to the serum-clot interface during centrifugation and it forms a stable barrier separating serum from blood clot. This barrier provides stability of certain parameters of the tubes under the recommended conditions for up to 48 hours, used for serum determinations in biochemical, immunological and serological antibody screening, indirect anti-globulin test, cross matching, antigen typing and drug assays, etc. The storage condition is: 4-25℃ in well-ventilated, environment with relative humidity less than 80%.

It is critical to take care when an individual is dealing with blood since blood is abiohazardous material. The container must be stoppered to prevent spillage, contamination, etc. The container must be properly labeled, since samples from multiple patients might be dealt with and there is high chance of confusion while conducting the tests. A wrong diagnosis can have devastating effects! The clinician looking at the results can draw to wrong conclusion and thus make wrong diagnosis. At the end of the day, it puts the life of the patient "on the line".

New Words

suspension /sə'spenʃn/ *n.* 悬浮,暂停,停职

extracellular /ˌɛkstrə'sɛljʊlə/ *adj.* [生物](位于或发生于)细胞外的

matrix /'meɪtrɪks/ *n.* [生物]基质,母体,子宫

vacuum /'vækjuːm/ *n.* 真空,空间 *adj.* 真空的,利用真空的,产生真空的

predetermine /ˌpriːdɪ'tɜːrmɪn/ *vt.* 预先确定,预先决定,预先查明

lavender /'lævəndər/ *n.* 薰衣草,淡紫色 *adj.* 淡紫色的

citrate /'sɪtret/ *n.* 柠檬酸盐

heparin /'hɛpərɪn/ *n.* [生化]肝素(用于防治血栓形成等),肝磷脂

hemolyze /ˈhɛməlaɪz/ *vt.* 使(红细胞)溶解 *vi.* 发生溶血(等于 haemolyze)
icteric /ɪkˈtɛrɪk/ *n.* 治黄疸之药 *adj.* 黄疸的
invalidate /ɪnˈvælɪdeɪt/ *vt.* 使无效,使无价值
convalescent /ˌkɑːnvəˈlesnt/ *n.* 恢复中的病人,康复的人 *adj.* 康复的,恢复期的
immunotherapy /ɪˈmjənoˈθɛrəpi/ *n.* 免疫疗法

Phrases and Expressions

be composed of ...	由……组成
WHO Model List of Essential Medicines	WHO 基本药物示范目录
be separated from ...	从……分离出来
erythrocyte sedimentation rate	红细胞沉降率,红细胞沉降速度
micronized silica	二氧化硅微粒
specific gravity	比重
inert separator gel	惰性分离胶

Notes

1. The main functions of plasma are to transport nutrients, waste material, to provide an appropriate environment for different blood cells; to stop the blood from coagulating in the blood vessels, and to prevent blood from losing immediately after injury by the blood coagulation material and anticoagulant material; to prevent the body from infecting by containing antibodies and so on.

血浆主要的功能是运输营养物质、废物;为不同的血细胞提供适宜的环境;依靠血液凝固物质和抗凝固物质阻止血液在血管内凝固,并且在受伤之后及时阻止血液流失;依靠含有的抗体阻止身体感染。

2. Nowadays, the vacuum tubes are disposable blood collection tube made of plastic with vacuum system to facilitate the predetermined draw volume of blood.

目前,真空管是用塑料制成的一次性采血管,采用真空系统,方便抽取预定的血液量。

3. For example, the vacuum tubes EDTA-treated (lavender cap) can be used for complete blood count; citrate-treated (light blue cap) can be used for the detection of coagulation function; citrate-treated (black cap) can be used for the detection of erythrocyte sedimentation rate; heparinized tubes (green cap) are indicated for some other applications, such as the detection of some emergency biochemical and routine biochemical items.

例如,含有 EDTA 真空管(紫色帽)可用于全血细胞计数;含有枸橼酸盐的真空管(浅蓝色帽)可用于检测凝血功能;含有枸橼酸盐的真空管(黑色帽)可用于红细胞沉降率检测;含有枸橼酸盐的管(绿色帽)表明可用于其他一些用途,比如一些紧急和常规的生化项目检测。

4. Samples which are hemolyzed, icteric, or lipemic can invalidate certain tests. Therefore, we should pay attention to these factors that affect the test results when accepting specimens to ensure that we accept qualified specimens, and so as to ensure the authenticity and reliability of the results.

溶血、黄疸或血脂的样品可使某些试验无效。因此,在接受标本时要注意这些影响检测结果的因素,以确保我们接受合格的标本,从而确保结果的真实性和可靠性。

5. The serum of convalescent patients who successfully recover (or already recovered) from an infectious disease can be used as a biological medicine in the treatment of other people with that same disease, because the antibodies which generated by the successful recovery are potent fighters of the pathogen.

在传染病中成功康复(或已经康复)的恢复期病人的血清,可以作为治疗同一疾病的其他人的生物药物,因为通过成功康复产生的抗体是抵抗病原体的强有力战士。

6. The specific gravity makes the barrier gel move upward to the serum-clot interface during centrifugation and it forms a stable barrier separating serum from blood clot.

比重使分离凝胶在离心过程中向上移动到血清和凝血块界面,形成稳定的屏障将血清从血凝块中分离出来。

7. This barrier provides stability of certain parameters of the tubes under the recommended conditions for up to 48 hours, used for serum determinations in biochemical, immunological and serological antibody screening, indirect anti-globulin test, cross matching, antigen typing and drug assays, etc.

在要求条件下,这个障碍可在长达48h的时间内为试管内一定的参数提供稳定性,被用于生物化学、免疫学、血清学抗体筛查,间接抗体试验、交叉配血、抗原定型、药物分析的血清测定。

8. The container must be properly labeled, since samples from multiple patients might be dealt with and there is high chance of confusion while conducting the tests. A wrong diagnosis can have devastating effects!

容器必须正确贴上标签,因为可能要处理来自多个病人的样本,而且在进行测试时很有可能出现混淆。错误的诊断会带来毁灭性的后果!

Exercises

Ⅰ. Fill in the blanks according to the texts.

1. _____ is a yellowish colored liquid and composed of blood that normally holds the blood cells in suspension, for which we call it extracellular matrix. (Text A)

2. Nowadays, the _____ tubes are disposable blood collection tube made of plastic with vacuum system to facilitate the predetermined draw volume of blood. (Text A)

3. Citrate-treated (light blue cap) can be used for the detection of _____. (Text A)

4. Serum do not contain _____, although some clotting factors remained. (Text B)

5. The specific gravity make the barrier gel move upward to the serum-clot _____ during centrifugation and it forms a stable barrier separating serum from blood clot. (Text B)

Ⅱ. Translate the following into Chinese.

Now how do we separate serum from blood? If commercial the vacuum tubes are used, the researcher can use the tubes which with red cap contain no additives. After collection of the whole blood, allow the blood to clot by leaving it undisturbed at room temperature. It usually takes 15-30 minutes. Separate the clot by the centrifugal force of 1000-2000 ×g for 10 minutes in a centrifuge. We can use this serum for biochemistry, immunology and serology tests in medical inspection.

Lesson 7　Microscopy and Microscope Slide
显微镜技术与显微镜载物片

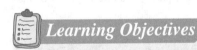
Learning Objectives

After studying this lesson, students are expected to be able to

1. master some medical terms about microscopy and microscope slide;

2. be familiar with the slides for pathological and biological research;

3. know about the "structural" components of a microscope;

4. use the microscope and slides properly.

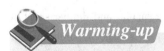
Warming-up

1. What are the branches of microscopy?

2. What is a microscope used for?

3. What is a microscope slide?

Text A   Brief Introduction to Microscopy
显微镜技术简介

Microscopy is the technical field of using microscopes to view samples and objects that cannot be seen with the unaided eyes. There are three well-known branches of microscopy, optical, electron and scanning probe microscopy.

A microscope is an instrument used to see objects that are too small for the naked eyes. The science of investigating small objects using such an instrument is called microscopy (figure 2-1). Microscopic means invisible to the eye unless aided by a microscope.

Optical and electron microscopy involve the diffraction, reflection, or refraction of electromagnetic radiation or electron beams interacting with the specimen, and the subsequent collection of this scattered radiation or another signal in order to create an image. This process may be carried out by wide-field irradiation of the sample (e.g., standard light microscopy and transmission electron microscopy) or by scanning of a fine beam over the sample (e.g., confocal laser scanning microscopy and scanning electron microscopy). Scanning probe microscopy involves the interaction of a scanning probe with the surface of the object of interest. The development of microscopy revolutionized biology and remains an essential technique in the life and physical sciences.

Microscope must accomplish three tasks: produce a magnified image of the specimen, separate the details in the image, and render the details visible to the human eye or camera. All modern optical microscopes designed for vie-

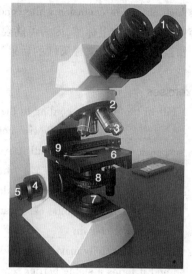

1. Ocular lens (eyepiece); 2. Objective turret or Revolver; 3. Objective; 4. Focus wheel to move the stage-coarse adjustment; 5. Focus wheel to move the stage-fine adjustment; 6. Frame to provide a mounting point for various microscope controls; 7. Light source, or a mirror; 8. Condenser and diaphragm; 9. Stage to hold the sample.

Figure 2-1   The Structure Map of a Microscope

wing samples by transmitted light share the same basic components of the light path. In addition, the vast majority of microscopes have the same "structural" components.

Text B   Microscope Slide
显微镜载物片

Microscope slide is a thin flat piece of glass, used to hold objects for examination under a microscope. Typically, the object is placed or secured (mounted) on the slide, and then both are inserted together in the microscope for viewing. This arrangement allows several slide-mounted objects to be quickly inserted and removed from the microscope, labeled, transported, and stored in appropriate slide cases or folders.

Microscope slides are often used together with a cover slip or cover glass, a smaller and thinner sheet of glass that is placed over the specimen. Slides are held in place on the microscope's stage by slide clips or slide clamps. A standard microscope slide measures about 75 mm by 25 mm and is about 1 mm thick. A range of other sizes are available for various special purposes.

For pathological and biological research, the specimen usually undergoes a complex histological preparation that may involve cutting it into very thin sections with a microtome, fixing it to prevent decay, removing any water contained in it, staining specific parts of it, and impregnating or infiltrating it with some transparent solid substance. As a result of this process, the specimen usually ends up firmly attached to the slide.

In a wet mount, the specimen is placed in a drop of water or other liquid held between the slide and the cover slip by surface tension. This method is commonly used, for example, to view microscopic organisms that grow in pond water or other liquid media, especially when studying their movement and behavior. It is also used to examine physiological liquids like blood, urine, saliva, semen, and vaginal discharge. Care must be taken to exclude air bubbles that would interfere with the viewing and hamper the organisms' movements.

Plain slides are the most common and there are several specialized types. A concavity slide has one or more shallow depressions ("wells"), designed to hold certain samples such as liquids and tissue cultures. Slides may have rounded corners for increased safety or robustness, or a cut-off corner for automated handling.

A graticule slide is marked with a grid of lines (e.g., a 1 mm grid) that allows the size of objects seen under magnification to be easily estimated and provides reference areas for counting minute objects. Sometimes one square of the grid will itself be subdivided into a finer grid. Slides for specialized applications, such as cell counting, may have various reservoirs, channels and barriers etched or ground on their upper surface.

New Words

optical /ˈɑːptɪkl/ *adj.* 光学的

diffraction /diˈfrækʃn/ *n.* 衍射

reflection /riˈflekʃn/ *n.* 反射

refraction /riˈfrækʃn/ *n.* 折射

electromagnetic /ɪˌlektroʊmægˈnetɪk/ *adj.* 电磁的

scattered /ˈskætərd/ *adj.* 散射的

irradiation /ɪˌreɪdiˈeɪʃn/ *n.* 照射

confocal /kɑnˈfokl/ *adj.* ［数］共焦的,同焦点的

revolutionize /ˌrevəˈluːʃənaɪz/ *vt.* 发动革命

ocular /ˈɑːkjələr/ *adj.* 眼睛的,视觉的,目击的 *n.* ［光］目镜

eyepiece /ˈaɪpiːs/ *n.* ［光］目镜,接目镜

turret /ˈtɜːrət/ *n.* 转台

revolver /rɪˈvɑːlvər/ *n.* 旋转器

condenser /kənˈdensər/ *n.* 冷凝器;［电］电容器;［光］聚光器

diaphragm /ˈdaɪəfræm/ *n.* 光圈

slide /slaid/ *n.* 载玻片

slip /slip/ *n.* 片

histological /ˌhɪstəˈlɔdʒɪkəl/ *adj.* 组织学的

microtome /ˈmaɪkrəˌtom/ *n.* 显微镜用薄片切片机

stain /steɪn/ *vt.* 给……着色

impregnate /ɪmˈpregneɪt/ *v.* 浸透

infiltrate /ˈɪnfɪltreɪt/ *v.* 使浸润

transparent /trænsˈpærənt/ *adj.* 透明的,显然的,坦率的,易懂的

concavity /kɑːnˈkævəti/ *n.* 凹面

cut-off /ˈkʌt ɔːf/ *n.* 截止,定点,界限

graticule /ˈgrætɪkjuːl/ *n.* 显微镜的计数线

reservoir /ˈrezərvwɑːr/ *n.* 储液槽

etch /etʃ/ *v.* 蚀刻

Phrases and Expressions

electromagnetic radiation	电磁辐射
electron beam	电子束
transmission electron microscopy	透射电子显微镜检查法
confocal laser scanning microscopy	共聚焦激光扫描显微镜检查法
objective turret	物镜转换器
focus wheel	调焦旋钮
microscope slide	显微镜载物片
cover slip / cover glass	盖玻片
vaginal discharge	阴道分泌物

Notes

1. Optical and electron microscopy involve the diffraction, reflection, or refraction of electromagnetic radiation or electron beams interacting with the specimen, and the subsequent collection of this scattered radiation or another signal in order to create an image.

光学显微镜和电子显微镜涉及与标本相互作用的电磁辐射或电子束的衍射、反射或折射，并且收集光散射以及其他的信号，以形成一个图像。

2. Scanning probe microscopy involves the interaction of a scanning probe with the surface of the object of interest.

扫描探针显微镜检查法涉及扫描探针与观察样品表面的相互作用。

3. Microscope must accomplish three tasks: produce a magnified image of the specimen, separate the details in the image, and render the details visible to the human eye or camera.

显微镜必须完成3项任务：产生放大的标本图像、分辨图像中的细节并将可视的图像细节呈现于人眼或照相机。

4. This arrangement allows several slide-mounted objects to be quickly inserted and removed from the microscope, labeled, transported, and stored in appropriate slide cases or folders.

这种排布能使多个置于载玻片上的标本，快速插入或移出显微镜，并能快速标记、运输和存储在合适的玻片盒或玻片夹中。

5. For pathological and biological research, the specimen usually undergoes a complex histological preparation that may involve cutting it into very thin sections with a microtome, fixing it to prevent decay, removing any water contained in it, staining specific parts of it, and impregnating or infiltrating it with some transparent solid substance.

对于病理学和生物学研究，标本通常要经过复杂的组织学制备。它可包括用薄片切片机将标本切成极薄的薄片，固定标本以防止腐烂，脱去标本中的水分，染色标本的特殊部分，以及用一些透明固体物质浸渍或透明标本。

6. A graticule slide is marked with a grid of lines (e. g. , a 1 mm grid) that allows the size of objects seen under magnification to be easily estimated and provides reference areas for counting minute objects.

带计数线的载物片以网格线标示（例如，1毫米网格），网格使得被放大的观察物体很容易估算出大小，而且提供的参考面积能用于微小物体的计数。

Exercises

Ⅰ. Fill in the blanks according to the texts.

1. There are three well-known branches of microscopy, optical, _____ and scanning probe microscopy. (Text A)

2. A microscope is an instrument used to see objects that are too small for the naked eye. The science of investigating small objects using such an instrument is called _____. (Text A)

3. Microscope slides are often used together with a _____ or cover glass, a smaller and thinner sheet of glass that is placed over the specimen. (Text B)

4. In a wet mount, the specimen is placed in a drop of water or other liquid held between the slide and the cover slip by_____. (Text B)

5. A concavity slide has one or more shallow depressions, designed to hold certain samples such as liquids and _____. (Text B)

Ⅱ. Translate the following into Chinese.

The actual power or magnification of a compound optical microscope is the product of the powers of the ocular (eyepiece) and the objective lens. Typical magnification values for eyepieces include ×2, ×5 and ×10. Typical magnification values for objective range from ×5 to ×100. The maximum normal magnifications of the ocular and objective are ×10 and ×100 respectively giving a final magnification of 1000×.

Lesson 8　Centrifugation and Electrophoresis Technology
离心分离与电泳技术

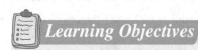 **Learning Objectives**

After studying this lesson, students are expected to be able to

1. master the definition of centrifugation and electrophoresis;
2. be familiar with the processes of centrifugation and electrophoresis;
3. know about the function of the centrifuge;
4. list the factors that influence molecular separation.

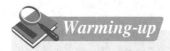 **Warming-up**

1. What is centrifugation?
2. What is electrophoresis technology?

Text A　Centrifugation
离心分离

Decantation is a process for the separation of mixtures. This is achieved by carefully pouring a solution from a container to leave the precipitate (sediments) in the bottom of the original container. A centrifuge may be useful in decanting a solution successfully.

Centrifugation is a process where the sedimentation of mixtures can be produced by the centrifugal force with a centrifuge, used in laboratory settings. More-dense components of the mixture migrate away from the axis of the centrifuge, while less-dense components of the mixture migrate towards the axis. Chemists and biologists may increase the effective gravitational force on a test tube so as to more rapidly and completely cause the precipitate to gather on the bottom of the tube. The remaining solution is properly called the "supernate" or "supernatant liquid". The supernatant liquid is then either quickly decanted from the tube without disturbing the precipitate or withdrawn with a Pasteur pipette. Pasteur pipettes, also known as droppers or eye droppers, are used to transfer small quantities of liquids. They are usually glass tubes tapered to a narrow point and fitted with a rubber bulb at the top.

Centrifuge is a piece of equipment, generally driven by an electric motor, which puts an object in rotation around a fixed axis, applying a force perpendicular to the axis. The centrifuge works according to the sedimentation principle, where the centripetal acceleration causes denser substances to separate out along the radial direction (the bottom of the tube). By the same token, lighter objects will tend to move to the top (of the tube).

The rotating unit, called the rotor, has fixed holes drilled at an angle (to the vertical). Test tubes are placed in these slots and the motor is spun. As the centripetal force is in the horizontal plane and the tubes are fixed at an angle, the particles have to travel only a little distance before they hit the wall and drop down to the bottom. These angle rotors are very popular in the lab for routine use.

Text B Electrophoresis
电泳

Electrophoresis, also called cataphoresis, is the motion of dispersed particles relative to a fluid under the influence of a spatially uniform electric field. Electrophoresis is a technique used to separate biological molecules, such as nucleic acids, carbohydrates, and amino acids, based on their movement due to the influence of a direct electric current in a buffered solution. Positively charged molecules move toward the negative electrode, while negatively charged molecules move toward the positive electrode.

In electrophoresis, the electric charge is often passed through what is known as a support medium. Under the influence of an electrical field, charged molecules can be separated from one another as they pass through a gel. The degree of separation and rate of molecular migration of mixtures of molecules depends upon a variety of factors, which can be tailored depending upon the intent of the separation. The factors that influence molecular separation include the individual size and shape of the molecules, their molecular charge, strength of the electric field, the type of support medium used (e. g. , cellulose acetate, starch, paper, agarose, polyacrylamide) and the conditions of the medium (e. g. , ion strength and concentration, pH, viscosity, temperature).

In general, the medium is mixed with a chemical mixture called a buffer. The buffer carries the electric charge that is applied to the system. The medium or buffer matrix is placed in a tray. Samples of molecules to be separated are loaded into wells or slots that have been formed at one end of the matrix. As electrical current is applied to the tray, the matrix takes on this charge and develops positively and negatively charged ends. As a result, molecules that are negatively charged such as deoxyribonucleic acid (DNA), ribonucleic acid (RNA), and protein are pulled toward the positive end of the gel.

Molecules have differing shapes, sizes and charges, and they are pulled through the matrix at different rates, which results in intermolecular separation of the molecules. In general, the smaller the molecule is and the more charges the molecule has, the faster the molecule moves through the matrix.

New Words

decantation /ˌdiːkænˈteɪʃən/ n. ［化工］倾析，倾注

sedimentation /ˌsedɪmenˈteɪʃn/ n. 沉淀

axis /ˈæksɪs/ n. 轴

supernate /ˈsjuːpəneit/ n. ［免疫］上清液

dropper /ˈdrɑːpər/ n. 滴管

tapered /ˈtepəd/ adj. 锥形的

rotation /roʊˈteɪʃn/ n. 旋转

centripetal /sen'trɪpɪtl/ *adj.* 向心的

acceleration /ək,selə'reɪʃn/ *n.* 加速度

drill /drɪl/ *v.* 钻孔

slot /slɑːt/ *n.* 位置

cataphoresis /,kætəfə'riːsɪs/ *n.* ［化学］电泳，阳离子电泳，电透法

positive /'pɑːzətɪv/ *adj.* ［医］［化学］阳性的

charge /tʃɑːrdʒ/ *n.* 电荷

negative /'negətɪv/ *adj.* ［医］［化学］阴性的

electrode /ɪ'lektroʊd/ *n.* ［电］电极

medium /'miːdɪəm/ *n.* 介质

starch /stɑːrtʃ/ *n.* 淀粉

polyacrylamide /'pɔli,ækri'læmaɪd/ *n.* ［高分子］聚丙烯酰胺

viscosity /vɪ'skɑːsəti/ *n.* 黏性，黏度

tray /treɪ/ *n.* 电泳槽

Phrases and Expressions

centrifugal force	离心力
supernatant liquid	上层液体
Pasteur pipette	巴斯德吸管
by the same token	出于同样原因
nucleic acid	核酸
amino acid	氨基酸
buffered solution	缓冲液
cellulose acetate	醋酸纤维素
deoxyribonucleic acid（DNA）	脱氧核糖核酸
ribonucleic acid（RNA）	核糖核酸

Notes

1. More-dense components of the mixture migrate away from the axis of the centrifuge, while less-dense components of the mixture migrate towards the axis.

混合物中密度较高的成分朝远离离心机轴的方向移动，而混合物中密度较低的成分则朝离心机轴方向移动。

2. The supernatant liquid is then either quickly decanted from the tube without disturbing the precipitate or withdrawn with a Pasteur pipette.

然后，可以迅速地从试管内倾泻出上层液体，不扰动沉淀物；也可以用巴斯德吸管吸去上层液体。

3. The degree of separation and rate of molecular migration of mixtures of molecules depends upon a variety of factors, which can be tailored depending upon the intent of the separation.

分子混合物被分离的程度和分子移动速率取决于多种因素，这些因素可以根据分离的目的进行调整。

4. Samples of molecules to be separated are loaded into wells or slots that have been formed at one end of the matrix.

将待分离的分子样品加入基质一端的加样孔或加样槽内。

5. In general, the smaller the molecule is and the more charges the molecule has, the faster the molecule moves through the matrix.

一般而言，分子越小，电荷越多，通过基质的速度就越快。

Exercises

Ⅰ. Fill in the blanks according to the texts.

1. _____ is a process for the separation of mixtures. (Text A)

2. Centrifugation is a process where the _____ of mixtures can be produced by the centrifugal force with a centrifuge, used in laboratory settings. (Text A)

3. The _____ liquid is then either quickly decanted from the tube without disturbing the precipitate or withdrawn with a Pasteur pipette. (Text A)

4. Electrophoresis, also called _____, is the motion of dispersed particles relative to a fluid under the influence of a spatially uniform electric field. (Text B)

5. As electrical current is applied to the tray, the _____ takes on this charge and develops positively and negatively charged ends. (Text B)

Ⅱ. Translate the following into Chinese.

The centrifuge works according to the sedimentation principle, where the centripetal acceleration causes denser substances to separate out along the radial direction (the bottom of the tube). By the same token, lighter objects will tend to move to the top (of the tube).

Lesson 9　Absorption Spectroscopy
吸收光谱分析技术

Learning Objectives

After studying this lesson, students are expected to be able to

1. master the definition of spectroscopy;

2. be familiar with the function of spectrophotometry;

3. know about the spectrophotometer;

4. list the factors that influence the determination of concentration.

Warming-up

1. What does the word "spectroscopy" mean?

2. What is the spectrophotometer used for?

Text A　Ultraviolet-Visible Spectrophotometry
紫外可见分光光度法

The word "spectroscopy" is used as a collective term for all the analytical techniques based on the interaction of light and matter. Spectroscopy consists of many different applications such as atomic absorption spectroscopy, atomic emission spectroscopy, nuclear magnetic resonance spectroscopy, ultraviolet-visible (UV-Vis) spectroscopy, and so on.

Spectrophotometry is one of the branches of spectroscopy where we measure the absorption of light by molecules that are in a gas or vapour state, or dissolved molecules or ions. Spectrophotometry investigates the absorption of the different substances with the wavelength limits of 190-780 nm (visible spectroscopy is restricted to the wavelength limits of electromagnetic radiation detectable by the human eye, that is above 360 nm; ultraviolet spectroscopy is used for shorter wavelengths). In this wavelength range the absorption of the electromagnetic radiation is caused by the excitation (i. e., transition to a higher energy level) of the bonding and non-bonding electrons of the ions or molecules. A graph of absorbance against wavelength gives the sample's absorption spectrum. Modern spectrophotometers draw this automatically. The measured spectrum is continuous, due to the fact that the different vibration and rotation states of the molecules make the absorption band wider.

Spectrophotometry is used for both qualitative and quantitative investigations of samples. The wavelength at the maximum of the absorption band will give information about the structure of the molecule or ion and the extent of the absorption is proportional with the amount of the species absorbing the light. An absorption spectrum can be quantitatively related to the amount of material present using the Beer-Lambert law. Determining the absolute concentration of a compound requires knowledge of the compound's absorption coefficient. The absorption coefficient for some compounds is available from reference sources, and it can also be determined by measuring the spectrum of a calibration standard with a known concentration of the target.

Text B   Spectrophotometer
分光光度计

The qualitative or quantitative analysis techniques of a substance by the absorption of light is called spectrophotometry, which is based on the Beer-Lambert law. The instrument used for the determination of substances by spectrophotometry is called "spectrophotometer".

The instrument consists of a light source, a monochromator, a cuvette (a sample tube), a detector and a readout. The light source emits a compound light, and the function of monochromator is to change the compound light into a monochromatic light with a particular wavelength. The cuvette is used to hold sample solution. When the cuvette is irradiated by the monochromatic light, a part of light is absorbed by the solution in the cuvette, and the other light penetrates through the cuvette and is measured by the detector, converting the light signal into an electric signal which is displayed as a certain absorbance on the readout.

Depending on the wavelength of light emitted by the light source, the spectrophotometer can be divided into visible spectrophotometer (wavelength limits of 400-760 nm) and ultraviolet-visible spectrophotometer (wavelength limits of 200-760 nm).

According to the Beer-Lambert law: $A = KLC$ (A for absorbance, K for the absorption coefficient, L for the thickness or path length of sample solution, C for the solution concentration), we can measure the absorbance of a substance for a particular wavelength (which is usually identical with the maximum absorption wavelength of the analyte), calculate the concentration from the determination results by using the molar absorptivity found in the literatures, and the unknown concentration can also be determined by comparing the determination results with a working curve (calibration curve) of absorbance and concentration.

However, the determination of substances concentration could be influenced by the following factors even in the simplest cases:

• Substance interference: Other substances or the existing substances might interfere with the determination of the absorbance value of the substances to be measured. Such interference could be eliminated (or at least reduced) by the extraction or dual wavelength methods.

• Non-monochromatic light: If the instrument is unable to extract the monochromatic light within the allowable error limits, it will cause the concentration of the substances to be measured to deviate from the standard curve.

New Words

spectroscopy /spek'trɑːskəpi/ *n.* [光] 光谱学

graph /græf/ *n.* 图表

absorbance /əb'sɔːrbəns/ *n.* [物化] 吸光度,吸收率

calibration /ˌkælɪˈbreɪʃn/ n. 校准

spectrophotometer /ˌspɛktrofoˈtamətə/ n. ［光］分光光度计

spectrophotometry /ˌspektrəufəuˈtɔmitri/ n. ［分化］［光］分光光度(测定)法

monochromator /ˌmɔnəuˈkrəumeitə/ n. ［光］单色仪，单色器，单色光镜

cuvette /kjʊˈvɛt/ n. ［生化］(分光光度计等仪器中盛样液用的)比色皿，比色杯

readout /ˈridˌaʊt/ n. 显示器，读出器，示值读数

emit /iˈmɪt/ vt. 发出，放射

irradiate /ɪˈreɪdieɪt/ vt. 辐射，辐照，照射，放射

penetrate /ˈpenətreɪt/ vt. & vi. 渗透，穿透，刺入

convert /kənˈvɜːrt/ vt. & vi. 转变，转换，变换

analyte /ˈænəlait/ n. ［分化］分析物，被分析物

absorptivity /ˌæbsɔrpˈtɪvɪti/ n. 吸收率，吸收能力，吸收性

eliminate /ɪˈlɪmɪneɪt/ vt 消除，排除

extraction /ɪkˈstrækʃn/ n. 取出，抽出，拔出，萃取

deviate /ˈdiːvieɪt/ vt. & vi. 偏离，脱离，越轨

Phrases and Expressions

atomic absorption spectroscopy	原子吸收光谱法
atomic emission spectroscopy	原子发射光谱法
nuclear magnetic resonance spectroscopy	核磁共振光谱法
ultraviolet-visible spectroscopy	紫外可见光光谱法
wavelength limits	波长范围
Beer-Lambert law	比尔-朗伯定律
absorption coefficient	吸收系数
calibration standard	校准标准
compound light	复合光
monochromatic light	单色光
molar absorptivity	摩尔吸光系数
calibration curve	校准曲线
extraction method	萃取法
dual wavelength method	双波长法
allowable error limits	误差允许范围

Notes

1. Spectrophotometry is one of the branches of spectroscopy where we measure the absorption of light by molecules that are in a gas or vapour state or dissolved molecules or ions.

分光光度法是光谱学的一个分支，主要用气体、蒸汽分子或溶解的分子或离子来测量光的吸收度。

2. Spectrophotometry investigates the absorption of the different substances with the wavelength limits of 190-780 nm (visible spectroscopy is restricted to the wavelength range of electromagnetic radiation detectable by the human eye, that is above 360 nm; ultraviolet spectroscopy is used for shorter wavelengths).

分光光度法研究不同物质在波长190nm至780nm的光的吸收度(可见光谱限于人眼可觉察的电磁辐射的波长范围，即360nm以上波长；紫外光谱则用于更短的波长)。

3. The qualitative or quantitative analysis techniques of a substance by the absorption of light is called spectrophotometry, which is based on the Beer-Lambert law.

利用对光的吸收作用对物质进行定性或定量分析的技术称为分光光度技术。它基于的原理是比尔-朗伯定律。

4. The instrument consists of a light source, a monochromator, a cuvette (a sample tube), a detector and a readout. The light source emits a compound light, and the function of monochromator is to change the compound light into a monochromatic light with a particular wavelength.

仪器由光源、单色器、比色皿(试样管)、检测器和显示器组成。光源发出的是复合光,单色器的功能是将复合光变成特定波长的单色光。

5. When the cuvette is irradiated by the monochromatic light, a part of light is absorbed by the solution in the cuvette, and the other light penetrates through the cuvette and is measured by the detector, converting the light signal into an electric signal which is displayed as a certain absorbance on the readout.

当单色光照射比色皿时,一部分光可以被比色皿中的溶液所吸收,一部单色光穿透比色皿,被检测器所检测到,将光信号转化为电信号,并通过显示器以一定吸光度显示出来。

Exercises

Ⅰ. Fill in the blanks according to the texts.

1. _____ is used as a collective term for all the analytical techniques based on the interaction of light and matter. (Text A)

2. An absorption spectrum can be quantitatively related to the amount of material present using the ____ _____law. (Text A)

3. The absorption _____ for some compounds is available from reference sources, and it can also be determined by measuring the spectrum of a calibration standard with a known concentration of the target. (Text A)

4. The instrument used for the determination of substances by spectrophotometry is called "_____ ____". (Text B)

5. Depending on the wavelength of light _____ by the light source, the spectrophotometer can be divided into visible spectrophotometer and ultraviolet-visible spectrophotometer. (Text B)

Ⅱ. Translate the following into Chinese.

Spectrophotometry is used for both qualitative and quantitative investigations of samples. The wavelength at the maximum of the absorption band will give information about the structure of the molecule or ion and the extent of the absorption is proportional with the amount of the species absorbing the light. An absorption spectrum can be quantitatively related to the amount of material present using the Beer-Lambert law.

Lesson 10 Electrochemical Analysis
电化学分析

Learning Objectives

After studying this lesson, students are expected to be able to

1. master the definitions of electrochemical cell and potentiometry;

2. be familiar with the electroanalytical methods;

3. know about the four main types of ion-selective membrane;

4. tell the structure of an electrochemical cell.

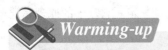

Text A   Electrochemical Cell and Potentiometry
电化学电池与电位计

An electrical cell is a device that is used to generate electricity or one that is used to make chemical reactions possible by applying electricity. An electrochemical cell consists of two half-cells. The two half-cells may use the same electrolyte, or they may use different electrolytes. Each half-cell consists of an electrode, and an electrolyte. In a full electrochemical cell, ions, atoms, or molecules from one half-cell lose electrons (oxidation) to their electrode while ions, atoms, or molecules from the other half-cell gain electrons (reduction) from their electrode. A salt bridge is often employed to provide electrical contact between two half-cells with very different electrolytes-to prevent the solutions from mixing.

Each half-cell has a characteristic voltage. Different choices of substances for each half-cell give different potential differences. Each reaction is undergoing an equilibrium reaction between different oxidation states of the ions — when equilibrium is reached the cell, it cannot provide further voltage. The cell potential can be predicted through the use of electrode potentials (the voltages of each half-cell). The difference in voltage between electrode potentials gives a prediction for the potential measured.

Electroanalytical methods are a class of techniques in analytical chemistry which study an analyte by measuring the potential (volts) and / or current (amperes) in an electrochemical cell containing the analyte. These methods can be categorized according to which aspects of the cell are controlled and which are measured. The three main categories are potentiometry (the difference in electrode potentials is measured), coulometry (the cell's current is measured over time), and voltammetry (the cell's current is measured while actively altering the cell's potential).

Potentiometry passively measures the potential of a solution between two electrodes, affecting the solution very little in the process. The potential is then related to the concentration of one or more analytes. The cell structure used is often referred to as an electrode even though it actually contains two electrodes: an indicator electrode and a reference electrode (distinct from the reference electrode used in the three electrode systems). Potentiometry usually uses electrodes that are sensitive to the selectivity of ions, such as a fluoride-selective electrode. The most common potentiometric electrode is the glass-membrane electrode used in a pH meter.

Text B   Ion-selective Electrode
离子选择电极

An ion-selective electrode (ISE), also known as a specific ion electrode (SIE), is a transducer (or sensor) that converts the activity of a specific ion dissolved in a solution into an electrical potential, which can be measured by a voltmeter or pH meter. The voltage is theoretically dependent on the logarithm of the ionic activity, according to the Nernst Equation. The sensing part of the electrode is usually made as an ion-specific membrane, along with a reference electrode. Ion-selective electrodes are used in biochemical and biophysical research, where measurements of ionic concentration in an aqueous solution are required, usually on a real time basis.

Any electrode (or microelectrode) can respond in a reproducible manner to changes in the concentration (strictly, in the activity) of a specific kind of ion in the solution. Yet the electrode is insensitive, or essentially so, to changes in the concentrations (strictly, in the activities) of any other kinds of ion in the solution. The electrode has at its surface a thin membrane of electrically conducting material, separating the internal and external solutions. Across the membrane an electric potential difference develops. The membrane consists of or contains an electroactive material responsive to the ions to be determined.

There are four main types of ion-selective membrane used in ion-selective electrodes: glass, solid state, liquid based and compound electrode. A very common example of ion-selective membrane is glass membrane. Glass membranes are made from an ion-exchange type of glass (silicate). This type of ISE has good selectivity, but only for several single-charged cations, mainly H^+, Na^+ and Ag^+.

These electrodes are prepared from glass capillary tubing approximately 2 millimeters in diameter, a large batch at a time. Polyvinyl chloride is dissolved in a solvent and plasticizers (typically phthalates) added. In order to provide the ionic specificity, a specific ion channel or carrier is added to the solution; this allows the ion to pass through the vinyl, which prevents the passage of other ions and water.

New Words

electrochemical /ɪˌlektrəuˈkemɪkəl/ *adj.* ［物化］电化学的,电气化学的

potentiometry /pəˌtenʃiˈɔmitri/ *n.* ［电］电势测定法,电位测定法

half-cell /ˈhɑːfsel/ *n.* ［物化］半电池

volt /voult/ *n.* 伏特(电压单位)

ampere /æmˈpɪr/ *n.* 安培(计算电流强度的标准单位)

coulometry /kuːˈlɔmɪtri/ *n.* 电量分析,库仑分析法

voltammetry /voulˈtæmitri/ *n.* ［分化］伏安法

meter /ˈmiːtər/ *n.* 仪表,计量器

transducer /trænzˈduːsər/ *n.* ［自］传感器；［电子］变换器,换能器

voltmeter /ˈvoultmiːtər/ *n.* 伏特计,电压表

logarithm /ˈlɔːgərɪðəm/ *n.* ［数］对数

microelectrode /ˌmaɪkrəuiˈlektrəud/ *n.* 微电极

reproducible /ˌriːprəˈduːsəbl/ *adj.* 可再生的

electroactive /ɪˌlektrəuˈæktɪv/ *adj.* 电活性

silicate /ˈsɪlɪkeɪt/ *n.* ［矿物］硅酸盐

plasticizer /ˈplæstəˌsaɪzɚ/ *n.* 塑化剂

phthalate /ˈ(f)θælˌet/ *n.* 邻苯二甲酸酯

vinyl /ˈvaɪnl/ *n.* 乙烯基(化学)

Phrases and Expressions

salt bridge	盐桥
indicator electrode	指示电极
reference electrode	参比电极
fluoride-selective electrode	氟离子电极
glass-membrane electrode	玻璃膜电极
ion-selective electrode	离子选择电极
Nernst Equation	能斯特方程
capillary tubing	毛细管
polyvinyl chloride	聚氯乙烯

Notes

1. Electrical cell is a device that is used to generate electricity, or one that is used to make chemical reactions possible by applying electricity.

电池是用来产生电流或利用施加的电流使化学反应得以实现的一种装置。

2. In a full electrochemical cell, ions, atoms, or molecules from one half-cell lose electrons (oxidation) to their electrode while ions, atoms, or molecules from the other half-cell gain electrons (reduction) from their electrode.

在完整电化学电池中,一个半电池的离子、原子或分子失去电子(氧化作用)给它们的电极,而另一半电池的离子、原子或分子从它们的电极获得电子(还原作用)。

3. Ion-selective electrodes are used in biochemical and biophysical research, where measurements of ionic concentration in an aqueous solution are required, usually on a real time basis.

离子选择性电极被用于生物化学和生物物理学研究。在研究中,需要对水溶液中的离子浓度进行检测,且这种检测通常是实时性的。

4. The electrode has at its surface a thin membrane of electrically conducting material, separating the internal and external solutions, across which an electric potential difference develops.

电极表面有一层导电材料的薄膜,将内外溶液分隔开,膜内外形成电势差。

5. There are four main types of ion-selective membrane used in ion-selective electrodes: glass, solid state, liquid based and compound electrode.

离子选择性电极主要有4类离子选择膜:玻璃膜、固态膜、液基膜和复合电极膜。

Exercises

Ⅰ. Fill in the blanks according to the texts.

1. An ＿＿＿＿＿＿ cell consists of two half-cells. The two half-cells may use the same electrolyte, or they may use different electrolytes. (Text A)

2. ＿＿＿＿＿＿ methods are a class of techniques in analytical chemistry which study an analyte by measuring the potential (volts) and / or current (amperes) in an electrochemical cell containing the analyte. (Text A)

3. The cell structure used is often referred to as an electrode even though it actually contains two electrodes: an indicator electrode and a ＿＿＿＿＿＿ electrode (distinct from the reference electrode used in the three electrode systems). (Text A)

4. Potentiometry usually uses electrodes that are sensitive to the selectivity of ions, such as a ＿＿＿＿＿＿ electrode. (Text B)

5. An ＿＿＿＿＿＿ electrode (ISE), also known as a specific ion electrode (SIE), is a transducer (or sensor) that converts the activity of a specific ion dissolved in a solution into an electrical potential, which can be measured by a voltmeter or pH meter. (Text B)

Ⅱ. Translate the following into Chinese.

Each half-cell has a characteristic voltage. Different choices of substances for each half-cell give different potential differences. Each reaction is undergoing an equilibrium reaction between different oxidation states of the ions — when equilibrium is reached the cell, it cannot provide further voltage.

笔记

Lesson 11　Validation of Laboratory
实验室确认

Learning Objectives

After studying this lesson, students are expected to be able to

1. master performance characteristics of validation test;
2. be familiar with two criteria of the results of tests with low efficiency;
3. know about the importance of equipment calibration.

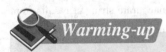

Warming-up

1. Do you agree with this sentence "a miss is as good as a mile"?
2. Talk about the necessity of equipment calibration.
3. Discuss the characteristics of validation test.

Text A　Equipment Calibration
设备校正

Analysis of a specimen in a laboratory involves a number of stepwise procedures. They use different equipment, processes, in vitro devices, software, etc. The "correctness" of results depends upon the correct functioning of all procedures involved. It is therefore essential to validate the equipment, processes, in vitro devices, software, etc. ISO 9001 defines validation as "the attaining and documenting of sufficient evidence to give reasonable assurance, given the current state of science and the art of manufacture, which the process, system and test method under consideration consistently does and / or will do what it is expected to do".

Validation must be done just after calibration of the system with the use of appropriate control material. This provides reassurance that the system and operator are working correctly. Thereafter, validation is done periodically according to user requirements and as written in the standard operating procedure (SOP) manual.

Calibration of equipment is a process which is applied to quantitative measuring or metering of equipment to assure its accurate operation throughout its measuring limits. Calibration of equipment refers to hardware calibration which will be performed by the company engineer. Subsequently it will be validated by checking QC or reference material. Equipment calibration must include technical aspects such as checking of optical systems, temperature, pipette probe, voltage. The company engineer should provide a calibration certificate with relevant details. Correct QC or reference material values indicate that the calibration of the equipment is according to the prescribed standards. If the results are beyond the acceptable limits, the source of error should be identified, and the equipment recalibrated.

Text B　Validation Test
确认试验

Performance characteristics with reference to validation are: accuracy, precision, efficiency and linearity.

The accuracy of a measurement system is the degree of closeness of the mean of observed values to true value. This can be quantitatively expressed as Bias

65

$$Bias = \frac{Observed\ value - True\ value}{True\ value} \times 100$$

Good accuracy means minimum bias.

Precision is closeness of results with each other ofa large number of successive observations in a measurement process, under prescribed conditions. This can be quantitatively expressed as percentage of coefficient of variation (%CV). Good precision means minimum % CV. It can be calculated using the formula given below:

$$CV\% = \frac{s}{\bar{x}} \times 100$$

A measurement system can be accurate but not precise, precise but not accurate, neither, or both. For example, if an experiment contains a systematic error, then increasing the sample size generally increases precision but does not improve accuracy. The end result would be a consistent yet inaccurate string of results from the flawed experiment. Eliminating the systematic error improves accuracy but does not change precision.

Precision is sometimes stratified into:

(a) Repeatability — Closeness of the agreement between the successive measurements of the same specimen and with the following conditions: The same measurement procedure; the same analyst; the same measurement systems used under the same conditions; the same location;

(b) Reproducibility — Closeness of the agreement between the results of successive measurements of the same specimen and with the following conditions: The same measurement procedure; different analysts; different measuring systems; different locations and at different times.

Efficiency of tests is the ability of a test to give the correct diagnosis of a disease or condition. The clinician requesting for a particular test must keep this in mind when interpreting the results of tests with low efficiency. This is measured by two criteria:

(a) Diagnostic sensitivity: The proportion of subjects with disease who have positive test results. The greater the sensitivity of a test, the fewer the number of false-negative results.

$$Sensitivity = \frac{True\ Positives}{True\ Positives + False\ Negatives}$$

(b) Diagnostic specificity: The proportion of subjects without disease who have negative test results. The ability of a test to give fewer false positive results.

$$Specificity = \frac{True\ Negatives}{False\ Positives + True\ Negatives}$$

Linearity of a test determines the upper and lower limit of reporting range of a test.

New Words

validation /ˌvælɪˈdeɪʃn/ n. 确认,批准,生效

stepwise/ˈstepwaɪz/ adv. 逐步地,阶梯式地

assurance /əˈʃʊrəns/ n. 保证,担保

reassurance /ˌriːəˈʃʊrəns/ n. 使安心,再保证,放心

subsequently/ˈsʌbsɪkwəntli/ adv. 随后,其后,后来

pipette /paɪˈpet/ n. 移液管,吸移管

probe /proʊb/ n. 探针,调查

voltage /ˈvoʊltɪdʒ/ n. [电] 电压

recalibrate /riˈkælɪbreɪt/ v. 重新校准

efficiency/ɪˈfɪʃnsɪ/ n. 效率,效能

linearity/ˌlɪnɪˈærəti/ *n.* 线性,直线性

closeness /ˈkloʊsnəs/ *n.* 接近,严密

quantitatively/ˈkwɔːntəteɪtɪvli/ *adv.* 数量上,分量上

bias /ˈbaɪəs/ *n.* 偏倚,偏差

repeatability/riˈpiːtəˈbiliti/ *n.* 重复性;[计] 可重复性,再现性

reproducibility/riprəˌdjuːsəˈbiliti/ *n.* [自] 再现性

Phrases and Expressions

standard operating procedure（SOP）　　　　　标准操作程序

observed value　　　　　　　　　　　　　　观测值

systematic error　　　　　　　　　　　　　系统误差

Notes

1. ISO 9001 defines validation as "the attaining and documenting of sufficient evidence to give reasonable assurance, given the current state of science and the art of manufacture, that the process, system and test method under consideration consistently does and/ or will do what it is expected to do".

ISO 9001 将"确认"定义为"获得和记录足够的证据,以提供合理的保证,考虑到目前的科学和制造技术,并始终如一地考虑到操作过程、系统和检验方法所做的和/或将要做的与所期望做的相一致"。

2. Calibration of equipment is a process which is applied to quantitative measuring or metering of equipment to assure its accurate operation throughout its measuring limits.

设备校准是一种用于设备定量测量或计量的过程,以保证设备在它的整个测定范围内精确运行。

3. Calibration of equipment refers to hardware calibration which will be performed by the company engineer. Subsequently it will be validated by checking QC or reference material.

设备校准是指公司工程师对硬件校准,随后通过校验质量控制或参照物进行确认。

4. Precision is closeness of results with each other of a large number of successive observations in a measurement process, under prescribed conditions.

精密度是在规定条件下,测量过程中大量连续观察的结果相互之间的接近程度。

5. Reproducibility — Closeness of the agreement between the results of successive measurements of the same specimen and with the following conditions: The same measurement procedure; different analysts; different measuring systems; different locations and at different times.

再现性——同一样品在不同的时间、不同的位置、不同的测量系统,不同的分析师用相同的测量步骤进行连续测量,其测量结果的接近程度。

6. Diagnostic sensitivity: The proportion of subjects with disease who have positive test results. The greater the sensitivity of a test, the fewer the number of false-negative results.

诊断的敏感性:检测为阳性结果的患病人数的比例。测试的敏感性越大,假阴性结果的数量就越少。

Exercises

Ⅰ. Fill in the blanks according to the texts.

1. The "correctness" of results depends upon the correct functioning of all procedures involved. It is therefore essential to ＿＿＿＿＿＿ the equipment, processes, in vitro devices, software, etc. (Text A)

2. Equipment calibration must include technical aspects such as checking of ＿＿＿＿＿＿ temperature, pipette probe, voltage. (Text A)

3. Performance characteristics with reference to validation are: accuracy,＿＿＿＿＿, efficiency and linearity. (Text B)

4. Good accuracy means minimum _____ . (Text B)

5. Diagnostic specificity: The proportion of subjects with disease who have positive test results. The greater the sensitivity of a test, the fewer the number of _____ results. (Text B)

Ⅱ. Translate the following into Chinese.

Efficiency of tests is the ability of a test to give the correct diagnosis of a disease or condition. The clinician requesting for a particular test must keep it in mind when interpreting the results of tests with low efficiency. This is measured by two criteria.

Lesson 12   Laboratory Automation Technology
实验室自动化技术

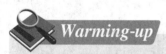

Learning Objectives

After studying this lesson, students are expected to be able to

1. master some medical words and terms about Laboratory Automation Technology;
2. be familiar with the applications of LIS and Auto Analyzers;
3. know about clinical significance of LIS and Auto Analyzers;
4. independently consult relevant professional literatures.

Warming-up

1. Do you know the current situation and development trend of the laboratory?
2. What is the practical significance of establishing LIS?

Text A   Laboratory Information System
实验室信息系统

Laboratory informatics is a professional application of information technology, aiming at optimizing laboratory operation. It includes electronic laboratory notebooks, sample management, data acquisition, data processing, reporting and scientific data management. Some people think that a closely related field is laboratory automation.

The laboratory information (management) systems (LIS or LIMS) is usually part of an integrated information science solution, involving many disparate applications. A laboratory information system is a kind of software to receive process and store the information generated by medical laboratory process. These systems often must interface with instruments and other information systems such as hospital information systems (HIS). A LIS is a highly configurable application according to the needs of users, so as to maximize the convenience of various laboratory work processes. Vendor selection typically takes months of research and planning. Installation takes from a few months to a few years depending on the complexity of the organization. There are many different types of LIS, which are compatible with different working modes in the laboratory. Some vendors provide a full range of service solutions to meet the needs of large hospital laboratories, while others provide specific specialized modules. LIS-supported laboratory disciplines include hematology, chemistry, immunology, blood banks, surgical pathology, anatomical pathology, flow cytometry, and microbiology. This system covers clinical laboratories, including hematology, chemistry and immunology.

The application of LIS is an important part of clinical IT (Information Technology) spectrum of systems, and contributes greatly to the overall care given to patients. The LIS is applied to inpatient and outpatient departments. In many cases, LIS supports two departments simultaneously. From an outpatient or ambulatory perspective, LIS begins frequent interaction after initial diagnosis from doctors. For example, a patient enters the hospital looking pale and complaining of fatigue. The doctor intends to diagnose anemia and may apply for a complete blood count (CBC). For the treatment of inpatients, when the patient is admitted to hospital, the system is usually applied for the laboratory test, providing sample preparation, receiving the results from analyzers, and delivering the laboratory reports to the attending physician. The application form is usually entered into the system by a doctor or laboratory scientist. The application or laboratory request contains a series of tests to be performed on one or more patient specimens (e. g. , blood or urine). In many cases, each application is tracked with a unique identifier. This identifier, which is usually a number, is often referred to as Lab ID. In this hypothetical case, the CBC application form is a combination of multiple tests, including white blood cell counts, red cell blood counts, and other related blood tests.

Text B　Auto Analyzer
自动分析仪

Modern laboratory application technologies need to keep pace with the times and remain competitive. Laboratories devoted to activities such as high-throughput screening, combinatorial chemistry, automated clinical and analytical testing, diagnostics, and many others, would not exist without advancements in laboratory automation. Automation is the application of control systems and information technology, which aims to reduce the labor of people in goods and services products.

An automatic analyzer is a medical laboratory instrument designed to quickly measure different chemical substances and other characteristics in many biological samples, with minimal human assistance. These are instruments that deal with a large portion of the samples going into a hospital or private medical laboratory. Automated inspection processes reduce test time, many of which are shortened from days to minutes.

Biochemical Auto Analyzers, for example, were used primarily for routine, repetitive medical laboratory analysis, but over the past few years, they have been increasingly replaced by discrete working systems, resulting in reduced reagent consumption. These instruments usually measure serum or other body specimens of albumin, alkaline phosphatase (ALP), aspartate transaminase (AST), blood urea nitrogen, bilirubin, calcium, cholesterol, creatinine, glucose, inorganic phosphorus, protein and uric acid. Automated analyzers automate the process of repetitive sample analysis manually performed by technicians, such as those previously mentioned in the medical inspection program. Thus, a technician can analyze hundreds of specimens every day with an Auto Analyzer.

Many methods have been invented to send specimens into the analyzer. This involves placing specimens tube into racks, moving the test tube along the track, or inserting the test tube into the rotating disk to rotate to a specific location to facilitate the collection of specimens. Some analyzers need to transfer specimens to the specimen cup. However, in order to protect the health and safety of laboratory workers, many manufacturers have been prompted to develop analyzers using closed tube sampling to prevent the operator from direct contact with specimens. Samples can be treated separately, in batches or continuously.

New Words

integrate /ˈɪntɪɡreɪt/ v. 使……成整体

disparate /ˈdɪspərət/ adj. 不同的,全异的

interface /ˈɪntərfeɪs/ v. 相互作用,交流

configurable /kənˈfɪɡjərəbl/ adj. 可配置的,结构的

vendor /ˈvendər/ n. 供应商,销售商

discipline /ˈdɪsəplɪn/ n. 学科,纪律,训练,惩罚

ambulatory /ˈæmbjələtɔːri/ *adj.* 流动的，走动的

perspective /pərˈspektɪv/ *n.* 观点，远景

complain /kəmˈpleɪn/ *v.* 抱怨

fatigue /fəˈtiːg/ *n.* 疲劳，疲乏

identifier /aɪˈdentɪfaɪər/ *n.* 标识符，认同者

hypothetical /ˌhaɪpəˈθetɪkl/ *adj.* 假设的

competitive /kəmˈpetətɪv/ *adj.* 竞争的

combinatorial /kəmˌbaɪnəˈtɔrɪəl/ *adj.* 组合的

repetitive /rɪˈpetətɪv/ *adj.* 重复的

rack /ræk/ n. 架子，样本架，行李架

Phrases and Expressions

urea nitrogen	尿素氮
inorganic phosphorus	无机磷
high-throughput screening	高通量筛选
combinatorial chemistry	组合化学
automated clinical and analytical testing	自动化临床检验和分析检验
alkaline phosphatase（ALP）	碱性磷酸酶
blood urea nitrogen	血尿素氮

Notes

1. A LIS is a highly configurable application according to the needs of users, so as to maximize the convenience of various laboratory work processes.

LIS 可根据用户的需求来配置，以求最大限度地方便各种实验室的工作流程。

2. The application of LIS is an important part of clinical IT（Information Technology）spectrum of systems, and contributes greatly to the overall care given to patients.

LIS 的应用是临床多部门信息系统的重要组成部分，并且大大有助于病人的整体护理。

3. In many cases, each application is tracked with a unique identifier.

许多病例中，每份申请单用唯一标识追踪。

4. Modern laboratory application technology needs to keep pace with the times and remain competitive.

现代实验室应用技术需要与时俱进和保持竞争性。

5. Laboratories devoted to activities such as high-throughput screening, combinatorial chemistry, automated clinical and analytical testing, diagnostics, and many others, would not exist without advancements in laboratory automation.

实验室致力于的活动，例如高通量筛选、组合化学、自动化临床检验和分析检验、诊断，以及其他许多方面，没有实验室自动化的进步将都不存在。

6. Automated Analyzers automate the process of repetitive sample analysis manually performed by technicians, such as those previously mentioned in the medical inspection program.

自动分析仪使技术员手工进行的重复样品分析步骤自动化，如前面所提及的那些医学检验项目。

7. This involves placing specimens tube into racks, moving the test tube along the track, or inserting the test tube into the rotating disk to rotate to a specific location to facilitate the collection of specimens.

这涉及放置标本试管到试管架，试管架可沿着轨道移动，或将试管插入旋转盘旋转至特定位置，以方便标本的取用。

Exercises

Ⅰ. Fill in the blanks according to the texts.

1. Laboratory informatics is a professional application of information technology, aiming at＿＿＿＿＿＿ laboratory operation. (Text A)

2. The laboratory information system (LIS) is usually part of an＿＿＿＿＿＿information science solution, involving many different applications. (Text A)

3. In many cases, each application is tracked with a＿＿＿＿＿＿ identifier. (Text A)

4. Automated biochemical analyzers, for example, were used primarily for routine,＿＿＿＿＿＿ medical laboratory analysis. (Text B)

5. However, in order to protect the health and safety of laboratory workers, many manufacturers have been prompted to develop analyzers using closed tube sampling to prevent the operator from＿＿＿＿＿＿ contact with specimens. (Text B)

Ⅱ. Translate the following into Chinese.

Some analyzers need to transfer specimens to the specimen cup. However, in order to protect the health and safety of laboratory workers, many manufacturers have been prompted to develop analyzers using closed tube sampling to prevent the operator from direct contact with specimens. Samples can be treated separately, in batches or continuously.

Lesson 13　Quality Assurance
质量评价

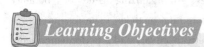

Learning Objectives

After studying this lesson, students are expected to be able to

1. master some medical words and terms about quality assurance;

2. know about the benefits of EQA or PT

3. independently consult relevant professional literatures.

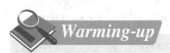

Warming-up

1. Do you think it is important to guarantee the quality of laboratory reports?

2. In your opinion, what are the consequences of incorrect laboratory results?

3. What are the benefits of quality assurance with a high level?

Text A　Quality Assurance Programme
质量评价程序

Quality assurance (QA) is the process in which the quality of laboratory reports can be guaranteed. Incorrect laboratory results may be due to errors occurring during specimen collection (pre-analytical stage), testing (analytical stage) and / or while reporting and interpreting (post-analytical stage) test results. However, Internal Quality Control (IQC) refers to the process of minimizing analytical errors, QA includes procedures adopted for minimizing errors that may occur at any stage. Provision of precise and accurate laboratory results optimize medical management. Inappropriate test selection, unnecessary investigations and incorrect test results not only have serious health implications but are also a financial burden to the individual and community. Reports with a high level of QA will help the physician to arrive rapidly at a correct diagnosis. To provide QA, all laboratories must have a proper quality assurance programme (QAP).

QUALITY ASSURANCE PROGRAMME（QAP）

1. QAP is a managerial process to maintain high standards of performance and to improve standards where necessary. The concept is best illustrated by Deming's cycle of Planning（P）, Doing（D）, Checking（C）, and Acting（A）. If any of the four components of the cycle lag behind, then the quality declines. it is important to put effort into preventing, detecting and correcting errors in each step while planning a QAP.

2. Quality Manager or designee or competent authorized person should review the quality control data and maintain record of evaluation.

3. The two important tools toward maintaining laboratory quality are as follows：

（1）Internal Quality Control（IQC）— for detection and minimization of immediate errors；

（2）External Quality Assessment（EQA）— for monitoring long term precision and accuracy of results.

Text B   External Quality Assessment
室间质量评价

External quality assessment（EQA）, using anonymous and coded performance evaluation samples, is used to help a laboratory in assessing its results and provide laboratory-to-laboratory comparisons. EQA is also known as proficiency testing（PT）.

EQA or PT refers to a system in which the performance of a laboratory is assessed periodically and retrospectively by an independent external agency to indicate to the laboratory staff of any shortcomings in performance. It indicates a need for improving and / or changing IQC procedures. An organizing agency or laboratory sends same specimens to all participating laboratories for testing by their routine methods. The results are received by the organizing agency and compared with a "correct" answer retrospectively and a performance score is assigned. All the participating laboratories are identified by a code and reports issued to the participants contain the performance score of all participating laboratories including its own score. This allows a comparison of quality between laboratories and thus describes the "state of the art" of laboratory work included by an external quality assessment programme（EQAP）.

The benefits of EQA or PT are：

1. Provide staff with an insight into their laboratory's performance；

2. Provide a comparison of performance with that of other laboratories, nationally and / or internationally；

3. Improve the standard of examinations；

4. Identify areas where there may be problems；

5. Demonstrate to clients, colleagues and accreditation bodies that there is a commitment to quality；

6. Educate staff to provide a better understanding of the impact of incorrect results.

New Words

Provision /prə'vɪʒn/ *n.* 供应，规定

designee /ˌdezɪg'niː/ *n.* 被指派者，被任命者

anonymous /ə'nɑːnɪməs/ *adj.* 匿名的，无名的

proficiency /prə'fɪʃnsi/ *n.* 精通，熟练

periodically /ˌpɪri'ɑːdɪklɪ/ *adv.* 定期地，周期性地

retrospectively /ˌretrə'spektɪvli/ *adv.* 回顾地

colleague /'kɑːliːg/ *n.* 同事，同僚

accreditation /əˌkredɪ'teɪʃn/ *n.* 认证，鉴定合格，委派

commitment /kə'mɪtmənt/ *n.* 承诺，保证

demonstrate /'demənstreɪt/ *vt.* 证明，展示，论证

Phrases and Expressions

quality assurance（QA）	质量保证,质量评价
quality assurance programme（QAP）	质量保证计划
pre-analytical stage	分析前阶段
post-analytical stage	分析后阶段
Deming's cycle	戴明循环或 PDCA 循环
proficiency testing（PT）	能力比对验证,能力验证
state of the art	当前发展状况
external quality assessment programme（EQAP）	室间质量评价计划
insight into …	深刻理解……,洞察……
accreditation body	认证机构,认可机构

Notes

1. Incorrect Laboratory results may be due to errors occurring during specimen collection (pre-analytical stage), testing (analytical stage) and / or while reporting and interpreting (post-analytical stage) test results.

不正确的实验结果可能是由于在样品采集期(分析前阶段)、检测期(分析阶段)和/或报告与解释检测结果时(分析后阶段)所出现的误差而导致的。

2. Inappropriate test selection, unnecessary investigations and incorrect test results not only have serious health implications but are also a financial burden to the individual and community.

不合适的检验项目选择、不必要的调查和不正确的检验结果,不仅严重影响健康,而且对个人和社会也是经济负担。

3. QAP is a managerial process to maintain high standards of performance and to improve standards where necessary.

质量评价程序是一个保证操作高标准、在需要之处提高标准的管理过程。

4. External quality assessment (EQA), using anonymous and coded performance evaluation samples, is used to help a laboratory in assessing its results and provide laboratory-to-laboratory comparisons.

室间质量评价通过匿名和代码方式评价样品,用来帮助一个实验室评估其实验结果,并提供实验室-实验室之间的比对。

5. EQA or PT refers to a system in which the performance of a laboratory is assessed periodically and retrospectively by an independent external agency to indicate to the laboratory staff of any shortcomings in performance.

室间质量评价或能力比对验证,是指一个系统。此系统由一个独立的外部机构对实验室性能进行周期性和回顾性评估,向实验室工作人员指出操作上的所有不足之处。

6. An organizing agency or laboratory sends same specimens to all participating laboratories for testing by their routine methods.

一个组织机构或实验室将相同的样本送给所有参加测试的实验室,以其常规方法进行测试。

7. The results are received by the organizing agency and compared with a "correct" answer retrospectively and a performance score is assigned.

所有检测结果由组织机构回收,并且回顾性地与一个"正确"结果比对,得到测评分数。

8. All the participating laboratories are identified by a code and reports issued to the participants contain the performance score of all participating laboratories including its own score.

所有参评实验室都可以通过代码识别,发给参评实验室的报告包含所有参评实验室的测评分数,也包括它自己的测评分数。

Exercises

Ⅰ. Fill in the blanks according to the texts.

1. Incorrect laboratory results may be due to errors occurring during _____ collection (pre-analytical stage) , testing (analytical stage) and / or while reporting (post-analytical stage) test results. (Text A)

2. The two important tools toward maintaining laboratory quality are as follows: (1) Internal Quality Control (IQC) — for detection and minimization of immediate errors; (2) _____ Quality Assessment (EQA) — for monitoring long term precision and accuracy of results. (Text A)

3. External quality assessment (EQA) , using anonymous and coded performance evaluation samples, is used to help a laboratory in assessing its results and provide laboratory-to-laboratory comparisons. EQA is also known as _____ testing (PT) . (Text B)

4. EQA or PT _____ a system in which the performance of a laboratory is assessed periodically and retrospectively by an independent external agency to indicate to the laboratory staff of any shortcomings in performance. (Text B)

5. An organizing _____ or laboratory sends same specimens to all participating laboratories for testing by their routine methods. (Text B)

Ⅱ. Translate the following into Chinese.

QAP is a managerial processto maintain high standards of performance and to improve standards where necessary. The concept is best illustrated by Deming's cycle of Planning (P) , Doing (D) , Checking (C) , and Acting (A) . If any of the four components of the cycle lag behind then the quality declines. it is important to put effort into preventing, detecting and correcting errors in each step while planning a QAP.

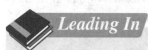

Chapter Ⅲ Clinical Laboratory Techniques
临床检验技术

Leading In

Through the study of this chapter, you will learn some general laboratory techniques in clinical hematology and osology, clinical chemistry, clinical immunology, clinical microbiology and clinical molecular biology. These techniques can be applied for many clinical testing items, such as blood cell analysis, coagulation function testing, blood group identification, cross matching, body fluids testing, electrolyte analysis, arterial blood gas analysis, enzyme activity assay, cardiac and tumor markers testing, etc. The functional status of the cardiovascular system, respiratory system, digestive system, genitourinary system and endocrine system can be judged respectively according to the testing results. Antigen antibody detection can assist the diagnosis of infectious diseases, and antibiotic susceptibility testing can provide the reference frame for selecting clinical antibiotics. In addition, polymerase chain reaction (PCR) and biochip technology are also introduced in this chapter, which will provide the basis for the diagnosis and treatment of diseases on the molecular biology level.

Lesson 1 PPT

Lesson 1   Complete Blood Count
全血细胞计数

Learning Objectives

After studying this lesson, students are expected to be able to

1. master the definition and clinical significance of complete blood count;

2. be familiar with the types and medical significance of blood cells;

3. know about the advantages and disadvantages of manual counting, the procedures of complete blood count by using an automated cell counter;

4. use complete blood cell count results to diagnose disease.

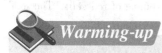

Warming-up

1. What are the main cells in the blood?
2. Can blood counting machines replace manual counting thoroughly?

笔记

Text A   Full Blood Count
全血细胞计数

The cells that circulate in the bloodstream are generally divided into three types: white blood cells (leukocytes), red blood cells (erythrocytes) and platelets (thrombocytes). Abnormally high or low counts may indicate the presence of many forms of disease. Therefore, the blood counts are among the most commonly performed blood tests in medicine, as they can provide an overview of a patient's general health status.

The clinical laboratory test that evaluates the three main cellular components of peripheral blood (red cells, white cells, and platelets) is called the "complete blood count" (CBC), also known as full blood count (FBC), or full blood exam (FBE), or blood panel. It is used commonly to assess whether a patient is anemic (low red cell count), has an infection (increased white blood cells), or has abnormal blood coagulation (platelet levels).

A phlebotomist collects the sample, drawing the blood into a test tube containing an anticoagulant (EDTA, sometimes citrate) to stop it from clotting. The sample is then transported to a laboratory. A scientist or lab technician performs the requested testing and provides the requesting medical professional with the results of the CBC. In the past, counting the cells in a patient's blood was performed manually, by viewing a slide prepared with a sample of the patient's blood under a microscope (a blood film, or peripheral smear). Nowadays, this process is generally automated by using an automated analyzer, with only approximately 30% of the samples being examined manually.

In manual counting, counting chambers that hold a specified volume of diluted blood (as there are far too many cells if it is not diluted) are used to calculate the number of red and white cells per litre of blood. Manual counting is useful in cases where automated analyzers cannot reliably count abnormal cells, such as those cells that are not present in normal patients and are only seen in peripheral blood with certain haematological conditions. Manual counting is subject to sampling error because so few cells are counted compared with automated analysis.

Text B   Automated Blood Count
自动化血液计数

The blood is well mixed (though not shaken) and placed on a rack in the automated analyzer. This instrument has many different components to analyze different elements in the blood. The cell counting component counts the numbers and types of different cells within the blood. The results are printed out or sent to a computer for review.

Blood counting machines aspirate a very small amount of the specimen through narrow tubing. Sensors count the number of cells passing through the tubing, and can identify the type of cell. The two main sensors used are light detectors and electrical impedance. One way the instrument can tell what type of blood cell is present is by size. Other instruments measure different characteristics of the cells to categorize them. The CBC examines the total number of red blood cells (RBC) and the RBC indices, including the mean corpuscular volume (MCV), the concentration of hemoglobin measured by the mean corpuscular hemoglobin (MCH) and its concentration (MCHC), and the hematocrit which is the mean packed-cell volume of red cells. The total white blood cell count, the various types of leukocytes (lymphocytes, monocytes, neutrophils, eosinophils, and basophils), and platelets are also measured.

Because an automated cell counter samples and counts so many cells, the results are very precise. However, certain abnormal cells in the blood may not be identified correctly, requiring manual review of the instrument's results and identification of any abnormal cells the instrument could not categorize.

In addition to counting, measuring and analyzing red blood cells, white blood cells and platelets, automated hematology analyzers also measure the amount of hemoglobin in the blood and within each red blood cell. This information can be very helpful to a physician who, for example, is trying to identify the cause of a patient's anemia. If the red cells are smaller or larger than normal, or if there is a lot of variation in the size of the red cells, these data can help guide the direction of further testing and expedite the diagnostic process so patients can get the treatment they need quickly.

New Words

circulate /ˈsɜːrkjəleɪt/ v. 循环

panel /ˈpænl/ n. 仪表板,嵌板

anemic /əniːmɪk/ adj. 贫血的

infection /ɪnˈfekʃn/ n. 感染

clot /klɑːt/ n. 凝块,黏团(尤指血块)v. (使)凝结成块,覆以黏性物质

manually /ˈmænjuəli/ adv. 手动地

chamber /ˈtʃeɪmbər/ n. (身体或器官内的)室,膛

haematological /ˌhiːmətəuˈlɒdʒikəl/ adj. 血液学的

aspirate /ˈæspərət/ v. 抽吸

sensor /ˈsensər/ n. 传感器

detector /dɪˈtɛktər/ n. 探测器

impedance /ɪmˈpiːdns/ n. [电] 阻抗

categorize /ˈkætəgəraɪz/ v. 将……分类

indices /ˈɪndɪsiːz/ n. 指标(index 的复数)

corpuscular /kəˈpʌskjulə/ adj. 血细胞的

hematocrit /hɪˈmætəkrɪt/ n. 血细胞比容

precise /prɪˈsaɪs/ adj. 精确的

expedite /ˈekspədaɪt/ v. 加快

Phrases and Expressions

peripheral blood	外周血
blood film	血涂片
electrical impedance	电阻抗
mean corpuscular volume (MCV)	平均红细胞体积
packed-cell volume	血细胞比容
automated hematology analyzers	自动血液分析仪
MCHC	平均红细胞血红蛋白浓度

Notes

1. The cells that circulate in the bloodstream are generally divided into three types: white blood cells (leukocytes), red blood cells (erythrocytes) and platelets (thrombocytes).

血流中循环的细胞大体上分成三类:白细胞、红细胞和血小板(也称凝血细胞)。

2. The clinical laboratory test that evaluates the three main cellular components of peripheral blood (red cells, white cells, and platelets) is called the "complete blood count" (CBC), also known as full blood count (FBC), or full blood exam (FBE), or blood panel.

评估外周血液中三类主要细胞(红细胞、白细胞和血小板)的临床实验室检查,称为全血细胞计数(CBC),或全血检查(FBE),或血液组合项目检查。

3. Nowadays, this process is generally automated by using an automated analyzer, with only approximately 30% of the samples being examined manually.

现在,这一过程(血细胞计数)普遍使用自动分析仪进行自动计数,仅有 30% 左右的样本仍由手工

计数。

4. Manual counting is useful in cases where automated analyzers cannot reliably count abnormal cells, such as those cells that are not present in normal patients and are only seen in peripheral blood with certain haematological conditions.

当自动分析仪不能可靠地计数异常细胞时,就需要用到手工计数,例如需要计数普通病人不存在的异常细胞,以及计数仅见于某些血液学状态的外周血液的异常细胞。

5. One way the instrument can tell what type of blood cell is present is by size.

仪器通过细胞大小区别所存在的血细胞种类。

6. The CBC examines the total number of red blood cells (RBC) and the RBC indices, including the mean corpuscular volume (MCV), the concentration of hemoglobin measured by the mean corpuscular hemoglobin (MCH) and its concentration (MCHC), and the hematocrit which is the mean packed-cell volume of red cells.

全血细胞计数检测红细胞(RBC)总数及其相关指标,包括平均红细胞体积(MCV),血红蛋白浓度,以及血细胞比容。血红蛋白浓度是由平均红细胞血红蛋白(MCH)与平均红细胞血红蛋白浓度(MCHC)测得。血细胞比容是红细胞的平均比容。

7. However, certain abnormal cells in the blood may not be identified correctly, requiring manual review of the instrument's results and identification of any abnormal cells the instrument could not categorize.

然而,血液中某些异常细胞可能无法被正确识别,需要手工复核仪器的检测结果,确认仪器不能分类的所有异常细胞。

8. In addition to counting, measuring and analyzing red blood cells, white blood cells and platelets, automated hematology analyzers also measure the amount of hemoglobin in the blood and within each red blood cell.

除计数、测量和分析红细胞、白细胞、血小板之外,全自动血液分析仪也测定血液中和每个红细胞内的血红蛋白量。

Exercises

Ⅰ. Fill in the blanks according to the texts.

1. The clinical laboratory test that _____ the three main cellular components of peripheral blood (red cells, white cells, and platelets) is called the "complete blood count" (CBC). (Text A)

2. Nowadays, this process is generally_____ by using an automated analyzer, with only approximately 30% of samples now being examined manually. (Text A)

3. In manual counting, counting chambers that hold a specified volume of_____ blood are used to calculate the number of red and white cells per litre of blood. (Text A)

4. Blood counting machines_____ a very small amount of the specimen through narrow tubing. (Text B)

5. Because an automated cell counter samples and counts so many cells, the results are very_____ ____. (Text B)

Ⅱ. Translate the following into Chinese.

The CBC examines the total number of red blood cells (RBC) and the RBC indices, including: the mean corpuscular volume (MCV); the concentration of hemoglobin, measured by the mean corpuscular hemoglobin (MCH) and its concentration (MCHC); and the hematocrit, which is the mean packed-cell volume of red cells.

Lesson 2 Urine and Stool Examination
尿液和粪便检验

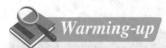

After studying this lesson, students are expected to be able to

1. master the definition of urinalysis and stool analysis;
2. be familiar with the methods of urinalysis and stool analysis;
3. know about the two basic procedures in modern urinalysis;
4. direct patients to collect urine and stool samples and handle the samples in the right way.

Warming-up

1. What are the two kinds of urinalysis? What is the difference between them?
2. What are the two basic procedures in modern urinalysis?
3. What kind of tests are included in stool analysis?

Text A Methods of Urinalysis
尿液检验方法

A urinalysis (UA) is an array of tests performed on urine, and one of the most common methods of medical diagnosis. The word is a portmanteau of the words urine and analysis.

When a doctor orders a urinalysis they will request either a routine urinalysis or a R&M urinalysis. The difference between the two is that rountine urinalysis does not include microscopy or culture whereas the R&M is a Routine urinalysis plus Microscopy. Modern urinalysis can be divided into two basic procedures: macroscopic and chemical examination, and microscopic analysis.

Macroscopic and chemical examination

Macroscopic examination includes noting the color and clarity of the urine. Normal urine is pale yellow or straw colored and is usually transparent or clear; abnormal urine may vary greatly in color and may show varying degrees of cloudiness. The specific gravity of urine, that is, the ratio of the weight of a volume of urine to that of the same volume of water, is measured routinely. Specific gravity is an indicator of the kidney's ability to concentrate or dilute the urine and thus of renal tubular function. The normal range is 1.003-1.032.

Most routine chemical urinalysis is now carried out by dipstick testing, which involves the use of plastic strips, or dipsticks, bearing pads embedded with chemical reactants and color indicators. The reaction of each pad represents a separate chemical test for a specific product in the urine. Dipstick testing includes the following categories: protein, glucose, ketone bodies, blood and bile.

Microscopic analysis

The urine normally contains a wide variety of formed elements that can be identified by using a light microscope. Together these elements form the urinary sediment.

Cells in the urine originate in the bloodstream or in the epithelium lining the urinary tract. The main types of epithelial cells are renal tubular cells, transitional (urothelial) cells, and squamous cells. All three types occur in relatively small numbers in the normal sediment. Blood cells occur normally in the urine in small numbers, and consist mainly of polymorphonuclear neutrophils and red blood cells.

Casts, the proteinaceous products of kidney, are of major importance when present in increased numbers or seen in abnormal forms, because they usually indicate intrinsic renal disease. Casts are cylindrical and are named on the basis of their microscopic appearance and the cells they contain.

Normally, urine is sterile, and the urinary sediment should not contain microorganisms. However, in patients with serious urinary tract infections, microorganisms are usually present in the urine in considerably greater numbers.

Mucus is frequently found in urine sediment and man has not known its pathological significance. A wide variety of crystals appear in the urine; their presence may be normal or may indicate an abnormal state.

Text B Stool Analysis
粪便检验

A stool analysis is a series of tests done on a stool (feces) sample to help diagnose certain conditions affecting the digestive tract. These conditions can include infection (from parasites, viruses, bacteria, etc.), poor nutrient absorption, or cancer.

For a stool analysis, a stool sample is collected in a clean container and then sent to the laboratory immediately. A stool laboratory analysis includes microscopic examination, chemical tests, and microbiological tests. The stool will be checked for color, consistency, amount, shape, odor, and the presence of mucus. The stool may be examined for hidden (occult) blood, fat, meat fibers, bile, white blood cells, and sugars called reducing substances. The pH of the stool also may be measured. A stool culture is done to find out if bacteria may be causing an infection.

Feces are solid bodily waste discharged from the colon through the anus during defecation. Normal feces are 75% water. The rest is about 30% dead bacteria, 30% indigestible food matter, 10%-20% cholesterol and other fats, 10%-20% inorganic substances, and 2%-3% protein. The colour and odour are produced by bacterial action on chemical constituents.

Human fecal matter varies significantly in appearance, depending on diet and health. Normally it is semisolid, with a mucus coating. Its brown coloration comes from a combination of bile and bilirubin, which comes from dead red blood cells. In newborn babies, fecal matter is initially yellow or green after the meconium. This coloration comes from the presence of bile alone.

Throughout the life of an ordinary human, one may experience many types of feces. A "green" stool is from rapid transit of feces through the intestines (or the consumption of certain blue or green food dyes in quantity), and "clay-like" appearance to the feces is the result of a lack of bilirubin. Bile overload is very rare, and not a health threat. Problems as simple as serious diarrhea can cause blood in one's stool. Black stools caused by blood usually indicate a problem in the intestines (the black is digested blood), whereas red streaks of blood in stool are usually caused by bleeding in the rectum or anus.

Food may sometimes make an appearance in the feces. Common undigested foods found in human feces are seeds, nuts, corn and beans, mainly because of their high dietary fiber content. Beets may turn feces different hues of red. Artificial food coloring in some processed foods such as highly colorful packaged breakfast cereals can also cause unusual feces coloring if eaten in sufficient quantities.

The laboratory examination of feces, also termed as stool examination or stool test, is usually conducted for the sake of diagnosis, for example, to detect the presence of parasites (e.g., pinworms and their ova) or disease-spreading bacteria.

New Words

portmanteau /pɔːrtˈmæntoʊ/ n. 混成词

indicator /ˈɪndɪkeɪtər/ n. 指标,标志,迹象,指示器;[试剂]指示剂

tubular /ˈtuːbjələr/ adj. 管状的

dipstick /ˈdɪpstɪk/ n. 试纸条

epithelium /ˌɛpəˈθilɪəm/ n. ［组织］上皮细胞

urothelial /jʊˈrɑːˈθilɪəl/ adj. 泌尿道上皮的

squamous /ˈskwemǝs/ adj. 鳞状的（等于 squamosa 或 squamose）

cast /kæst/ n. 管型

proteinaceous /proʊtiːˈneɪʃǝs/ adj. 蛋白质的

cylindrical /sǝˈlɪndrɪkl/ adj. 圆柱形的

pathological /ˌpæθǝˈlɒːdʒɪkl/ adj. 病理学的（等于 pathologic）

digestive /daɪˈdʒestɪv/ n. 助消化药 adj. 消化的，助消化的

consistency /kǝnˈsɪstǝnsi/ n. 浓度，稠度，一致性，相容性

mucus /ˈmjuːkǝs/ n. 黏液

occult /ǝˈkʌlt/ adj. 被掩蔽的

defecation /ˌdefǝˈkeɪʃn/ n. 排便

indigestible /ˌɪndɪˈdʒestǝbl/ adj. 难消化的

cholesterol /kǝˈlestǝrɔːl/ n. ［生化］胆固醇

inorganic /ˌɪnɔːrˈgænɪk/ adj. ［无化］无机的

semisolid /ˌsemɪˈsɒlɪd/ n. 半固体

coloration /ˌkʌlǝˈreɪʃn/ n. 着色

meconium /mǝˈkonɪǝm/ n. 胎便

intestine /ɪnˈtestɪn/ n. 肠

diarrhea /ˌdaɪǝˈriǝ/ n. 腹泻

streak /striːk/ n. 条纹，线条

rectum /ˈrektǝm/ n. 直肠（复数 rectums 或 recta）

ovum /ˈoʊvǝm/ n. ［细胞］［组织］卵子（复数 ova）

Phrases and Expressions

routine and microscopy（R&M）	常规与显微镜检验
ketone body	酮体
transitional cell	移行细胞
polymorphonuclear neutrophils	多形核中性粒白细胞
digestive tract	消化道
poor nutrient	营养不良
hidden blood	隐血
occult blood	潜血
reducing substances	还原物质
dietary fiber	膳食纤维

Notes

1. A urinalysis（UA）is an array of tests performed on urine, and one of the most common methods of medical diagnosis. The word is a portmanteau of the words urine and analysis.

尿液分析或尿液检验（UA）是对尿液进行的一系列检验，也是最常用的医学诊断方法之一。尿液分析或尿液检验这个词（urinalysis）是单词尿液（urine）和分析（analysis）的混成词。

2. When a doctor orders a urinalysis they will request either a routine urinalysis or a R&M urinalysis. The difference between the two is that rountine urinalysis does not include microscopy or culture whereas the R&M is a Routine urinalysis plus Microscopy. Modern Clirinalysis can be divided into two basic procedures: macroscopic and chemical examination, and microscopic analysis.

笔记

医生申请尿液分析时,会申请尿常规检验或者尿常规检验和显微镜检验(R&M)。二者的区别在于,尿常规检验不包括显微镜检验或细菌培养,而 R&M 是尿常规检验和显微镜检验。现代尿液分析可分成两个基本程序:外观检验和化学检验,以及显微镜分析。

3. Specific gravity is an indicator of the kidney's ability to concentrate or dilute the urine and thus of renal tubular function.

比重是肾脏浓缩或稀释尿液功能的指征,因此也是肾小管功能的指征。

4. Most routine chemical urinalysis is now carried out by dipstick testing, which involves the use of plastic strips, or dipsticks, bearing pads embedded with chemical reactants and color indicators. The reaction of each pad represents a separate chemical test for a specific product in the urine.

现在大多数常规化学尿检验采用试纸条检验。试纸条检验用到塑料试纸条,塑料试纸条装有嵌入化学反应剂和颜色指示剂的药垫。每个药垫的反应代表针对尿液中一种特定产物的独立化学检验。

5. The urine normally contains a wide variety of formed elements that can be identified by using a light microscope. Together these elements form the urinary sediment.

尿液通常含有种类繁多的组成成分,这些成分能用光学显微镜鉴定。这些成分的总和构成尿沉渣。

6. Casts, the proteinaceous products of kidney, are of major importance when present in increased numbers or seen in abnormal forms, because they usually indicate intrinsic renal disease. Casts are cylindrical and are named on the basis of their microscopic appearance and the cells they contain.

管型是肾脏的蛋白质产物,当其数量增加或形态异常时具有极其重要的临床意义,因为它们通常指示内在的肾脏疾病。管型为圆柱体,根据其显微外观和所含细胞而得名。

7. For a stool analysis, a stool sample is collected in a clean container and then sent to the laboratory immediately. A stool laboratory analysis includes microscopic examination, chemical tests, and microbiological tests. The stool will be checked for color, consistency, amount, shape, odor, and the presence of mucus. The stool may be examined for hidden (occult) blood, fat, meat fibers, bile, white blood cells, and sugars called reducing substances. The pH of the stool also may be measured. A stool culture is done to find out if bacteria may be causing an infection.

对于粪便检验,粪便样品要收集在干净的容器中,然后立刻送到实验室。实验室粪便检验包括显微镜学检查、化学检验和微生物学检验。粪便检验对粪便的颜色、稠度、重量(体积)、形状、气味和黏液进行检验;还检验粪便的潜血、脂肪、肌肉纤维、胆汁、白细胞,以及被称为还原物质的糖类。粪便的 pH 值也可以被检测。粪便培养旨在发现是否有细菌引起感染。

8. Human fecal matter varies significantly in appearance, depending on diet and health. Normally it is semisolid, with a mucus coating. Its brown coloration comes from a combination of bile and bilirubin, which comes from dead red blood cells.

人的粪便物外观差异明显,这取决于饮食和健康。正常情况下,人的粪便为带有黏液覆盖物的半固体。粪便的褐色来源于胆汁和胆红素的混合物,而后者(胆红素)来源于死亡的红细胞。

9. Black stools caused by blood usually indicate a problem in the intestines (the black is digested blood), whereas red streaks of blood in stool are usually caused by bleeding in the rectum or anus.

由血液造成的黑色粪便通常指示肠道问题(黑色物质是被消化的血液),而粪便中的红血丝通常是由直肠或肛门部位的出血造成的。

10. The laboratory examination of feces, also termed as stool examination or stool test, is usually conducted for the sake of diagnosis, for example, to detect the presence of parasites (e.g., pinworms and their ova) or disease-spreading bacteria.

粪便的实验室检验,也称为粪便检验,通常用于疾病诊断,例如,检测寄生虫的存在(如蛲虫及其虫卵等)或者传播疾病的细菌。

Exercises

Ⅰ. Fill in the blanks according to the texts.

1. Dipstick testing includes the following categories: protein, _____, ketone bodies, blood and bile. (Text A)

2. The main types of _____ cells are renal tubular cells, transitional (urothelial) cells, and squamous cells. (Text A)

3. Casts, the proteinaceous products of_____, are of major importance when present in increased numbers or seen in abnormal forms, because they usually indicate intrinsic renal disease. (Text A)

4. A stool laboratory analysis includes microscopic examination, chemical tests, and _____ tests. (Text B)

5. Human fecal matter varies significantly in appearance, depending on _____ and health. (Text B)

Ⅱ. Translate the following into Chinese.

A stool laboratory analysis includes microscopic examination, chemical tests, and microbiological tests. The stool will be checked for color, consistency, amount, shape, odor, and the presence of mucus. The stool may be examined for hidden (occult) blood, fat, meat fibers, bile, white blood cells, and sugars called reducing substances. The pH of the stool also may be measured. A stool culture is done to find out if bacteria may be causing an infection.

Lesson 3   Vaginal Discharge and Semen Examination
阴道分泌物和精液检验

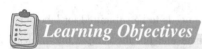
Learning Objectives

After studying this lesson, students are expected to be able to

1. master some medical words and terms about vaginal discharge and semen examination;

2. be familiar with methods and contents of vaginal discharge and semen examination;

3. know about the clinical significance of vaginal discharge and semen examination;

4. independently consult relevant professional literatures.

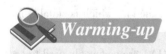
Warming-up

1. Do you know how to make vaginal discharge examinations?

2. What's the purpose of vaginal discharge examinations?

Text A   Vaginal Discharge Examination
阴道分泌物检验

The consistency, texture, taste, color and smell of vaginal lubricants can vary, which depends on sexual arousal, the stage of the menstrual cycle, the presence of an infection, certain medications, genetic factors and diet. A vaginal wet mount (or vaginal smear) is a gynecological examination method that contains a vaginal sample. A vaginal smear does not occur during menstruation because menstrual blood on a slide can confuse the results.

Vaginal smears may be considered when vaginal inflammation, whose symptoms include vaginal itching, burning, rash, odor or secretions, is suspectd. It may help diagnose vaginal yeast infection, trichomoniasis and bacterial vaginosis. Infections such as chlamydia, genital warts, syphilis, herpes simplex and gonorrhea can also affect the vagina, but these diseases can be found by other tests.

Usually, vaginal fluids are slightly acidic and can become more acidic for certain sexually transmitted diseases. The normal pH of vaginal fluid is between 4.0 and 4.5, while the pH of male semen is generally between 7.2 and 8.0. No yeast, bacteria, trichomonas or clue cells should be found in normal vaginal discharge section. White blood cells usually do not exist or are in small quantities.

Yeast infections in the vagina usually result in white, blocky secretions which look like cottage cheese. Trichomoniasis causes vaginal discharge to be yellow-green, foamy and has an unpleasant smell. Bacterial vaginal diseases generally produce vaginal discharge, thin and milky, with a strong fishy taste. In addition, clue cells can also be seen in bacterial vaginosis. The clue cell is the epithelial cell of the vagina, which is covered by bacteria to form a distinctive stippled appearance. At the same time, they are also the medical symbol of bacterial vaginitis (BV), especially vaginitis caused by Gardnerella vaginalis, a Gram-variant bacterium. This bacterial infection emits a stench of vaginal vaginal discharge, fishy yellow or gray foam secretions, and the vaginal pH increases to above 5.5. In addition, the presence of white blood cells is a general sign of infection.

Text B Semen Examination
精液检验

Semen is an organic liquid, which may contain sperms. Besides sperms, there are some other components in semen, such as proteolytic enzymes, other enzymes and fructose. Semen can promote sperm survival and provide sperm with a medium for exercise or "swimming".

In order to determine a man's fertility or infertility, a semen sample needs to be submitted for laboratory analysis. The most common way to collect a semen sample is to masturbate and put the sample into a clean cup. During sexual intercourse, a sample can also be collected using a special type of condom, known as a collection condom. It is more effective to obtain the sample in a doctor's office or laboratory to ensure safe and rapid analyses. Otherwise, the sample must be sent to the laboratory quickly and stored at room temperature and under light until delivery. Some doctors recommend not having sex one week before the test.

The parameters measured in semen analysis include: volume, sperm count, activity, morphology, fructose level, and pH. The volume can be determined by measuring the weight of the sample container and knowing the mass of the empty container. Sperm count and morphology can be calculated with a microscope. Sperm count can also be estimated by measuring the number of sperm related proteins in the kit, which is suitable for home use.

Computer Aided Semen Analysis (CASA) and Sperm Quality Analyzer (SQA) are commonly used to assess sperm concentration and fluidity characteristics, such as velocity and linear velocity. There are already CASA systems based on image analysis and new technologies, which can achieve near-perfect results and complete adequate analysis in a matter of seconds. With some techniques, sperm concentration and motion measurement are at least as reliable as current manual methods. SQA is a semen analysis instrument integrated with photoelectric technology, computer technology and micro video technology. It can evaluate the quality of semen directly, objectively and quickly, but cannot completely replace the traditional manual microscope examination.

New Words

texture /ˈtekstʃər/ *n.* 质地,质感

lubricant /ˈluːbrɪkənt/ *n.* 润滑剂,润滑油

arousal /əˈraʊzl/ *n.* 唤起,觉醒

menstrual /ˈmenstruəl/ *adj.* 月经的

gynecologic /ˌɡaɪnɪkəˈlɒdʒɪk/ *adj.* 妇科的,妇产科医学的

inflammation /ˌɪnfləˈmeɪʃn/ *n.* ［病理］炎症;［医］发炎,燃烧,发火

itch /ɪtʃ/ *n.* 痒,疥疮 *vt. & vi.* (使)发痒

rash /ræʃ/ *n.* (皮肤)皮疹

yeast /jiːst/ *n.* 泡沫,酵母,酵母片

trichomoniasis /ˌtrɪkəuməˈnaɪəsis/ *n.* 滴虫病

chlamydia /kləˈmɪdiə/ *n.* 衣原体

genital /ˈdʒenɪtl/ *n.* 生殖器 *adj.* 外阴部,生殖的

wart /wɔːrt/ *n.* ［皮肤］疣(等于 verruca)

herpes /ˈhəːpiz/ *n.* ［皮肤］疱疹

gonorrhea /ˌɡɒnəˈrɪə/ *n.* ［性病］淋病

cheese /tʃiːz/ *n.* ［食品］乳酪,干酪

milky /ˈmɪlkɪ/ *adj.* 乳状的,乳白色的

fishy /ˈfɪʃɪ/ *adj.* 鱼的

distinctive /dɪˈstɪŋktɪv/ *adj.* 独特的,有特色的,与众不同的

stippled /ˈstɪpld/ *adj.* 带有小圆点的,布满斑点的

gardnerella /ɡɑːdnɪrələ/ *n.* 加德纳菌属

foam /foum/ *n.* 泡沫

sperm /spɜːrm/ *n.* 精子,精液

proteolytic /ˌprəutiəuˈlɪtɪk/ *adj.* ［生化］蛋白水解的,解蛋白的

fructose /ˈfrʌktous/ *n.* ［有化］果糖

fertility /fərˈtɪləti/ *n.* 生育力

masturbate /ˈmæstərbeɪt/ *vi.* 手淫 *vt.* 对……行手淫

intercourse /ˈɪntərkɔːrs/ *n.* 性交

condom /ˈkɑːndəm/ *n.* 避孕套

Phrases and Expressions

menstrual cycle	月经周期
vaginal smear	阴道涂片
genital warts	生殖器疣
herpes simplex	单纯疱疹
clue cell	线索细胞
gardnerella vaginalis	阴道加德纳菌
cottage cheese	白软干酪
proteolytic enzyme	蛋白水解酶

Notes

1. A vaginal wet mount (or vaginal smear) is a gynecological examination method that contains a vaginal sample.

阴道湿涂片(或阴道分泌物涂片)是从阴道取样所进行的妇产科检验。

2. No yeast, bacteria, trichomonas or clue cells should not be found in normal vaginal discharge section.

正常阴道液涂片应该见不到任何的酵母、细菌、滴虫或线索细胞。

3. The clue cell is the epithelial cell of the vagina, which is covered by bacteria to form a distinctive stippled appearance. At the same time, they are also the medical symbol of bacterial vaginitis (BV), especially vaginitis caused by Gardnerella vaginalis, a Gram-variant bacterium.

线索细胞是布满细菌、呈现出特征性点状外观的阴道上皮细胞。同时,线索细胞也是细菌性阴道炎,尤其是阴道加德纳菌阴道炎的医学征象。阴道加德纳菌是一组革兰氏染色不定的细菌。

4. Besides sperms, there are some other components in semen, such as proteolytic enzymes, other enzymes and fructose. Semen can promote sperm survival and provide sperm with a medium for exercise or "swimming".

除精子外,精液中还含有其他几种成分,如蛋白水解酶、其他酶类、果糖等。精液促进精子存活,并为精子运动或"游泳"提供媒介。

5. Otherwise, the sample must be sent to the laboratory quickly and stored at room temperature and under light until delivery.

否则,标本必须尽快递交实验室,并在递交前保持室温,避光的环境。

6. Sperm count can also be estimated by measuring the number of sperm related proteins in the kit, which is suitable for home use.

精子计数也可以用测量精子相关蛋白质的试剂盒进行评价,这种试剂盒适合于家用。

7. There are already CASA systems based on image analysis and new technologies, which can achieve near-perfect results and complete adequate analysis in a matter of seconds.

基于图像分析的 CASA 系统通过使用新技术,能得到近于完美的结果,并在几秒钟之内完成全部分析。

Exercises

Ⅰ. Fill in the blanks according to the texts.

1. A_____ does not occur during menstruation because menstrual blood on a slide can confuse the results. (Text A)

2. Vaginal smears may be considered when vaginal inflammation, such as vaginal itching, burning, rash, odor or_____. (Text A)

3. Semen is an organic liquid, which may contain_____. (Text B)

4. In order to determine male_____ or infertility, semen samples need to be submitted for laboratory analysis. (Text B)

5. There are already CASA systems_____ image analysis and new technologies, which can achieve near-perfect results and completed adequate analysis in a matter of seconds. (Text B)

Ⅱ. Translate the following into Chinese.

Yeast infections in the vagina usually result in white, blocky secretions which look like cottage cheese. Trichomoniasis causes vaginal discharge to be yellow-green, foamy and has an unpleasant smell. Bacterial vaginal disease generally produces vaginal discharge, thin and milky, with a strong fishy taste.

Lesson 4　Cerebrospinal Fluid and Sputum Examination
脑脊液和痰液检验

 Learning Objectives

After studying this lesson, students are expected to be able to

1. master some medical words and terms about cerebrospinal fluid and sputum examination;

2. be familiar with methods and contents of cerebrospinal fluid and sputum examination;

3. know the clinical significance of cerebrospinal fluid and sputum examination;

4. independently consult relevant professional literatures.

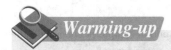

1. What is the purpose of cerebrospinal fluid examinations?
2. How do we properly collect the cerebrospinal fluid sample?

Text A   Routine Examination of Cerebrospinal Fluid
脑脊液常规检验

Cerebrospinal fluid (CSF) is a kind of transparent and colorless body fluid. This liquid is the ultrafiltrate of plasma. CSF analysis is a set of laboratory tests used to examine fluid samples around the brain and spinal cord. The CSF is produced at the rate of 500 mL per day. It includes glucose, electrolytes, amino acids, and other small molecules found in plasma, but has very little protein and few cells.

Routine examination of CSF includes the naked eye observation of color and transparency, as well as testing of glucose, protein, lactic acid, lactate dehydrogenase, red blood cell count, white blood cell count and difference, syphilis serology (detection of antibodies indicating syphilis), Gram staining and bacterial culture. Further testing may be required based on initial test results and presumptive diagnosis.

Color and clarity are important diagnostic features of CSF. Pigments of straw, pink, yellow or amber are abnormal, indicating the presence of bilirubin, hemoglobin, red blood cells, or increased protein. Turbidity indicates an increase in the number of cells. Visual inspection is helpful in differentiating subarachnoid hemorrhage from penetrating puncture. Puncture wound infiltration in the collection of cerebrospinal fluid, the fluid is often sequential to clarify, or other clarified liquids have bloodshot, or solidified samples.

A series of laboratory tests analyze various substances in the CSF in order to rule out malignancy or other central nervous system diseases. The following are reference values for commonly tested substances:

CSF pressure: 50-180 mmH$_2$O;

Glucose: 40-85 mg/dL;

Protein: 15-50 mg/dL;

Leukocytes (white blood cells) total less than 5 per mL;

Lymphocytes (specific type of white blood cell): 60%-70%;

Monocytes (a kind of white blood cell): 30%-50%;

Neutrophils (another kind of white blood cell): none.

Under normal circumstances, there is no red blood cell in the CSF unless the needle passes through the blood vessels to the CSF. If so, the red blood cells in the first tube should be more than those in the last one.

Text B   Sputum Macro-examination
痰液外观检验

Sputum is mucus or phlegm that is coughed out of the lungs, bronchi and trachea, which is excreted by humans through the mouth. It is commonly used for microbiological investigation of respiratory infections. When a sputum specimen is plated out, it is best to take most of the parts that look like pus to the cotton swabs. If there is any blood in the sputum, this should also be on the swab. The best sputum samples contain very little saliva, as it contaminates the sample with oral bacteria. Clinical microbiologists assess this event by examining the Gram stain of sputum. More than 25 squamous epithelial cells at low enlargement indicates salivary contamination.

Purulent sputum contains a large amount of pus, consisting of white blood cells, cell fragments, dead tissue, serous liquids, and viscous liquids (mucus). In most cases, it's yellow in color, as well as green. That is often seen in case of bronchiectasis, lung abscess, or advanced stage of bronchitis, acute upper respiratory tract infection (cold, laryngitis) .

No pathogenic microorganisms exist in a normal sputum specimen. If the sputum sample is abnormal, the results are called "positive." Identifying organisms that cause diseases may be helpful for the diagnosis of:

1. Hematoma (hemoptysis)

(1) Blood-streaked sputum: tuberculosis, lung cancer, bronchiectasis;

(2) Pink phlegm evenly mixed with blood, from alveoli, bronchioles;

(3) Large area of blood cavity pulmonary tuberculosis, pulmonary abscess, bronchiectasis, infarction, embolism.

2. Rusty colored- usually caused by pneumococcus (pneumonia) .

3. Pus-containing purulent fluid. This color can provide hints for effective treatment of chronic bronchitis patients.

(1) yellow-green (mucopurulent) color indicates that antibiotic therapy can alleviate symptoms. Green is caused by neutrophil myeloperoxidase;

(2) white, milky or opaque (mucoid) appearance usually means that antibiotics are ineffective in treating symptoms. (This information may be associated with the presence of a bacterial or viral infection, although current research does not support such a generalization) .

4. Foamy white-may come from obstruction or even edema.

5. Frothy pink-pulmonary edema.

New Words

ultrafiltrate /ˌʌltrəˈfiltreit/ *n.* [化学] 超滤液

spinal /ˈspaɪnl/ *adj.* 脊髓的,脊柱的

cord /kɔːrd/ *n.* 绳索,束缚

lactate /ˈlækteɪt/ *n.* 乳酸,乳酸盐

dehydrogenase /ˌdihaɪˈdrɑdʒəˌnes/ *n.* [生化] 脱氢酶

syphilis /ˈsɪfɪlɪs/ *n.* [性病] 梅毒

subarachnoid /ˌsʌbəˈræknɔɪd/ *adj.* 蛛网膜下的

nervous /ˈnɜːrvəs/ *adj.* 神经的

phlegm /flem/ *n.* 痰,黏液

bronchi /ˈbrɑnkai/ *n.* 细支气管(bronchus 的复数)

trachea /ˈtreɪkiə/ *n.* [脊椎] [解剖] 气管;[植] 导管

purulent /ˈpjʊrələnt/ *adj.* 化脓的,脓的

bronchiectasis /ˌbrɑŋkɪˈɛktəsɪs/ *n.* [内科] 支气管扩张

abscess /ˈæbses/ *n.* 脓疮

laryngitis /ˌlærɪnˈdʒaɪtɪs/ *n.* [耳鼻喉] 喉炎

hemoptysis /hɪˈmɑptəsɪs/ *n.* [临床] 咯血,咳血

alveoli /ælˈviəlaɪ/ *n.* 肺泡(alveous 的复数)

embolism /ˈembəlɪzəm/ *n.* 栓塞,闰日

pneumococcus /ˌnjʊməˈkɑkəs/ *n.* [微] [基医] 肺炎球菌

pneumonia /nuːˈmoʊniə/ *n.* 肺炎

mucopurulent /ˌmjuːkəʊˈpjuərulənt/ *adj.* 黏脓性的

myeloperoxidase /ˌmaɪələʊpəˈrɔksideis/ *n.* 髓过氧化物酶

opaque /oʊˈpeɪk/ *adj.* 不透明的

obstruction /əbˈstrʌkʃn/ *n.* 阻塞,障碍

edema /iˈdimə/ *n.* [病理] 水肿,瘤腺体(等于 oedema)

Phrases and Expressions

cerebrospinal fluid	脑脊液
spinal cord	脊髓, 脊椎神经
lactate dehydrogenase	乳酸脱氢酶
syphilis serology	梅毒血清学
reference value	参考值
pulmonary abscess	肺脓肿
advanced stage	晚期

Notes

1. CSF analysis is a set of laboratory tests used to examine fluid samples around the brain and spinal cord.

脑脊液分析是对脑和脊髓周围液体的样本进行多项目检验的实验室检查。

2. Visual inspection is helpful in differentiating subarachnoid hemorrhage from penetrating puncture. Puncture wound infiltration in the collection of cerebrospinal fluid, the fluid is often sequential to clarify, or other clarified liquids have bloodshot, or solidified samples.

目测有助于区别蛛网膜下腔出血与穿刺伤渗血。穿刺伤渗血在收集脑脊液时，液体常常逐渐变为澄清，澄清液体中或有血丝，或有凝固的样本。

3. A series of laboratory tests analyze various substances in the CSF in order to rule out malignancy or other central nervous system diseases.

一系列的实验室检验分析脑脊液中的各种物质，以便于排除中枢神经系统的恶性肿瘤或其他中枢神经系统疾病。

4. Sputum is mucus or phlegm that is coughed out of the lungs, bronchi and trachea, which is excreted by humans through the mouth.

痰是从肺、支气管和气管经人体口腔吐出的黏液或痰液。

5. When a sputum specimen is plated out, it is best to take most of the parts that look like pus to the cotton swabs.

当取得痰液标本时，最好是取拭子上看上去最像脓液的部分。

Exercises

Ⅰ. Fill in the blanks according to the texts.

1. Cerebrospinal fluid (CSF) is a kind of transparent and colorless body fluid. This fluid is the ultrafiltrate of_____. (Text A)

2. Color and_____ are important diagnostic characteristics of CSF. (Text A)

3. Sputum is mucus or phlegm that is coughed out of the lungs, bronchi and trachea, which is_____ _____ by humans through the mouth. (Text B)

4. Purulent sputum contains a large amount of_____. (Text B)

5. If the sputum sample is abnormal, the results are called "_____". (Text B)

Ⅱ. Translate the following into Chinese.

Color and clarity are important diagnostic features of CSF. Pigments of straw, pink, yellow or amber are abnormal, indicating the presence of bilirubin, hemoglobin, red blood cells, or increased protein. Visual inspection is helpful in differentiating subarachnoid hemorrhage from penetrating puncture. Puncture wound infiltration in the collection of cerebrospinal fluid, the fluid is often sequential to clarify, or other clarified liquids have bloodshot, or solidified samples.

Lesson 5　White Blood Cell
白细胞

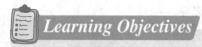

Learning Objectives

After studying this lesson, students are expected to be able to

1. master some medical terms about white blood cells and the characteristics of neutrophils and lymphocytes;

2. be familiar with the main types of white blood cells and their major functions;

3. know about the clinical significance of white blood cell count;

4. independently consult relevant professional literatures.

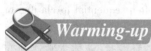

Warming-up

1. What are the five main types of white blood cells?

2. What is the primary function of white blood cells?

3. What is the normal range of white blood cell count?

Text A　Types of White Blood Cell
白细胞分类

White blood cells (abbreviated as WBCs) are also called leukocytes or leucocytes. The name derives from the fact that after centrifugation of a blood sample, the white cells are found in the buffy coat, a thin, typically white layer of nucleated cells between the sedimented red blood cells and the blood plasma. The scientific term *leukocyte* is derived from the Greek roots *leuk-*, which means "white" and *cyt-*, which means "cell".

White blood cells can be classified in different ways. Two pairs of broadest categories classify them either by structure (granulocytes or agranulocytes) or by cell lineage (myeloid cells or lymphoid cells). These broadest categories can be further categorized into five main types: neutrophils, eosinophils, basophils, lymphocytes, and monocytes. These types are distinguished by their physical and functional characteristics. Monocytes and neutrophils are phagocytic. Although there are diverse types of leukocytes, they are all produced and derived from a multipotent cell in the bone marrow called the hematopoietic stem cell. They all have nuclei, which distinguishes them from the other blood cells, the anucleated red blood cells (RBCs) and platelets.

The primary function of leukocytes is to protect the body against infectious diseases or foreign invaders. Therefore, the abnormal number of leukocytes in the blood is often indication of diseases, and thus the white blood cell count is an important subset of the complete blood count. To identify the numbers of different white cells, a blood film is made, and a large number of white cells (at least 100) are counted. This gives the percentage of cells that are of each type. By multiplying the percentage with the total number of white blood cells, the absolute number of each type of white cell can be obtained. There are normally between 4×10^{9} and 1.1×10^{10} white blood cells in a litre of blood. An increase in the number of leukocytes over the upper limit is called leukocytosis. It is occasionally abnormal, when it is neoplastic or autoimmune in origin. A decrease below the lower limit is called leukopenia, which indicates a weakened immune system.

The different types of leukocytes are often characterized as granulocytes or agranulocytes.

1. Granulocytes (polymorphonuclear leukocytes): leukocytes characterized by the presence of differently staining granules in their cytoplasm when viewed under light microscopy. These granules are membrane-bound enzymes which primarily act in the digestion of endocytosed particles. There are three types of granulocytes: neutrophils, basophils, and eosinophils, which are named according to their staining properties.

2. Agranulocytes (mononuclear leukocytes): leukocytes characterized by the apparent absence of granules in their cytoplasm. Although the name implies a lack of granules, these cells do contain non-specific azurophilic granules, which are lysosomes. The cells include lymphocytes, monocytes and macrophages.

Text B   Neutrophils and Lymphocytes
中性粒细胞和淋巴细胞

Neutrophil granulocytes (neutrophils), or polymorphonuclear neutrophils (or PMNs), belong to the granulocyte group, while lymphocytes fall into the agranulocyte category.

Neutrophils are the most abundant type of white blood cells in mammals and form an essential part of the innate immune system. The name, neutrophil, derives from staining characteristics on hematoxylin and eosin (H&E) histological or cytological preparations. Whereas basophils stain dark blue and eosinophils stain bright red, neutrophils stain a neutral pink. Normally neutrophils contain a nucleus divided into 2-5 lobes.

Neutrophils are normally found in the blood stream. Neutrophils can recruit and activate other cells of the immune system. They also play a key role in the front-line defense against invading pathogens. Neutrophils have three methods for directly attacking micro-organisms: phagocytosis (ingestion), degranulation (release of soluble anti-microbials), and generation of neutrophil extracellular traps (NETs). During the beginning (acute) phase of inflammation, particularly as a result of bacterial infection, environmental exposure, and some cancers, neutrophils are one of the first-responders of inflammatory cells to migrate towards the site of inflammation. They migrate through the blood vessels, then through interstitial tissue, following chemical signals such as interleukin-8 (IL-8), complement component C5a (C5a), and leukotriene B4 in a process called chemotaxis. They are the predominant cells in pus, accounting for its whitish or yellowish appearance.

A lymphocyte is one of the subtypes of leukocyte in a vertebrate's immune system. They are the main type of cell found in lymph, which prompted the name "lymphocyte". Lymphocytes include three major types: T cells (for cell-mediated, cytotoxic adaptive immunity), B cells (for humoral, antibody-driven adaptive immunity), and natural killer cells (which function in cell-mediated, cytotoxic innate immunity). Mammalian stem cells differentiate into several kinds of blood cell within the bone marrow. All lymphocytes originate, during this process, from a common lymphoid progenitor before differentiating into their distinct lymphocyte types.

Under microscope, in a Wright's stained peripheral blood smear, a normal lymphocyte has a large, dark-staining nucleus with little to no eosinophilic cytoplasm. In normal situations, the coarse, dense nucleus of a lymphocyte is approximately the size of a red blood cell (about 7 μm in diameter). Some lymphocytes show a clear perinuclear zone (or halo) around the nucleus or could exhibit a small clear zone to one side of the nucleus. Polyribosomes are a prominent feature in the lymphocytes and can be viewed with an electron microscope. The ribosomes are involved in protein synthesis allowing the generation of large quantities of cytokines and immunoglobulins by these cells.

A lymphocyte count is usually part of a peripheral complete blood cell count and is expressed as the percentage of lymphocytes to the total number of white blood cells counted. A general increase in the number of lymphocytes is known as lymphocytosis, whereas a decrease is known as lymphocytopenia. An increase in lymphocyte concentration is usually a sign of a viral infection. A high lymphocyte count with a low neutrophil count might be caused by lymphoma.

New Words

centrifugation /senˌtrɪfjuˈgeiʃən/ *n.* 离心法,离心过滤

buffy /ˈbʌfi/ *adj.* 淡黄色的

nucleate /ˈnjʊklɪɪt/ *v.* (使)成核 *adj.* 有核的

sediment /ˈsedɪmənt/ *n.* 沉淀物,沉积物,沉渣

diverse /daɪˈvɜːrs/ *adj.* 不同的

multipotent /mʌlˈtipətənt/ *adj.* 多能的

granulocyte /ˈgrænjələˌsaɪt/ *n.* [组织]粒细胞,粒性白细胞

agranulocyte /eiˈgrænjuləʊsait/ *n.* [组织]无颗粒白细胞

granule /ˈgrænjuːl/ *n.* 颗粒

lysosome /ˈlaɪsəˌsom/ *n.* [细胞](细胞中的)溶酶体

mammal /ˈmæml/ *n.* [脊椎]哺乳动物

cytological /saiˈtɔlədʒikl/ *adj.* 细胞学的

neutral /ˈnuːtrəl/ *adj.* 中性的,中立的

migrate /ˈmaɪgreɪt/ *v.* 迁移,移居

leukotriene /ˌljuːkəʊˈtraiən/ *n.* [生化]白三烯

pus /pʌs/ *n.* 脓,脓汁

vertebrate /ˈvɜːrtɪbrət/ *adj.* 脊椎动物的 *n.* 脊椎动物

differentiate /ˌdɪfəˈrenʃieɪt/ *v.* 分化,区分

progenitor /proʊˈdʒenɪtər/ *n.* 祖先,起源

perinuclear /ˌpɛrəˈnjʊklɪɚ/ *adj.* 细胞核周围的

cytokine /ˈsaɪtəˌkaɪn/ *n.* [细胞]细胞因子,细胞激素

lymphocytosis /ˌlɪmfosaɪˈtosɪs/ *n.* [内科]淋巴球增多,淋巴细胞(球)过多症

lymphocytopenia /ˌlimfəsaitəˈpiːniə/ *n.* [内科]淋巴球减少,淋巴细胞(球)减少症

Phrases and Expressions

derive from …	源出……,来自……
peripheral blood smear	外周血涂片
be involved in …	包括在……中
bone marrow	骨髓
play a key role in …	在……中起关键作用
as a result of …	作为……的结果
fall into the category	归为……(类别)
be characterized as …	被描述为……
immune system	免疫系统
stem cell	干细胞

Notes

1. The scientific term leukocyte is derived from the Greek roots *leuk-*, which means "white" and *cyt-*, which means "cell".

"leukocyte"这一科学术语来自希腊语词根"*leuk-*"(意为"白色")和"*cyt-*"(意为"细胞")。

2. Although there are diverse types of leukocytes, they are all produced and derived from a multipotent cell in the bone marrow called the hematopoietic stem cell.

尽管存在多种类型的白细胞,但它们都是由骨髓中称为造血干细胞的多能干细胞产生和分化的。

3. Granulocytes (polymorphonuclear leukocytes): leukocytes characterized by the presence of differently staining granules in their cytoplasm when viewed under light microscopy. These granules are membrane-bound

enzymes which primarily act in the digestion of endocytosed particles.

粒细胞(多形核白细胞):以光镜下观察到胞浆内存在不同染色颗粒为特征。这些颗粒由质膜包裹酶形成,主要作用于消化细胞内吞的颗粒。

4. Agranulocytes (mononuclear leukocytes): leukocytes characterized by the apparent absence of granules in their cytoplasm.

无颗粒白细胞(单核细胞):即细胞的胞浆内无明显颗粒为其特征的白细胞。

5. They migrate through the blood vessels, then through interstitial tissue, following chemical signals such as interleukin-8 (IL-8), complement component C5a (C5a), and leukotriene B4 in a process called chemotaxis.

在被称之为化学趋化(Chemotaxis)的过程中,中性粒细胞受到一些化学信号,如白介素-8(IL-8)、补体成分 C5a(C5a)以及白三烯 B4 等的吸引,穿过血管,通过间质组织向炎症部位迁移。

6. Polyribosomes are a prominent feature in the lymphocytes and can be viewed with an electron microscope. The ribosomes are involved in protein synthesis allowing the generation of large quantities of cytokines and immunoglobulins by these cells.

多聚核糖体是淋巴细胞的一个显著特征,可用电子显微镜观测到。核糖体参与蛋白质合成,使淋巴细胞能产生大量细胞因子和免疫球蛋白。

Exercises

Ⅰ. Fill in the blanks according to the texts.

1. An increase in the number of leukocytes over the upper limits is called＿＿＿＿＿＿＿. (Text A)

2. ＿＿＿＿＿＿＿ are characterized by the presence of differently staining granules in their cytoplasm when viewed under light microscopy. (Text A)

3. Agranulocytes include lymphocytes, ＿＿＿＿＿＿＿ and macrophages. (Text A)

4. ＿＿＿＿＿ have three methods for directly attacking micro-organisms: phagocytosis (ingestion), degranulation (release of soluble anti-microbials), and generation of neutrophil extracellular traps (NETs). (Text B)

5. An increase in lymphocyte concentration is usually a sign of a＿＿＿＿＿＿＿infection. (Text B)

Ⅱ. Translate the following into Chinese.

A lymphocyte is one of the subtypes of leukocyte in a vertebrate's immune system. They are the main type of cell found in lymph, which prompted the name "lymphocyte". Lymphocytes include three major types: T cells (for cell-mediated, cytotoxic adaptive immunity), B cells (for humoral, antibody-driven adaptive immunity), and natural killer cells (which function in cell-mediated, cytotoxic innate immunity).

Lesson 6　Related Tests of Blood Coagulation
凝血相关检测

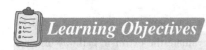 **Learning Objectives**

After studying this lesson, students are expected to be able to

1. master some medical terms about Related Tests of Blood Coagulation;

2. be familiar with the clinical significance of platelet count, PT and APTT;

3. know about the commonly used tests of blood coagulation.

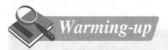

1. What do you know about platelet?
2. What are the commonly used tests of blood coagulation?
3. Do you know how to perform a platelet count?

Text A   Platelet Count
血小板计数

Platelets, also called thrombocytes, are small, irregularly shaped clear cell fragments (i. e., cells that do not have a nucleus containing DNA), 2-3 μm in diameter, which are derived from fragmentation of precursor megakaryocytes of the bone marrow, and then enter the circulation. The average lifespan of a platelet is normally 5-9 days. They circulate in the blood of mammals and are involved in hemostasis, leading to the formation of blood clots.

A normal platelet count in a healthy individual is between 150,000 and 450,000 per μl (microlitre) of blood (150×10^9/L-450×10^9/L). Ninety-five percent of healthy people will have platelet counts in this range. If the number of platelets is too low, excessive bleeding can occur. Low platelet concentration is thrombocytopenia and is due to either decreased production or increased destruction. By contrast, if the number of platelets is too high, blood clots can form (thrombosis), which may obstruct blood vessels and result in such events as a stroke, myocardial infarction, pulmonary embolism or the blockage of blood vessels to other parts of the body, such as the extremities of the arms or legs. Elevated platelet concentration is thrombocytosis and is either congenital, reactive (to cytokines), or due to unregulated production: one of the myeloproliferative neoplasms or certain other myeloid neoplasms. A disorder of platelet function is a thrombocytopathy.

Platelet counts use a freshly collected blood specimen to which a chemical called EDTA has been added to prevent the blood from clotting before the test begins. About 5 mL of blood are drawn from a vein in the patient's inner elbow region, or other area. Blood drawn from a vein helps to produce a more accurate count than blood drawn from a fingertip. Collection of the sample takes only a few minutes. After collection, the mean platelet volume of EDTA-blood will increase over time. This increase is caused by a change in the shape of the platelets after removal from the body. The changing volume is relatively stable for a period of one to three hours after collection. This period is the best time to count the sample when using electronic instruments, because the platelets will be within a standard size range.

Text B   Prothrombin Time and Activated Partial Thromboplastin Time
凝血酶原时间与活化部分凝血活酶时间

Prothrombin Time (PT)

PT and its derived measures of prothrombin ratio (PR — the PT for a patient, divided by the result for control plasma) and international normalized ratio (INR) are assays to evaluate the extrinsic pathway of coagulation. They are used to determine the clotting tendency of blood, in the measure of warfarin dosage, liver damage, and vitamin K status. PT measures factors Ⅰ, Ⅱ, Ⅴ, Ⅶ and Ⅹ.

A one-stage clotting test based on the time required for clotting to occur after the addition of tissue thromboplastin and calcium to decalcified plasma. Blood is drawn into a test tube containing liquid citrate, which acts as an anticoagulant by binding the calcium in a sample. The blood is mixed and then centrifuged to obtain plasma. An excess of calcium is added, (thereby reversing the effects of citrate), which enables the blood to clot again. Tissue factor is added to activate the extrinsic clotting pathway, and the time the sample takes to clot is measured optically. Some laboratories use a mechanical measurement, which eliminates interference from lipemic and icteric samples.

The results (in seconds) for a PT performed on a normal individual will vary according to the type of analytical system employed. This is due to the variations between different batches of manufacturer's tissue factor used in the reagent to perform the test. The INR was devised to standardize the results. Each manufacturer assigns an International Sensitivity Index (ISI) value for any tissue factor they manufacture. The ISI value indicates how a particular batch of tissue factor compares to an international reference tissue factor. The INR is the ratio of a patient's PT to a normal (control) sample, raised to the power of the ISI value for the analytical system used.

$$INR = \left(\frac{PT_{test}}{PT_{nomal}} \right)^{ISI}$$

Activated Partial Thromboplastin Time（APTT）

APTT is used to measure the efficacy of both the "intrinsic" and the common coagulation pathways. The test is termed "partial" due to the absence of tissue factor from the reaction mixture.

First, blood is collected into a tube containing oxalate or citrate to arrest coagulation by binding the calcium in a sample. The specimen is then delivered to the laboratory. In order to activate the intrinsic pathway, an activator (such as silica, celite, kaolin, ellagic acid) and calcium (to reverse the anticoagulant effect of the oxalate) are mixed into the plasma sample. The time is measured until a thrombus forms. The typical reference range is between 30 s and 42 s (depending on laboratory).

APTT is also used to monitor the treatment effects with heparin. Shortening of APTT has little clinical relevance, but some research indicates that it might increase the risk of thromboembolism. Normal APTT times require the presence of the following coagulation factors: Ⅰ, Ⅱ, V, Ⅷ, Ⅸ, Ⅹ, Ⅺ and Ⅻ. Notably, deficiencies in factors Ⅶ or Ⅷ will not be detected with the APTT test. Prolonged APTT may indicate: (1) use of heparin (or contamination of the sample); (2) antiphospholipid antibody (especially lupus anticoagulant); (3) coagulation factor deficiency (e. g. , hemophilia).

New Words

platelet /ˈpleɪtlət/ n. ［组织］血小板, 薄片

fragmentation /ˌfrægmenˈteɪʃn/ n. 破碎, 分裂

precursor /priˈkɜːrsər/ n. 前体, 前体物

megakaryocyte /ˌmegəˈkæriəusait/ n. ［组织］巨核细胞

lifespan /ˈlaɪfspæn/ n. 寿命, 预期生命期限

hemostasis /ˌhiːməʊˈsteɪsɪs/ n. ［医］止血, 止血法

thrombocytopenia /ˌθrɑmbəˌsaɪtəˈpiniə/ n. ［内科］血小板减少（症）

stroke /stroʊk/ n. 中风

extremity /ɪkˈstreməti/ n. 末端, 极端, 手足

thrombocytosis /ˌθrɒmbəʊsaiˈtəusis/ n. ［内科］血小板增多（症）

neoplasm /ˈnioplæzm/ n. ［医］赘生物, 瘤, 新生物

thrombocytopathy /θrɑmbəˈsitəpəθi/ n. ［内科］血小板病

prothrombin /proˈθrɑmbɪn/ n. 凝血素, 凝血酶原

anticoagulant /ˌæntɪkoʊˈægjələnt/ n. （助剂）抗凝剂 adj. 抗凝血的

thromboplastin /ˌθrɑmbəˈplæstɪn/ n. ［生化］促凝血酶原激酶, 血栓形成质

coagulation /koʊˌægjuˈleɪʃn/ n. 凝固, 凝结, 凝结物

thromboembolism /ˌθrɒmbəʊˈembəlɪzəm/ n. ［病理］血栓栓塞

antiphospholipid /ˈæntiˌfɒsfə(ʊ)ˈlɪpɪd/ n. ［医］抗磷脂

Phrases and Expressions

blood clot	血凝块,血块
myocardial infarction（MI）	心肌梗死
pulmonary embolism	肺栓塞,肺血管阻塞症
reference range	参考范围
be detected with …	被检测到……
be devised to …	被设计来……
coagulation factor	凝血因子

Notes

1. Platelets, also called thrombocytes, are small, irregularly shaped clear cell fragments (i. e., cells that do not have a nucleus containing DNA), 2-3 μm in diameter, which are derived from fragmentation of precursor megakaryocytes of the bone marrow, and then enter the circulation.

血小板（也称血栓细胞）是一些小而形态不规则和透亮的细胞碎片（即缺乏含 DNA 核的细胞），直径 2～3μm，以骨髓的巨核细胞为前体，经破裂形成碎片后，进入血液循环形成。

2. Elevated platelet concentration is thrombocytosis and is either congenital, reactive (to cytokines), or due to unregulated production: one of the myeloproliferative neoplasms or certain other myeloid neoplasms.

血小板浓度升高称为血小板增多症，或是先天性的、反应性的（对细胞因子的反应），或是由于生成的失调：某种骨髓增殖性肿瘤或某些其他髓系肿瘤导致。

3. Platelet counts use a freshly collected blood specimen to which a chemical called EDTA has been added to prevent the blood from clotting before the test begins.

血小板计数用新鲜收集血标本，加入乙二胺四乙酸（EDTA）；该化学品用于防止血液在计数前就发生凝固。

4. The INR is the ratio of a patient's PT to a normal (control) sample, raised to the power of the ISI value for the analytical system used.

国际标准化比值（INR）是病人凝血酶原时间（PT）与正常对照 PT 之比的 ISI 次方。

5. The test is termed "partial" due to the absence of tissue factor from the reaction mixture.

该测试被称为"部分"测试是由于反应体系中缺乏组织因子。

Exercises

Ⅰ. Fill in the blanks according to the texts.

1. Platelets, also called_____, are small, irregularly shaped clear cell fragments (i. e., cells that do not have a nucleus containing DNA), 2-3 μm in diameter, which are derived from fragmentation of precursor megakaryocytes of the bone marrow, and then enter the circulation. (Text A)

2. Platelets circulate in the blood of mammals and are involved in_____, leading to the formation of blood clots. (Text A)

3. PT and its derived measures of prothrombin ratio (PR) and international normalized ratio (INR) are assays to evaluate the_____ pathway of coagulation. (Text B)

4. APTT is used to measure the efficacy of both the "_____" and the common coagulation pathways. (Text B)

5. Shortening of APTT has little clinical relevance, but some research indicates that it might increase risk of _____. (Text B)

Ⅱ. Translate the following into Chinese.

Low platelet concentration is thrombocytopenia and is due to either decreased production or increased destruction. By contrast, if the number of platelets is too high, blood clots can form (thrombosis), which may obstruct blood vessels and result in such events as a stroke, myocardial infarction, pulmonary embolism or the blockage of blood vessels to other parts of the body, such as the extremities of the arms or legs.

Lesson 7   Blood Group System and Cross-matching
血型系统与交叉配血

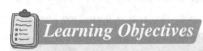

After studying this lesson, students are expected to be able to

1. master some medical words and terms about blood group systems;
2. be familiar with the usage of attributive clause;
3. know about the notices of cross-matching blood in transfusion medicine.

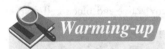

1. Where are the antigens of blood group?
2. Who established the ABO blood group system first?
3. What do the red cells and serum contain respectively in the Type A blood?

Text A   Blood Group System
血型系统

The International Society of Blood Transfusion (ISBT) currently recognizes 30 major blood group systems (including the ABO and Rh systems). Thus, in addition to the ABO antigens and Rhesus antigens, many other antigens are expressed on the red blood cell surface membrane. For example, an individual can be AB RhD positive, and at the same time M and N positive (MNS system), K positive (Kell system) and Le^a or Le^b positive (Lewis system). Many of the blood group systems were named after the patients in whom the corresponding antibodies were initially encountered.

The ABO blood group system is the most important blood type system (or blood group system) in human blood transfusion. The A, B and O blood groups were first established by Austrian immunologist Karl Landsteiner in 1901.

The ABO blood group system, the classification of human blood based on the inherited properties of red blood cells (erythrocytes) as determined by the presence or absence of the antigens A and B, which are carried on the surface of the red cells. Persons may thus have Type A, Type B, Type O or Type AB blood. Blood containing red cells with type A antigen on their surface has in its serum (fluid) antibodies against Type B red cells. If, in transfusion, Type B blood is injected into persons with Type A blood, the red cells in the injected blood will be destroyed by the antibodies in the recipient's blood. In the same way, Type A red cells will be destroyed by anti-A antibodies in Type B blood. Type O blood can be injected into persons with Type A, B or O blood unless there is incompatibility with respect to some other blood group system also present. Persons with Type AB blood can receive Type A, B or O blood.

The Rh (Rhesus) blood group system (including the Rh factor) is one of thirty current human blood group systems. Clinically, it is the most important blood group system after ABO. At Present, the Rh blood group system consists of 50 defined blood-group antigens, among which the 5 antigens D, C, c, E and e are the most important. The commonly-used terms Rh factor, Rh positive and Rh negative refer to the D antigen

97

only. Besides its role in blood transfusion, the Rh blood group system, the D antigen, in particular, is a relevant cause of the hemolytic disease of the newborn or erythroblastosis fetalis, for which prevention is the key.

Text B   Cross-matching Blood
交叉配血

Before a recipient receives a transfusion, compatibility testing between donor and recipient blood must be done. Cross-matching blood, in transfusion medicine, refers to the complex testing that is performed prior to a blood transfusion, to determine if the donor's blood is compatible with the blood of an intended recipient. Blood compatibility has many aspects, and is determined not only by the blood types (O, A, B, AB), but also by blood factors (Rh, Kell, etc.). Cross-matching blood is done by a certified laboratory technologist, in a laboratory. It can be done electronically, with a computer database, or serologically.

Electronic cross-matching is essentially a computer-assisted analysis of the data entered from testing done on the donor unit and blood samples drawn from intended recipient. This includes ABO or Rh typing of the unit and of the recipient, and an antibody screen of the recipient. Electronic cross-matching can only be used if a patient has a negative antibody screen, which means that they do not have any active red blood cell atypical antibodies, or the atypical antibodies are below the detectable level of current testing methods. If all of the data entered is compatible, the computer will print a compatibility label stating that the unit is safe to transfuse.

Cross-matching blood falls into two categories:

Major Cross-match: Recipient serum is tested against donor packed cells to determine if the recipient has preformed antibodies against any antigens on the donor's cells. This is the required cross-match prior to release of a unit of packed cells.

Minor Cross-match: Recipient red cells are tested against donor serum to detect donor antibodies directed against a patient's antigens. This is no longer required. It is assumed that the small amount of donor serum and antibodies left in a unit of packed cells will be diluted in a recipient.

New Words

recognize /'rekəgnaɪz/ v. 承认,认可,识别
corresponding /ˌkɔːrəˈspɑːndɪŋ/ adj. 相当的,相应的,一致的
recipient /rɪˈsɪpiənt/ n. 接受者,容纳者
incompatibility /ˌɪnkəmˌpætəˈbɪləti/ n. 不相容,不一致
hemolytic /hiːˈmɒlitik/ adj. [生理][免疫]溶血的
erythroblastosis /ɪˌrɪθroblæsˈtosɪs/ n. 骨髓成红血细胞增多症
fetalis /ˈfetəlɪs/ n. 胎儿
donor /ˈdoʊnər/ n. 捐赠者,供者
intended /ɪnˈtendɪd/ adj. 有意的,打算中的
certified /ˈsɝtəˌfaɪd/ adj. 被证明的,具有证明文件的
serologically /siˈrɔlədʒikli/ adv. 血清学地
atypical /ˌeɪˈtɪpɪkl/ adj. 非典型的,不合规则的
assumed /əˈsuːmd/ adj. 假定的,假装的

Phrases and Expressions

international society of blood transfusion (ISBT)	国际输血学会
rhesus antigens	恒河猴抗原
kell system	凯尔系统
Lewis system	路易斯系统

Karl Landsteiner	卡尔·兰德斯坦纳(人名)
compatibility testing	兼容性测试
cross-matching blood	交叉配血
major cross-match	主侧配血
packed cells	浓集细胞
minor cross-match	次侧配血

Notes

1. Many of the blood group systems were named after the patients in whom the corresponding antibodies were initially encountered.

许多血型系统是依据最初被鉴定出相应抗体的病人而命名。

2. The ABO blood group system, the classification of human blood based on the inherited properties of red blood cells (erythrocytes) as determined by the presence or absence of the antigens A and B, which are carried on the surface of the red cells.

ABO 血型系统,血细胞基于红细胞的遗传特性进行分类,这一特性由红细胞表面是否存在 A、B 抗原决定。

3. Blood containing red cells with Type A antigen on their surface has in its serum (fluid) antibodies against Type B red cells.

在红细胞表面存在 A 型抗原的血液中,其血清(液体)有抗 B 型红细胞的抗体。

4. Type O blood can be injected into persons with Type A, B, or O blood unless there is incompatibility with respect to some other blood group system also present.

O 型血可以注入 A 型、B 型或者 O 型血的人,除非存在有其他一些不相容性的血型系统。

5. Besides its role in blood transfusion, the Rh blood group system, the D antigen, in particular, is a relevant cause of the hemolytic disease of the newborn or erythroblastosis fetalis for which prevention is the key.

Rh 血型系统,特别是 D 抗原,除了输血中的作用,还与新生儿溶血病或胎儿成红细胞增多病有关联,是预防的关键。

6. Cross-matching blood, in transfusion medicine, refers to the complex testing that is performed prior to a blood transfusion, to determine if the donor's blood is compatible with the blood of an intended recipient.

输血医学中,交叉配血是复杂的检验。检验于输血之前进行,以确定献血者的血液是否与预定受血者的血液匹配。

7. Electronic cross-matching is essentially a computer-assisted analysis of the data entered from testing done on the donor unit and blood samples drawn from intended recipient.

电子交叉配血本质上是计算机辅助数据分析,输入数据为供血单位标本和预定受血者血液标本的检验结果。

8. Electronic cross-matching can only be used if a patient has a negative antibody screen, which means that they do not have any active red blood cell atypical antibodies, or the atypical antibodies below the detectable level of current testing methods.

电子交叉配血只能用于抗体筛检为阴性的病人,这意味着他们没有任何活跃红细胞非典型的抗体,或者其水平低于当前测试方法的可检测水平。

9. Major Cross-match: Recipient serum is tested against donor packed cells to determine if the recipient has preformed antibodies against any antigens on the donor's cells. This is the required cross-match prior to release of a unit of packed cells.

主侧配血:受血者的血清与供血者的浓集红细胞进行配合实验,确定是否受血者体内预先存在抗供血者细胞表面任何抗原的抗体。输入一个单位浓集红细胞之前必需做这种交叉配血。

10. Minor Cross-match: Recipient red cells are tested against donor serum to detect donor antibodies di-

rected against a patient's antigens.

次侧配血:受血者的红细胞与供血者的血清进行配合试验,检测供血者的抗体与病人抗原的反应情况。

Exercises

Ⅰ. Fill in the blanks according to the texts.

1. Many of the blood group systems were_____the patients in whom the corresponding antibodies were initially encountered. (Text A)

2. The ABO blood group system is the most important blood type system (or blood group system) in human blood _____. (Text A)

3. Besides its role in blood transfusion, the Rh blood group system, the D antigen, in particular, is a relevant cause of the _____ disease of the newborn or erythroblastosis fetalis for which prevention is key. (Text A)

4. Before a recipient receives a transfusion,_____ testing between donor and recipient blood must be done. (Text B)

5. Cross-matching blood, in transfusion medicine, refers to the complex testing that is performed _____ _____ a blood transfusion, to determine if the donor's blood is compatible with the blood of an intended recipient. (Text B)

Ⅱ. Translate the following into Chinese.

The International Society of Blood Transfusion (ISBT) currently recognizes 30 major blood group systems (including the ABO and Rh systems). Thus, in addition to the ABO antigens and Rhesus antigens, many other antigens are expressed on the red blood cell surface membrane. For example, an individual can be AB RhD positive, and at the same time M and N positive (MNS system), K positive (Kell system) and Le^a or Le^b positive (Lewis system).

Lesson 8   Electrolytes in Body Fluids
体液电解质

Learning Objectives

After studying this lesson, students are expected to be able to

1. master some medical words and terms about electrolytes and electrolyte analyzer;
2. be familiar with how electrolytes work in living species;
3. know about the characteristics of Fully Automatic Electrolyte Analyzer.

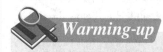

Warming-up

1. Can you tell some electrolytes in nature?
2. What roles do electrolytes play in the body?
3. What is the electrolyte analyzer used for?

Text A   Important Electrolytes in Human Body
人体重要的电解质

Electrolytes are ions that form when salts dissolve in water or fluids. These ions have an electric charge. The electric charge symbols of plus (+) and minus (−) indicate that the substance in question is ionic in nature and has an imbalanced distribution of electrons. Positively charged ions are called cations. Negatively charged ions are called anions.

In physiology, the primary ions of electrolytes are sodium (Na^+), potassium (K^+), calcium (Ca^{2+}), magnesium (Mg^{2+}), chloride (Cl^-), hydrogen phosphate (HPO_4^{2-}), and hydrogen carbonate (HCO_3^-).

As it is known to all, human body requires a subtle and complex electrolyte balance between the intracellular and extracellular environment. In particular, the maintenance of precise osmotic gradients of electrolytes is important. Such gradients affect and regulate the hydration of the body as well as blood pH and are critical for nerve and muscle function. Various mechanisms exist in living species that keep the concentrations of different electrolytes under tight control.

Both muscle tissue and neurons are considered as electric tissues of the body. Muscles and neurons are activated by electrolyte activity between the extracellular fluid or interstitial fluid, and intracellular fluid. Electrolytes may enter or leave the cell membrane through ion channels. Ion channels are specialized protein structures embedded in the plasma membrane. For example, muscle contraction is dependent upon the presence of calcium (Ca^{2+}), sodium (Na^+) and potassium (K^+). Without sufficient levels of these key electrolytes, muscle weakness or severe muscle contraction may occur.

Electrolyte balance is maintained by oral, or in emergencies, intravenous (Ⅳ) intake of electrolyte-containing substances, and is regulated by hormones, generally with the kidneys flushing out excess levels. In human body, electrolyte homeostasis is regulated by hormones such as antidiuretic hormone, aldosterone and parathyroid hormone. Serious electrolyte disturbances, such as dehydration and overhydration, may lead to cardiac and neurological complications and will result in a medical emergency unless they are rapidly resolved.

Text B   Electrolyte Analyzer
电解质分析仪

Measurement of electrolytes is a commonly performed diagnostic procedure. Medical technologists accomplish it through blood testing with ion selective electrodes or urinalysis. The interpretation of these values is somewhat meaningless without analysis of the clinical history. it is often impossible to explain them without parallel measurement of renal function. One important test conducted on urine is the specific gravity test to determine the occurrence of electrolyte imbalance. Chloride levels are rarely measured except for arterial blood gas interpretation since they are inherently linked to sodium levels. Electrolytes measured most often are sodium and potassium.

Sodium Potassium Ionized Calcium and Chloride Electrolyte Analyzer introduces internationally advanced ion-selective electrode technology. Reliability, practicability and convenience make the instrument be able to test the sodium, potassium, ionized calcium and chloride in whole blood, plasma, serum and diluted urine.

Product Description:

1. Measurement Characteristics of Fully Automated Electrolyte Analyzer

- Compact, economical and easy to use;
- Long life, high performance, maintenance-free electrodes;
- Automatic sampling, probe wiping and calibration;
- Intelligent reagent pack with electronic chip;
- Battery back-up facility;
- Extremely low cost per test.

2. Technical specifications of the equipment

- Principle：Direct measurement with ION Selective Electrode（ISE）；
- Sample：120 μL for Whole Blood, Serum, Plasma, 700 μL for diluted（1∶5）Urine；
- Data Storage：100 Patients result；
- QC-up to 30 results of Normal, Low, and High each；
- Output：128×64 Graphics Display with Yes or No Numeric Keypad 24 column thermal printer USB port；
- Ambient conditions：Temperature 3-10℃, <85% noncondensing humidity；
- Input voltage：100/115 VAC, 50-60 Hz or 220 VAC, 50-60 Hz, 0.75 amp；
- Size and Weight：15 in. W×12 in. H × 7.0 in. D, 10 kg；
- Battery Option：Built in Lithium Ion Battery with Power back-up of 10 hours.

New Words

cation /ˈkætaɪən/ n. ［化学］阳离子,正离子

anion /ˈænaɪən/ n. ［化学］阴离子,负离子

potassium /pəˈtæsɪəm/ n. ［化学］钾,钾离子

magnesium /mægˈniːzɪəm/ n. ［化学］镁,镁离子

hydrogen /ˈhaɪdrədʒən/ n. ［化学］氢

carbonate /ˈkɑːrbənət/ n. 碳酸盐

osmotic /ɑːzˈmɑːtɪk/ adj. 渗透性的

gradient /ˈɡreɪdɪənt/ n. 梯度,坡度

hydration /haɪˈdreɪʃn/ n. ［化学］水合作用

mechanism /ˈmekənɪzəm/ n. 原理,机制

contraction /kənˈtrækʃn/ n. 收缩,紧缩

intravenous /ˌɪntrəˈviːnəs/ adj. 静脉内的

aldosterone /ælˈdɑstəˌron/ n. ［生化］醛固酮,醛甾酮

parathyroid /ˌpærəˈθaɪrɔɪd/ n. 甲状旁腺

disturbance /dɪˈstɜːrbəns/ n. 失调,紊乱（等于 disorder）

dehydration /ˌdiːhaɪˈdreɪʃn/ n. 脱水

homeostasis /ˌhoʊmiəˈsteɪsɪs/ n. ［生理］体内平衡（复数 homeostases）

neurological /ˌnʊrəˈlɑːdʒɪkl/ adj. 神经病学的,神经学上的

chip /tʃɪp/ n. 芯片,碎片

ambient /ˈæmbɪənt/ adj. 周围的,外界的

noncondensing /ˈnɒnkənˈdensiŋ/ adj. 不凝固的,不凝结的

humidity /hjuːˈmɪdəti/ n. ［气象］湿度,湿气

Phrases and Expressions

electric charge	电荷
ion channel	离子通道
antidiuretic hormone	抗利尿激素
parathyroid hormone	甲状旁腺素
ion selective electrode	离子选择性电极
renal function	肾功能
thermal printer	热敏印刷机
lithium ion battery	锂离子电池

Notes

1. As it is known to all, human body requires a subtle and complex electrolyte balance between the intracellular and extracellular environment. In particular, the maintenance of precise osmotic gradients of electrolytes is important.

众所周知,人体需要细胞内外环境之间处于精细和复杂的电解质平衡状态。特别是维持电解质的精确渗透梯度尤为重要。

2. Electrolytes may enter or leave the cell membrane through ion channels. Ion channels are specialized protein structures embedded in the plasma membrane.

电解质可通过离子通道进出细胞膜。离子通道为镶嵌于质膜的特殊蛋白质结构。

3. Electrolyte balance is maintained by oral, or in emergencies, intravenous (Ⅳ) intake of electrolyte-containing substances, and is regulated by hormones, generally with the kidneys flushing out excess levels.

电解质平衡通过口服或紧急情况下静脉注射(Ⅳ)含电解质的物质来维持,并受激素的调节,多余的电解质通常由肾脏排出。

4. Measurement of electrolytes is a commonly performed diagnostic procedure. Medical technologists accomplish it through blood testing with ion selective electrodes or urinalysis.

电解质测定是一种常用的诊断方法。医学技术人员通过用离子选择电极做血液检验或进行尿液分析来完成电解质测定。

5. The interpretation of these values is somewhat meaningless without analysis of the clinical history. it is often impossible to explain them without parallel measurement of renal function.

如果不分析临床病史,解释这些(电解质)测定值就没有多大意义。如果不同时测量肾脏功能,通常也不能对这些(电解质)测定值予以解释。

6. Reliability, practicability and convenience make the instrument be able to test the sodium, potassium, ionized calcium and chloride in whole blood, plasma, serum and diluted urine.

该仪器可靠、实用和方便,能够测定全血、血浆、血清和稀释尿液中的钠、钾、离子钙和氯。

Exercises

Ⅰ. Fill in the blanks according to the texts.

1. Positively charged ions are called _____ Negatively charged ions are called anions. (Text A)

2. Both muscle tissue and_____are considered electric tissues of the body. (Text A)

3. One important test conducted on urine is the specific gravity test to determine the occurrence of electrolyte _____. (Text B)

4. Chloride levels are rarely measured _____ arterial blood gas interpretation since they are inherently linked to sodium levels. (Text B)

5. Sodium Potassium Ionized Calcium and Chloride Electrolyte Analyzer introduces international advanced_____ technology. (Text B)

Ⅱ. Translate the following into Chinese.

Electrolyte balance is maintained by oral, or in emergencies, intravenous (Ⅳ) intake of electrolyte-containing substances, and is regulated by hormones, generally with the kidneys flushing out excess levels. In human body, electrolyte homeostasis is regulated by hormones such as antidiuretic hormone, aldosterone and parathyroid hormone. Serious electrolyte disturbances, such as dehydration and overhydration, may lead to cardiac and neurological complications, will result in a medical emergency unless they are rapidly resolved.

Lesson 9 Arterial Blood Gas Analysis
动脉血气分析

Learning Objectives

After studying this lesson, students are expected to be able to

1. master the basic knowledge of arterial blood gas;
2. be familiar with the techniques for Arterial Blood Gas Sample Collection;
3. know about the parameters of blood gas analysis.

Warming-up

1. Have you ever heard about Arterial Blood Gas Sample Collection?
2. Who can collect Arterial Blood Gas Sample?
3. Do you know the parameters of blood gas analysis?

Text A   Collection Techniques of Arterial Blood Gas Sample
动脉血气分析标本收集技术

Arterial blood is used for blood gas analysis. It is usually drawn by respiratory therapist, phlebotomist, nurse or doctor.

The radial artery, the femoral artery, the brachial artery and arterial catheter can be chosen for Arterial blood collection. As the radial artery at the wrist is easily accessible, can be compressed to control bleeding, and has less risk for occlusion, it is most commonly chosen. The femoral artery (or the brachial artery, seldomly used) is used only during emergency situations or with children. Blood can also be taken from an arterial catheter already placed in one of these arteries. For these puncture sites, two are available to laboratory personnel. One is the brachial artery above the crease of the elbow and, more preferably, the other one is the radial artery at its site of most palpable pulsation in the wrist. Laboratory personnel are not authorized to use the femoral artery. The patient's physician may use it or other sites.

In order to prevent blood coagulation, the syringe should be pre-packaged with a small amount of heparin. Or it needs to be heparinized by drawing up a small amount of heparin and squirting it out again. Once the sample is obtained, visible gas bubbles need to be eliminated, as these bubbles can dissolve into the sample and cause inaccurate results. Then the sealed syringe is taken to a blood gas analyzer. If the sample cannot be analyzed within 10-15 minutes, it must be placed on ice for valid results. Blood gas values may change within five to ten minutes if the sample remains at room temperature. Even when placed on ice, samples should still be analyzed within 1 hour.

Arterialized Capillary Sample Collection Technique:
- Warm capillary bed 5-10 minutes; vasodilation increases blood flow to near arterial rate.
- Puncture Sites: heel pad, ear lobe, and fingertip.
- Draw full heparinized capillary tubes, excluding air bubbles.
- Seal both ends of the tube.
- Place on ice and transport to the lab immediately.

Text B Parameters of Blood Gas Analysis
血气分析参数

Laboratory analyzes arterial blood gases and provides the following information.

pH — The normal range of pH is 7.35-7.45. As the pH decreases (pH<7.35; H^+>45 nmol/L (nM)), it implies acidosis, while if the pH increases (pH>7.45; H^+<35 nmol/L (nM)) it implies alkalosis.

HCO_3^- — The HCO_3^- ion indicates whether a metabolic problem is present (such as ketoacidosis). A low HCO_3^- indicates metabolic acidosis while a high HCO_3^- indicates metabolic alkalosis. As the HCO_3^- in blood gas results is often calculated by the analyzer, correlation between it and total CO_2 levels as directly measured should be checked as the following.

TCO_2 — This means the total amount of CO_2. It is the sum of HCO_3^- and PCO_2 by the following formula:
$TCO_2 = [HCO_3^-] + \alpha \times PCO_2$ ($\alpha = 0.226$ mM/kPa, HCO_3^- is expressed in millimolar concentration (mM) (mmol/L) and PCO_2 is expressed in kPa)

PCO_2 — The carbon dioxide partial pressure (PCO_2) is an indicator of CO_2 production and elimination, for a constant metabolic rate, the PCO_2 is determined entirely by its elimination through ventilation. A high PCO_2 (respiratory acidosis, alternatively hypercapnia) indicates underventilation (or, more rarely, a hypermetabolic disorder), a low PCO_2 (respiratory alkalosis, alternatively hypocapnia) indicates hyper- or overventilation.

PO_2 — Low PO_2 indicates that the patient is not oxygenating properly and is hypoxemic. (Note that a low PO_2 doesn't mean the patient has hypoxemia.) If PO_2 is less than 60 mmHg, supplemental oxygen should be administered. If PO_2 is less than 26 mmHg, the patient is at risk of death and must be oxygenated immediately.

CaO_2 — It is the sum of oxygen dissolved in plasma and chemically bound to hemoglobin as determined. It can be calculated by the formula: $CaO_2 = (PO_2 \times 0.003) + (SaO_2 \times 1.34 \times Hgb)$ (Hemoglobin concentration is expressed as g/dL).

SaO_2 or O_2 sats — Oxygen saturation, measure the percentage of hemoglobin binding sites in the bloodstream occupied by oxygen.

These parameters can be used for assessing a patient's acid-base balance. They reflect the ability of the lungs to exchange oxygen and carbon dioxide, the ability of the kidneys to control the retention or elimination of bicarbonate, and the effectiveness of the heart as a pump. Because the lungs and kidneys act as important regulators of the respiratory and metabolic acid-base balance, assessment of the status of a patient with any disorder of respiration and metabolism includes periodic blood gas measurements.

New Words

palpable /ˈpælpəbl/ *adj.* 明显的,可感知的,易觉察的

syringe /sɪˈrɪndʒ/ *vt.* 注射,冲洗 *n.* 注射器,洗涤器

bubble /ˈbʌbl/ *n.* 气泡,泡沫 *v.* 沸腾,冒泡

vasodilation /ˌveɪzoʊdaɪˈleɪʃn/ *n.* 血管舒张

acidosis /ˌæsɪˈdosɪs/ *n.* [内科] 酸中毒,酸毒症

alkalosis /ˌælkəˈlosɪs/ *n.* 碱毒症

calculate /ˈkælkjuleɪt/ *v.* 计算,预测,打算

formula /ˈfɔːrmjələ/ *n.* 公式,准则,配方

constant /ˈkɑːnstənt/ *adj.* 不变的,恒定的 *n.* [数] 常数,恒量

ventilation /ˌventɪˈleɪʃn/ *n.* 通风设备,空气流通

oxygenate /ˈɑːksɪdʒəneɪt/ *vt.* 氧化,充氧,以氧处理

hypoxemic /ˌhaɪpɔkˈsiːmik/ *adj.* 血氧过低的

笔记

supplemental /ˌsʌpləˈmɛntl/ *adj.* 补充的,追加的

bound /baʊnd/ *adj.* 有义务的 *v.* 束缚,限制 *n.* 界限,范围

retention /rɪˈtenʃn/ *n.* 保留,扣留,滞留,记忆力

bicarbonate /ˌbaɪˈkɑːrbənət/ *n.* 碳酸氢盐,重碳酸盐

periodic /ˌpɪriˈɑːdɪk/ *adj.* 周期的,定期的

Phrases and Expressions

respiratory therapist	呼吸治疗师
radial artery	桡动脉,桡骨动脉
femoral artery	股动脉,股骨动脉
brachial artery	肱动脉,臂动脉
respiratory acidosis	呼吸性酸中毒
acid-base balance	酸碱平衡

Notes

1. As the radial artery at the wrist is easily accessible, can be compressed to control bleeding, and has less risk for occlusion, it is most commonly chosen.

由于腕部桡动脉操作简单方便,可以通过压迫控制出血,闭塞风险小,所以多选择腕部桡动脉。

2. In order to prevent blood coagulation, the syringe should be pre-packaged with a small amount of heparin.

为了防止血液凝固,注射器需要事先包装并含有少量肝素。

3. HCO_3^- — The HCO_3^- ion indicates whether a metabolic problem is present (such as ketoacidosis). A low HCO_3^- indicates metabolic acidosis while a high HCO_3^- indicates metabolic alkalosis. As the HCO_3^- in blood gas results is often calculated by the analyzer, correlation between it and total CO_2 levels as directly measured should be checked as the following.

HCO_3^-——HCO_3^-离子含量反映机体是否存在代谢紊乱(如酮症酸中毒)。HCO_3^-含量低表示代谢性酸中毒,HCO_3^-含量高表示代谢性碱中毒。由于HCO_3^-的数值通常是分析仪给定的血气分析结果计算值,因此,该值与直接测得的CO_2总量之间的关联需要审核。

4. A high PCO_2(respiratory acidosis, alternatively hypercapnia) indicates underventilation (or, more rarely, a hypermetabolic disorder), a low PCO_2(respiratory alkalosis, alternatively hypocapnia) indicates hyper- or overventilation.

高PCO_2(呼吸性酸中毒或高碳酸血症)表明肺换气不足(或罕见的高代谢紊乱疾病),低PCO_2(呼吸性碱中毒或低碳酸血症)表明换气过度。

5. They reflect the ability of the lungs to exchange oxygen and carbon dioxide, the ability of the kidneys to control the retention or elimination of bicarbonate, and the effectiveness of the heart as a pump.

它们反映肺脏交换氧气和二氧化碳的能力,肾脏控制或消除碳酸氢盐的能力,以及心脏的泵血效力。

Exercises

Ⅰ. Fill in the blanks according to the texts.

1. It is usually drawn by respiratory _____ , phlebotomist, nurse or doctor. (Text A)

2. The radial artery, the _____ artery, the brachial artery and arterial catheter can be chosen for Arterial blood collection. (Text A)

3. In order to prevent blood _____, the syringe should be pre-packaged with a small amount of heparin. (Text A)

4. A low HCO_3^- indicates metabolic _____ while a high HCO_3^- indicates metabolic alkalosis. (Text B)

5. These parameters can be used for assessing a patient's _____ balance. (Text B)

Ⅱ. Translate the following into Chinese.

CaO_2— It is the sum of oxygen dissolved in plasma and chemically bound to hemoglobin as determined. It can be calculated by the formula: $CaO_2 = (PO_2 \times 0.003) + (SaO_2 \times 1.34 \times Hgb)$ (Hemoglobin concentration is expressed as g/dL).

SaO_2 or O_2 sats — Oxygen saturation, measure the percentage of hemoglobin binding sites in the bloodstream occupied by oxygen.

Lesson 10 Blood Lipids and Lipoproteins
血脂和脂蛋白

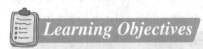

Learning Objectives

After studying this lesson, students are expected to be able to

1. master the concept of blood lipids and lipoproteins;
2. be familiar with some medical words and terms about blood lipids and lipoproteins;
3. know about the classifications of lipoproteins;
4. understand the sentence and grammar structures and the main idea of the texts.

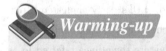

Warming-up

1. What is blood lipid? And how many components does it consist of?
2. What are the definition and functions of cholesterol?
3. What are the functions of lipoprotein in human body?

Text A Blood Lipids
血脂

Blood lipids are lipids in the blood, either free or bound to other molecules. Triacylglycerols, free and esterified cholesterol and phospholipids, present in the lipoproteins in blood plasma.

Triglycerides or simple fats and oils are fatty acid esters of glycerol. In chemistry, especially biochemistry, a fatty acid is a carboxylic acid with a long unbranched and aliphatic tail (chain), which is either saturated or unsaturated. Fatty acids are usually derived from triglycerides or phospholipids. When they are not attached to other molecules, they are known as "free" fatty acids. Blood fatty acids are in different forms in different stages in the blood circulation. They are taken in through the intestine in chylomicrons, but also exist in very low density lipoproteins and low density lipoproteins after processing in the liver. In addition, when released fromadipocytes, fatty acids exist in the blood as free fatty acids.

Cholesterol is an organic chemical substance classified as a waxy steroid of fat. It is an essential structural component of mammalian cell membranes and is required to establish proper membrane permeability and fluidity. In addition, cholesterol is an important component for the manufacture of bile acids, steroid hormones, and vitamin D. Although cholesterol is important and necessary for the aforementioned biological processes, high levels of cholesterol in the blood have been linked to damage to arteries and cardiovascular disease.

Phospholipid is composed of glycerol bonded to two fatty acids and a phosphate group. The resulting compound called phosphatidic acid contains a region (the fatty acid component) that is fat-soluble along with a region (the charged phosphate group) that is water-soluble. Most phospholipids also have an additional chemical group bound to the phosphate. For example, it can be connected with choline, the resulting phospholipid is called phosphatidylcholine, or lecithin. Other phospholipids include phosphatidylglycerol, phosphatidylinositol, phosphatidylserine, and phosphatidylethanolamine. The bipolar character of phospholipids is essential to their biological function in cell membranes. The fat-soluble portions associate with the fat-soluble portions of other phospholipids while the water-soluble regions remain exposed to the surrounding solve.

Text B   Lipoproteins
脂蛋白

Lipoproteins, classified based on the density and chemical quality, are the principal means by which lipids are transported in the blood. The interior of the lipoprotein contains triglycerides (glycerol esterified with three fatty acids) and cholesterol esterified with fatty acids. The covering membrane of a lipoprotein contains chemicals more easily soluble in blood than those in the interior, such as free cholesterol, phospholipids (e.g., lecithin), and apoproteins. Different lipoproteins contain different amounts of triglycerides and cholesterol, and can be separated by centrifuging them into particles with different densities. So lipoproteins generally fall into five categories, i.e., chylomicrons (CM), very low density lipoproteins (VLDL), intermediate density lipoproteins (IDL), low density lipoproteins (LDL) and high density lipoproteins (HDL).

CMs carry triglycerides (fat) from the intestines to the liver, the skeletal muscle, and the adipose tissue. VLDLs carry (newly synthesized) triacylglycerol from the liver to the adipose tissue. IDLs are intermediate between VLDLs and LDLs, and they are not usually detectable in the blood. LDLs carry cholesterol from the liver to cells of the body, so they are sometimes referred to as "the bad cholesterol" lipoprotein. HDLs collect cholesterol from the body's tissues and bring it back to the liver, so they are sometimes referred to as "the good cholesterol" lipoprotein.

Apolipoproteins are proteins that bind lipids (oil-soluble substances such as fat and cholesterol) to form lipoproteins and transport the lipids through the lymphatic and circulatory systems. There are six major classes of apolipoproteins and several sub-classes. Apolipoprotein B (APOB or ApoB) is the primary apolipoprotein of LDL. The protein presents in the plasma in 2 main isoforms, APOB48 and APOB100. The first is synthesized exclusively by the small intestine, the second by the liver. It is well established that APOB100 levels are associated with coronary heart diseases.

New Words

triacylglycerol /traiˈæsilglisərəul/ n. ［生化］三酰甘油,甘油三酯

esterify /ɛsˈtɛrɪˌfai/ v. (使)酯化

lipoprotein /ˈlɪpəprəutiːn/ n. ［生化］脂蛋白

esters /ˈestəs/ n. 酯类

unbranched /ˈʌnˈbraːntʃt/ adj. 无支链的

saturated /ˈsætʃəreɪtɪd/ adj. 饱和的,渗透的

chylomicrons /ˌkaɪləuˈmaɪkrɔns/ n. ［生化］乳糜微粒

waxy /ˈwæksi/ adj. 象蜡的

steroid /ˈsterɔɪd/ n. ［有化］类固醇,甾族化合物

permeability /ˌpɜːrmiəˈbɪləti/ n. 渗透性

fluidity /fluˈɪdəti/ n. ［流］流质,流动性(度),易变性

aforementioned /əˈfɔːrmenʃənd/ adj. 上述的,前面提及的

cardiovascular /ˌkɑːrdioʊˈvæskjələr/ *adj.* ［解剖］心血管的

choline /ˈkolin/ *n.* ［生化］胆碱

phosphatidylcholine /ˈfɔsfəˌtaidilˈkəuliːn/ *n.* ［生化］卵磷脂，磷脂酰胆碱

lecithin /ˈlesɪθɪn/ *n.* ［生化］卵磷脂，蛋黄素

phosphatidylglycerol /ˌfɔsfəˈtaidilˈglisərɔl/ *n.* ［生化］磷脂酰甘油

phosphatidylinositol /ˌfɔsfəˈtaidiliˈnəusitɔl/ *n.* ［生化］磷脂酰肌醇

phosphatidylserine /ˈfɔsfəˈtaidilsəriːn/ *n.* ［生化］磷脂酰丝氨酸

phosphatidylethanolamine /ˌfɔsfəˈtaidilˌeθəˈnɔləmiːn/ *n.* ［生化］磷脂酰乙醇胺

bipolar /ˌbaɪˈpoʊlər/ *adj.* 有两极的，双极的

interior /ɪnˈtɪrɪər/ *n.* 内部

apoprotein /ˌæpəˈprəutiːn/ *n.* ［生化］载脂蛋白

skeletal /ˈskelətl/ *adj.* 骨骼的

adipose /ˈædɪˈpous/ *adj.* 脂肪的

lymphatic /lɪmˈfætɪk/ *adj.* 淋巴的

isoform /ˈaisəufɔːm/ *n.* 亚型，同种型

Phrases and Expressions

carboxylic acid	羧酸
very low-density lipoprotein（VLDL）	极低密度脂蛋白
low-density lipoprotein（LDL）	低密度脂蛋白
bile acids	胆汁酸
phosphatidic acid	磷脂酸
steroid hormones	类固醇激素，甾体激素
oil-soluble	油溶的

Notes

1. In chemistry, especially biochemistry, a fatty acid is a carboxylic acid with a long unbranched aliphatic tail（chain）, which is either saturated or unsaturated.

在化学中，特别是生物化学中，脂肪酸是一种具有长的、无分支脂肪链的羧酸，可以是饱和脂肪酸或不饱和脂肪酸。

2. Blood fatty acids are in different forms in different stages in the blood circulation. They are taken in through the intestine in chylomicrons, but also exist in very low density lipoproteins and low density lipoproteins after processing in the liver.

血液脂肪酸在血液循环的不同阶段有不同的形式。经过小肠时以乳糜颗粒的形式被小肠吸收，但经过肝脏处理加工之后，以极低密度脂蛋白和低密度脂蛋白形式存在。

3. Cholesterol is an organic chemical substance classified as a waxy steroid of fat. It is an essential structural component of mammalian cell membranes and is required to establish proper membrane permeability and fluidity.

胆固醇是一种甾醇类的有机化合物。它是哺乳动物细胞膜的基本组成成分，具有建立适当的膜透性和流动性的功能。

4. The resulting compound called phosphatidic acid contains a region（the fatty acid component）that is fat-soluble along with a region（the charged phosphate group）that is water-soluble.

所产生的一种叫作磷脂酸的化合物包含一个脂溶性区域（脂肪酸成分）和一个水溶性的区域（带电荷的磷酸盐基团）。

5. Lipoproteins, classified based on the density and chemical quality, are the principal means by which lipids are transported in the blood.

脂蛋白是在血液中运输脂质的主要方式,可根据密度和化学性质进行分类。

6. Different lipoproteins contain different amounts of triglycerides and cholesterol, and can be separated by centrifuging them into particles with different densities. So lipoproteins generally fall into five categories, i. e., chylomicrons (CM), very low density lipoproteins (VLDL), intermediate density lipoproteins (IDL), low density lipoproteins (LDL) and high density lipoproteins (HDL).

由于不同的脂蛋白含有甘油三酯和胆固醇的量不同,并且可以通过离心分离成不同密度的颗粒。因此,脂蛋白总的来说可以分为五类:即乳糜颗粒(CM)、极低密度脂蛋白(VLDL)、中间密度脂蛋白(IDL)、低密度脂蛋白(LDL)和高密度脂蛋白(HDL)。

7. LDLs carry cholesterol from the liver to cells of the body, so they are sometimes referred to as "the bad cholesterol" lipoprotein. HDLs collect cholesterol from the body's tissues and bring it back to the liver, so they are sometimes referred to as "the good cholesterol" lipoprotein.

低密度脂蛋白(LDL)携带胆固醇经肝脏到身体的各细胞中,因此有时被称为"坏胆固醇"脂蛋白。高密度脂蛋白(HDL)从人体组织中收集胆固醇并将其带回肝脏,因此有时被称为"好胆固醇"脂蛋白。

Exercises

Ⅰ. Fill in the blanks according to the texts.

1. In chemistry, especially _____, a fatty acid is a carboxylic acid with a long unbranched and aliphatic tail (chain), which is either saturated or unsaturated. (Text A)

2. Phospholipid is composed of _____ bonded to two fatty acids and a phosphate group. (Text A)

3. The covering membrane of a lipoprotein contains chemicals more easily _____ in blood than those in the interior, such as free cholesterol, phospholipids (e.g., lecithin), and apoproteins. (Text B)

4. LDLs carry _____ from the liver to cells of the body. (Text B)

5. It is well established that APOB100 levels are associated with _____ heart disease. (Text B)

Ⅱ. Translate the following into Chinese.

Lipid profile or lipid panel, is the collective term given to the estimation of, typically, total cholesterol (TC), high-density lipoprotein cholesterol (HDL-C), low-density lipoprotein cholesterol (LDL-C), and triglycerides. An extended lipid profile may include very low-density lipoprotein. This is used to identify hyperlipidemia (various disturbances of cholesterol and triglyceride levels), many forms of which are recognized risk factors for cardiovascular disease and sometimes pancreatitis.

Lesson 11   Diagnostic Tests of Endocrine
内分泌诊断试验

 Learning Objectives

After studying this lesson, students are expected to be able to

1. master the concepts of endocrine and endocrine disorders;

2. be familiar with some medical words and terms about endocrine disorders;

3. know about the influences of endocrine disorders;

4. understand the sentence and grammar structures and the main idea of the texts.

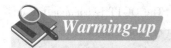

1. Why is the endocrine system so important?
2. What kinds of diseases are caused byendocrine disorders?
3. How do we test the diabetes through plasma glucose?

Text A　Endocrine Disorders
内分泌紊乱

Endocrinology is a branch of biology and medicine dealing with the endocrine system, its diseases, and its specific secretions called hormones, the integration of developmental events such as proliferation, growth, and differentiation (including histogenesis and organogenesis) and the coordination of metabolism, respiration, excretion, movement, reproduction, and sensory perception depend on chemical cues and substances synthesized and secreted by specialized cells.

The endocrine glands involved in the maintenance of normal body conditions are pituitary, thyroid, parathyroid, adrenal, pancreas, ovary, and testis. These hormones produced by endocrine glands are liberated directly into the bloodstream and transported to a distant part or parts of the body, where they exert a specific effect for the benefit of the body as a whole. Chemically, most hormones belong to one of three major groups: proteins and peptides, steroids (fat-soluble molecules whose basic structure is a skeleton of four carbon rings), or derivatives of the amino acid tyrosine.

Endocrine disorders may stem from over-secretion or under-secretion of a given hormone. Over-secretion may be due to a tumor either in the tissue normally producing the hormone or in one growing in an abnormal location — for example in the lung. It may alternatively be due to inappropriate secretion from the whole gland. There is, for example, an autoimmune disease of the thyroid: thyrotoxicosis or Graves' disease, in which antibodies stimulate the gland to over-secretion. Apparently under-activity of an endocrine gland may in fact be due to a failure of the target tissues to respond to a particular hormone. For example, those who develop diabetes later in life may have an elevated rather than a low concentration of insulin in the blood. This is because their tissues are relatively unresponsive to the hormone. The most common endocrine disorder is diabetes, with disorders of thyroid function coming second.

Most endocrine disorders can now be successfully treated. Diagnosis and treatment, however, require accurate measurement of blood hormone concentrations. Early assays were bioassays performed on animal tissues, and these are still used in checking the activity of hormone preparations made for medicinal purposes. However, routine determination in blood now involves the technique of enzyme immunoassay; when care is taken in setting this up, even very low concentrations of the hormone can be determined quite rapidly on a large number of samples.

Text B　Plasma Glucose Tests of Diabetes
糖尿病血糖检测

Clinical diagnosis of diabetes is based on symptoms and confirmed by blood tests that measure the level of glucose in blood plasma. Dipstick or reagent test strips that measure glucose in the urine can only detect glucose levels above 180 mg/dL and are non-specific, so they are not of use in the diagnosis of diabetes. However, they are a non-invasive way to obtain a fast and simple reading that a physician might use as a basis for ordering further diagnostic blood tests for diabetes, particularly in children.

Blood tests are the gold standard for the diagnosis of both Type1 and Type 2 diabetes in children and adults. The American Diabetes Association recommends that a random plasma glucose, fasting plasma glucose, or oral glucose tolerance test (OGTT) be used for diagnosis of diabetes. The OGTT is commonly used as a screening measure for gestational diabetes. Fasting plasma glucose is the test of choice unless a child is exhibiting classic symptoms of diabetes, in which case a random (or casual) plasma glucose test is acceptable.

Random Plasma Glucose Test: Blood is drawn at any time of day, regardless of whether the patient has eaten. A random plasma glucose concentration of 200 mg/dL (11.1 mmol/L) or higher in the presence of symptoms indicates diabetes.

Fasting Plasma Glucose Test: Blood is drawn from a vein in the child's arm following an eight-hour fast (i.e., no food or drink), usually in the morning before breakfast. The red blood cells are separated from the sample and the amount of glucose is measured in the remaining plasma. A fasting plasma glucose level of 126 mg/dL (7.0 mmol/L) or higher indicates diabetes (with a confirming retest on a subsequent day).

Oral Glucose Tolerance Test: Blood samples are taken both before and several times after patient drinks 75 grams of a glucose-based beverage. If plasma glucose levels taken two hours after the glucose drink is consumed are 200 mg/dL (11.1 mmol/L) or higher, the test is diagnostic of diabetes (and should be confirmed on a subsequent day if possible).

Although the same diagnostic blood tests are used for both types of diabetes, whether a child is diagnosed as Type 1 or Type 2 can typically be determined based on her personal and medical history. The majority of children diagnosed in childhood are Type 1, but if blood test results indicate prediabetes and a child is significantly overweight and has a history of Type 2 diabetes in her family, Type 2 is a possibility.

Further blood tests can help to differentiate between Type1 and Type 2 when the diagnosis is unclear. One of these is an assessment of C-peptide levels, a protein released along with insulin that can help a physician determine whether or not a patient is producing sufficient amounts of insulin. The other is a GAD (Glutamic Acid Decarboxylase) autoantibody test. The presence of GAD autoantibodies may indicate the beginning of the autoimmune process that destroys pancreatic beta cells.

New Words

endocrinology /ˌendoʊkrɪˈnɑːlədʒi/ n. 内分泌学

integration /ˌɪntɪˈgreɪʃn/ n. 集成

proliferation /prəˌlɪfəˈreɪʃn/ n. 增殖，扩散

histogenesis /ˌhɪstoˈdʒɛnɪsɪs/ n. ［胚］组织发生

organogenesis /ɔːˌgænoˈdʒɛnɪsɪs/ n. ［胚］器官发生，器官形成

coordination /koʊˌɔːrdɪˈneɪʃn/ n. 协调

sensory /ˈsensəri/ adj. 感觉的

perception /pərˈsepʃn/ n. 知觉

cues /kjuːz/ n. 线索

pituitary /pɪˈtuːəteri/ n. 脑垂体

adrenal /ædˈrinl/ n. 肾上腺

ovary /ˈoʊvəri/ n. ［解剖］卵巢（复数 ovaries）

testis /ˈtestɪs/ n. ［解剖］睾丸

under-secretion /ˈʌndə siˈkriːʃn/ n. 分泌低下

over-secretion /ˈəʊvə siˈkriːʃn/ n. 分泌过多

thyrotoxicosis /ˌθaɪroˌtɑksəˈkosɪs/ n. ［内科］甲状腺功能亢进，甲状腺毒症

unresponsive /ˌʌnrɪˈspɑːnsɪv/ adj. 反应迟钝的

bioassay /ˌbaɪoəˌse/ n. ［生物］生物测定，生物鉴定，活体检定

beverage /ˈbevərɪdʒ/ n. 饮料

prediabetes /ˈpriˌdaɪəˈbitɪs/ n. ［内科］前驱糖尿病

insulin /ˈɪnsəlɪn/ n. ［生化］［药］胰岛素

Phrases and Expressions

endocrine disorder	内分泌紊乱
sensory perception	感官知觉
stem from ...	来自……
Graves' disease	毒性弥漫性甲状腺肿,格雷夫斯病
random plasma glucose	随机血糖
fasting plasma glucose	空腹血糖
oral glucose tolerance test（OGTT）	口服葡萄糖耐量试验
gestational diabetes	妊娠糖尿病
glutamic acid decarboxylase	谷氨酸脱羧酶

Notes

1. Apparently under-activity of an endocrine gland may in fact be due to a failure of the target tissues to respond to a particular hormone.

很显然,内分泌腺体分泌不足实际上可能是由于靶组织对特定激素不反应。

2. The most common endocrine disorder is diabetes, with disorders of thyroid function coming second.

最常见的内分泌紊乱疾病是糖尿病,其次是甲状腺功能失调。

3. However, routine determination in blood now involves the technique of enzyme immunoassay; when care is taken in setting this up, even very low concentrations of the hormone can be determined quite rapidly on a large number of samples.

然而,现在的常规血液检测还包含酶联免疫分析技术。使用这种方法时,即使是非常低浓度的激素也可以在大样本中快速测定。

4. Blood samples are taken both before and several times after patient drinks 75 grams of a glucose-based beverage.

在病人饮用75g葡萄糖饮料前后分别抽取一次血液。

5. If plasma glucose levels taken two hours after the glucose drink is consumed are 200 mg/dL (11.1 mmol/L) or higher, the test is diagnostic of diabetes (and should be confirmed on a subsequent day if possible).

如果在病人饮用葡萄糖饮料2h以后血浆葡萄糖水平达到200mg/dL(11.1mmol/L)或更高时,可诊断为糖尿病(如有可能,应在随后一天确认)。

6. The majority of children diagnosed in childhood are Type 1, but if blood test results indicate prediabetes and a child is significantly overweight and has a history of Type 2 diabetes in her family, Type 2 is a possibility.

多数儿童期的孩子患糖尿病的话往往是1型糖尿病,但如果验血结果表明只是糖尿病前期,而且患儿体重显著超重,再加上患儿家族有2型糖尿病史的话,那么该患儿更可能为2型糖尿病。

Exercises

Ⅰ. Fill in the blanks according to the texts.

1. These hormones produced by endocrine glands are liberated directly into the _____ and transported to a distant part or parts of the body, where they exert a specific effect for the benefit of the body as a whole. (Text A)

2. For example, those who develop diabetes later in life mayhave an elevated rather than a low concentration of _____ in the blood. (Text A)

3. Early assays were _____ performed on animal tissue, and these are still used in checking the activity of hormone preparations made for medicinal purposes. (Text A)

4. Clinical diagnosis of diabetes is based on symptoms and confirmed by blood tests that measure the lev-

笔记

113

el of _____ in blood plasma. (Text B)

5. Although the same _____ blood tests are used for both whether types of diabetes, as a child is diagnosed typically Type 1 or Type 2 can be determined based on her personal and medical history. (Text B)

Ⅱ. Translate the following into Chinese.

Clearly elevated free thyroxine (T_4) levels support the clinical findings of a diagnosis of hyperthyroidism while clearly low free T_4 levels coupled with appropriate clinical findings, can establish a diagnosis of hypothyroidism. Measurement of free T_4 levels along with other thyroid tests and clinical findings can establish borderline hyperthyroidism and hypothyroidism diagnoses. Free T_4 is a better indicator than total T_4 in that it is not affected by levels of T_4 binding proteins.

Lesson 12   Liver and Renal Function Tests
肝肾功能检验

Learning Objectives

After studying this lesson, students are expected to be able to

1. master some medical words and terms about liver and renal function tests;

2. be familiar with the main methods for liver and renal function tests;

3. know about the useful expressions related to the diagnosis and treatment of liver and renal disease;

4. have comprehensive knowledge about liver and renal function tests.

Warming-up

1. What is the definition of Liver Function Tests?
2. What are the simple means of estimating renal function?
3. What is GFR?

Text A   Standard Liver Panel
标准肝功能组合

The liver function tests (LFT) are a group of blood assays, a kind of clinical biochemical tests, designed to detect the state of a patient's liver.

Albumin (Alb): Albumin is a protein made specifically by the liver, and can be measured cheaply and easily. It is the main constituent of total protein; the remaining fraction is called globulin (including the immunoglobulins). Albumin levels are decreased in chronic liver disease, such as cirrhosis. It is also decreased in nephrotic syndrome, where it is lost through the urine. Poor nutrition or states of impaired protein catabolism may also lead to hypoalbuminemia. The half-life period of albumin is approximately 20 days. Albumin is not considered to be an especially useful marker of liver synthetic function; coagulation factors are much more sensitive.

Alanine transaminase (ALT): ALT, also called Serum Glutamic Pyruvate Transaminase (SGPT) or Alanine aminotransferase (ALAT) is an enzyme present in hepatocytes (liver cells). When a cell is damaged, it leaks this enzyme into the blood, where it is measured. ALT rises dramatically in acute liver damage, such as viral hepatitis or paracetamol (acetaminophen) overdose, Elevations are often measured in multiples of the upper limit of normal.

Aspartate transaminase (AST): AST also called Serum Glutamic Oxaloacetic Transaminase (SGOT) or aspartate aminotransferase (ASAT) is similar to ALT in that it is another enzyme associated with liver parenchymal cells. It is raised in acute liver damage, but is also present in red blood cell, and cardiac and skeletal muscle and is therefore not specific to the liver. The ratio of AST to ALT is sometimes useful in differentiating between causes of liver damage. Elevated AST levels are not specific for liver damage, and AST has also been used as a cardiac marker.

Alkaline phosphatase (ALP): ALP is an enzyme in the cells lining the biliary ducts of the liver. ALP levels in plasma will rise with large bile duct obstruction, intrahepatic cholestasis or infiltrative diseases of the liver. ALP is also present in bone and placental tissue, so it is also higher in growing children and elderly patients with Paget's disease.

Total bilirubin (TBIL): Bilirubin is a breakdown product of heme (a part of hemoglobin in red blood cells). The liver is responsible for clearing the blood of bilirubin. It does this by the following mechanism: Bilirubin is taken up into hepatocytes, conjugated (modified to make it water-soluble), and secreted into the bile, which is excreted into the intestine. Increased total bilirubin causes jaundice.

Direct bilirubin (Conjugated Bilirubin): The diagnosis can be narrowed down further by looking at the level of direct bilirubin. If direct (i. e., conjugated) bilirubin is normal, then the problem is an excess of unconjugated bilirubin, and the location of the problem is upstream of bilirubin excretion. Hemolysis, viral hepatitis, or cirrhosis can be suspected. If direct bilirubin is elevated, then the liver is conjugating bilirubin normally, but is not able to excrete it. Bile duct obstruction by gallstones or cancer should be suspected.

Gamma glutamyl transpeptidase (GGT): Although reasonably specific to the liver and a more sensitive marker for cholestatic damage than ALP, GGT may be elevated with even minor, sub-clinical levels of liver dysfunction. It can also be helpful in identifying the cause of an isolated elevation in ALP (e. g., GGT is raised in chronic alcohol toxicity).

Text B   Renal Function Measurement
肾功能测定

A simple way of estimating renal function is to measure pH, blood urea nitrogen, creatinine, and basic electrolytes (including sodium, potassium, chloride, and bicarbonate). As the kidney is the most important organ in controlling these values, any derangement in these values could suggest renal impairment.

Another prognostic marker for kidney disease is an elevated level of protein in the urine. The most sensitive marker of proteinuria is elevated urine albumin. Persistence presence of more than 30 mg albumin per gram creatinine in the urine is diagnostic of chronic kidney disease. The level of albumin protein produced by microalbuminuria can be detected by special albumin-specific urine dipsticks. A microalbumin urine test determines the presence of the albumin in urine. In a properly functioning body, albumin is not normally present in urine because it is retained in the bloodstream by the kidneys. Microalbuminuria can be diagnosed from a 24-hour urine collection (30-300 mg/24 hours) or more commonly, from elevated concentrations in a spot sample (30-300 mg/L). Both must be measured on at least 2-3 times over a two-to-three-month period.

Most doctors use the plasma concentrations of the waste substances of creatinine and urea (U) as well as electrolytes (E), to determine renal function. These measures are adequate to determine whether a patient is suffering from kidney diseases. However, blood urea nitrogen (BUN) and creatinine will not be raised above the normal range until 60% of total kidney functions are lost. Hence, the more accurate Glomerular filtration rate (GFR) or its approximation of the creatinine clearance is measured whenever renal disease is suspected or careful dosing of nephrotoxic drugs is required.

GFR is the volume of fluid filtered from the renal glomerular capillaries into the Bowman's capsule per unit time. GFR can be calculated by measuring any chemical that has a steady level in the blood, and is freely filtered but neither reabsorbed nor secreted by the kidney. The rate therefore measured is the quantity of the substance in the urine that originated from a calculable volume of blood. The GFR is typically recorded in units of volume per time, such as milliliters per minute (mL/min).

$$GFR = \frac{Urine\ Concentration \times Urine\ Flow}{Plasma\ Concentration}$$

There are several different techniques used to calculate or estimate the GFR.

New Words

cirrhosis /sə'roʊsɪs/ n. ［内科］硬化,肝硬化(复数 cirrhoses)

impaired /ɪm'perd/ adj. 受损的

catabolism /kə'tæbəlizəm/ n. ［生化］分解代谢

hypoalbuminemia /ˌhaɪpəʊælˌbjuːməˈniːmiə/ n. ［内科］低白蛋白血症

hepatocyte /hɪ'pætəsaɪt/ n. ［细胞］肝细胞

paracetamol /ˌpærə'siːtəmɑːl/ n. 对乙酰氨基酚

acetaminophen /əˌsiːtə'mɪnəfen/ n. 对乙酰氨基酚

parenchymal /pərəŋ'kəməl/ adj. 薄壁组织的

intrahepatic /ˌɪntrəhi'pætik/ adj. ［解剖］肝内的

cholestasis /ˌkɒlə'stəsɪs/ n. 胆汁阻塞,胆汁淤积

infiltrative /ɪn'fɪltreɪtɪv/ adj. 渗透性的

placental /plə'sentl/ adj. 胎盘的

gallstone /'gɔːlstoʊn/ n. ［病理］胆石

cholestatic /ˌkəʊlə'stætɪk/ adj. 胆汁淤积的

dysfunction /dɪs'fʌŋkʃn/ n. 功能紊乱,功能障碍

toxicity /tɑːk'sɪsəti/ n. ［毒物］毒效

renal /'riːnl/ adj. ［解剖］肾脏的

prognostic /prɑːg'nɑːstɪk/ n. 预兆,预后症状 adj. 预后的,医学预测的

derangement /dɪ'reɪndʒmənt/ n. 精神错乱

proteinuria /ˌprotiin'jʊəriə/ n. ［泌尿］蛋白尿(症)

microalbuminuria /ˌmaɪkrəʊælˌbjʊmɪ'nʊriə/ n. 微白蛋白尿,微量白蛋白尿

accurate /'ækjərət/ adj. 精确的

nephrotoxic /ˌnefrə'tɔksɪk/ adj. ［医］对肾脏有害处的

Phrases and Expressions

nephrotic syndrome	肾病综合征
half-life period	半衰期
serum glutamic pyruvate transaminase (SGPT)	血清谷氨酰丙酮酸转氨酶
alanine aminotransferase (ALAT)	丙氨酸转氨酶
serum glutamic oxaloacetic transaminase (SGOT)	血清谷氨酰草酰乙酸转氨酶
aspartate aminotransferase (ASAT)	天冬氨酸转氨酶
biliary ducts	胆管
direct bilirubin	直接胆红素
conjugated bilirubin	结合胆红素
unconjugated bilirubin	未结合胆红素
gamma glutamyl transpeptidase	γ 谷氨酰转肽酶
glomerular filtration rate	肾小球滤过率

Notes

1. Elevations are often measured in multiples of the upper limit of normal.

测得的升高值常常数倍于正常上限。

2. Bilirubin is taken up into hepatocytes, conjugated (modified to make it water-soluble), and secreted into the bile, which is excreted into the intestine.

胆红素被摄入肝细胞,经结合(使其转变为水溶性的)后分泌入胆汁,随胆汁排泄到肠道中。

3. If direct bilirubin is elevated, then the liver is conjugating bilirubin normally, but is not able to excrete it. Bile duct obstruction by gallstones or cancer should be suspected.

如果直接胆红素升高,肝脏正常结合胆红素,但不能排泄。应怀疑胆结石或癌症所造成的胆管梗阻。

4. Although reasonably specific to the liver and a more sensitive marker for cholestatic damage than ALP, GGT may be elevated with even minor, sub-clinical levels of liver dysfunction. It can also be helpful in identifying the cause of an isolated elevation in ALP.

虽然 GGT 对肝脏有一定的特异性,是胆汁淤积损伤时比 ALP 更为敏感的标记物,但是,即便是轻微的、亚临床水平的肝功能不全也可能会使 GGT 升高。这也有助于确定 ALP 孤立升高的原因。

5. However, blood urea nitrogen (BUN) and creatinine will not be raised above the normal range until 60% of total kidney functions are lost.

然而,血尿素氮(BUN)和肌酐只有在肾功能丧失到60%的时候才会超过正常范围。

6. Most doctors use the plasma concentrations of the waste substances of creatinine and urea (U), as well as electrolytes (E), to determine renal function.

大多数医生使用肌酐、尿素(U)和电解质(E)的血浆浓度来测定肾功能。

7. GFR can be calculated by measuring any chemical that has a steady level in the blood, and is freely filtered but neither reabsorbed nor secreted by the kidneys.

GFR 可以通过测量血液中任何稳定水平的化学物质来计算,这些物质能被肾脏自由过滤,但不能被肾脏重吸收或分泌。

8. The rate therefore measured is the quantity of the substance in the urine that originated from a calculable volume of blood.

因此,测量所得出的速率就是尿液中物质的量,其源自可计算的血液量。

Exercises

Ⅰ. Fill in the blanks according to the texts.

1. The liver function tests (LFT) are a group of blood assays, a kind of clinical biochemical tests, designed to detect the _____ of a patient's liver. (Text A)

2. The liver is _____ for clearing the blood of bilirubin. (Text A)

3. Although reasonably specific to the liver and a more sensitive marker for cholestatic damage than ALP, GGT may be _____ with even minor, sub-clinical levels of liver dysfunction. (Text A)

4. As the kidney is the most important organ in _____ these values, any derangement in these values could suggest renal impairment. (Text B)

5. These measures are _____ to determine whether a patient is suffering from kidney disease. (Text B)

Ⅱ. Translate the following into Chinese.

GFR is the volume of fluid filtered from the renal glomerular capillaries into the Bowman's capsule per unit time. GFR can be calculated by measuring any chemical that has a steady level in the blood, and is freely filtered but neither reabsorbed nor secreted by the kidney. The rate therefore measured is the quantity of the substance in the urine that originated from a calculable volume of blood. The GFR is typically recorded in units of volume per time, such as milliliters per minute (mL/min).

Lesson 13 Cardiac and Tumor Markers
心肌与肿瘤标志物

Learning Objectives

After studying this lesson, students are expected to be able to

1. master the definition of Cardiac and Tumor Markers;
2. be familiar with the types of Cardiac and Tumor Markers;
3. know about how to use Cardiac and Tumor Markers to diagnose diseases.

Warming-up

1. What are Cardiac and Tumor Markers?
2. Can you tell the types of Cardiac and Tumor Markers?
3. How do we use cardiac and tumor markers to diagnose cancer?

Text A Types of Cardiac Markers
心肌标志物种类

Cardiac markers are biomarkers used to detect and evaluate heart function. They are commonly discussed in the context of myocardial infarction (MI). But cardiac marker level can also be elevated in other conditions. As most of the early markers identified were enzymes, the term "cardiac enzymes" is sometimes used. However, not all of the markers currently used are enzymes. Take troponin for example, it is not classified as a cardiac enzyme in formal use.

Generally, there are the following types of Cardiac markers:

Troponin

During the MI, troponin (Cardiac Troponin I and T) is released from thecytosolic pool of myocytes. Its subsequent release is prolonged with degradation of actin and myosin filaments. The differential diagnoses of troponin elevation include acute myocardial infarction, acute right cardiac overload caused by severe pulmonary embolism, heart failure, and myocarditis. Troponins can also be used to calculate infarct size. But for the peak, it must be measured in the 3rd day.

Creatine Kinase (CK-MB)

CK-MB resides in the cytoplasm and promotes the high-energy phosphoric acid into and out of the mitochondria. It is distributed in a large number of tissues even in the skeletal muscle. Since it has a short duration, it is not used for late diagnosis of acute myocardial infarction. If its level rises again, it can indicate an infarct extension. This condition usually returns to normal within 2-3 days.

Lactate Dehydrogenase (LDH)

LDH catalyzes the transformation of pyruvate into lactic acid. LDH-1 isozyme is usually distributed in myocardium while LDH-2 is mainly present in blood serum. Increasing level of LDH-1 relative to LDH-2 indicates MI. LDH level can also elevate during tissue destruction or hemolysis. It means cancer, meningitis, encephalitis or HIV. LDH is less specific than troponin.

Aspartate Transaminase (AST)

AST was used firstly. As it is one of the liver function test indicators, it is not specific to heart injury.

Myoglobin（Mb）

Mb is less often used than other markers. Mb is the primary oxygen-carrying pigment of muscle tissue. It will rise when muscle tissue is damaged but it lacks specificity. It has the advantage of responding very rapidly, rising and falling sooner than CK-MB or troponin. It also has been used in assessing reperfusion after thrombolysis.

Text B　Serum Tumor Markers
血清肿瘤标志物

Tumor markers are widely used for monitoring cancer patients and screening certain tumors. A tumor marker is a substance in the blood, urine, or body tissues that can be elevated in case of cancers. There are many different tumor markers, each of which represents a particular disease process. They are used in oncology to help detect the presence of cancer.

Oncofetal Antigens

There are two common oncofetal antigens, alpha fetoprotein (AFP) and carcinoembryonic antigen (CEA). CA 72-4 is newly discovered and just being used. The oncofetal antigens are usually produced during embryonic development and quickly decrease after birth. Cancer cells tend to dedifferentiate, or revert to less mature tissue and start producing oncofetal antigens again. CEA is nonspecific and can be expressed in many types of cancers. However, they can be used to monitor patients' disease progression and how responsive they are to treatment according to disease.

Cancer Antigen 15-3（CA 15-3）

It is produced by breast cells and its elevation is associated with breast cancer.

Cancer Antigen 125（CA 125）

Although many types of cells can produce CA 125, it is mainly produced by ovarian cells.

Cancer Antigen 19-9（CA 19-9）

CA 19-9 has been identified in patients with digestive tract or intraperitoneal cancers such as colorectal, pancreatic, gastric, and cholangiocarcinoma.

Prostate specific antigen（PSA）

PSA levels and digital rectal examination are used to screen prostate cancer. PSA is a protein produced by the prostate gland and can be overproduced in prostate cancer. PSA exists in the serum in the state of binding and swimming. At the same time, the measurement of both levels can improve the specificity of the test and reduce unnecessary biopsy.

Bence-Jones protein

Patients with plasmacytomas such as myeloma overproduce monoclonal immunoglobulin, also known as M protein. Bence-Jones protein belongs to immunoglobulin light chain and is the part of immunoglobulin. Bence-Jones protein is secreted into urine and can be detected in urine. It is the first identified tumor marker.

Human Chorionic Gonadotropin（HCG）

HCG is usually produced by the placenta during pregnancy. HCG produces two protein subunits. One is the β subunit and the other one is α subunit. It is the β subunit that elevates in women's serum during early pregnancy. It is also the beta subunit that elevates in some malignant tumors. Tumors secreting β-HCG are typical embryonic cell tumors such as teratoma.

Neuron-specific enolase（NSE）

NSE is a protein and can be mainly found in neurons and neuroendocrine cells. NSE of tumors derived from these tissues, including neuroblastoma and small cell lung cancer is elevated.

Other hormones and enzymes

Endocrine gland neoplasms overproduce corresponding hormones. Clues about cancer can be obtained by measuring specific hormones. For example, breast furuncle cells can secrete prolactin and estrogen. The determination of several serum enzymes can help detecting tumor metastases in cancer patients. For example, tumors that metastasize to the liver can cause the increase in serum alkaline phosphatase, gamma glutamyl transferase and transaminases.

New Words

evaluate /ɪˈvæljʊeɪt/ *vt. & vi.* 评价，评估

myocyte /ˈmaɪəsaɪt/ *n.* 肌细胞，肌丝层

mitochondria /ˌmaɪtoˈkɑndrɪr/ *n.* 线粒体（mitochondrion 的复数）

distribute /dɪˈstrɪbjuːt/ *vt.* 分配，散布，分开，把……分类

duration /duˈreɪʃn/ *n.* 持续，持续的时间，期间

isozyme /ˈaɪsəuzaim/ *n.* ［生化］同工酶（等于 isoenzyme）

serum /ˈsɪrəm/ *n.* （免疫）血清，浆液

myoglobin /ˈmaɪoˌglobɪn/ *n.* ［生化］肌红蛋白（等于 myohemoglobin）

pigment /ˈpɪgmənt/ *n.* ［物］［生化］色素，颜料

tumour /ˈtuːmər/ *n.* ［肿瘤］瘤，肿瘤，肿块

monitor /ˈmɑːnɪtər/ *n.* 监视器，监听器，班长 *vt.* 监控

oncology /ɑːnˈkɑːlədʒi/ *n.* ［肿瘤］肿瘤学

dedifferentiate /diːˌdifəˈrenʃieit/ *v.* （细胞或组织）去分化

ovarian /ouˈveriən/ *adj.* ［解剖］卵巢的，子房的

intraperitoneal /ˈintrəˌperitəuˈniːəl/ *adj.* 腹膜内的

rectal /ˈrektəl/ *adj.* 直肠的

prostate /ˈprɑːsteɪt/ *adj.* 前列腺的 *n.* 前列腺

secrete /sɪˈkriːt/ *vt.* 藏匿，私下侵吞，分泌

metastases /məˈtæstəsiːs/ *n.* 转移（metastasis 的复数）

transaminase /trænsˈæmɪnez/ *n.* ［生化］转氨酶，氨基转移酶

Phrases and Expressions

heart failure　　　　　　　　　　　　　心力衰竭

oncofetal antigens　　　　　　　　　　　癌胎抗原

alpha fetoprotein（AFP）　　　　　　　甲胎蛋白

prostate specific antigen（PSA）　　　　前列腺特异抗原

human chorionic gonadotropin（HGG）　人体绒毛膜促性腺激素

neuron-specific enolase（NSE）　　　　神经特异性烯醇

Notes

1. Cardiac markers are biomarkers used to detect and evaluate heart function. They are commonly discussed in the context of myocardial infarction（MI）.

心脏标志物是用于检测、评估心脏功能的生物标志，通常在心肌梗死（MI）的情况下被讨论。

2. During the MI, troponin（Cardiac Troponin I and T）is released from thecytosolic pool of myocytes.

心肌梗死过程中，肌钙蛋白（心脏肌钙蛋白 I 和肌钙蛋白 T）从肌细胞细胞质池中被释放出来。

3. The differential diagnoses of troponin elevation include acute myocardial infarction, acute right cardiac overload caused by severe pulmonary embolism, heart failure, and myocarditis.

肌钙蛋白升高的鉴别诊断包括急性心肌梗死、严重的肺动脉栓塞导致的急性右心负荷过重、心力衰竭、心肌炎。

4. CK-MB resides in the cytoplasm and promotes the high-energy phosphoric acid into and out of the mitochondria.

CK-MB 分布在细胞质,促进高能磷酸进出线粒体。

5. LDH-1 isozyme is usually distributed in myocardium while LDH-2 is mainly present in blood serum.

LDH-1 同工酶通常分布在心肌中,而 LDH-2 主要存在于血清中。

6. A tumor marker is a substance in the blood, urine, or body tissues that can be elevatedin case of cancers.

肿瘤标志物是在血液、尿液或身体组织中存在的一种物质,可在癌症中升高。

7. The oncofetal antigens are usually produced during embryonic development and quickly decrease after birth.

癌胚抗原通常在胚胎发育期产生,出生后很快减少。

8. CA 19-9 has been identified in patients with digestive tract or intraperitoneal tumors such as colorectal, pancreatic, gastric, and cholangiocarcinoma.

CA 19-9 已被确定存在于消化道或腹腔内肿瘤如结直肠癌、胰腺癌、胃癌、胆管癌的病人中。

9. Tumors secreting β-HCG are typical embryonic cell tumors such as teratoma.

分泌 β-HCG 的肿瘤是典型的胚细胞肿瘤如畸胎瘤。

10. NSE of tumors derived from these tissues, including neuroblastoma and small cell lung cancer is elevated.

源于这些组织的肿瘤,包括神经母细胞瘤和小细胞肺癌,其 NSE 升高。

Exercises

Ⅰ. Fill in the blanks according to the texts.

1. During the MI, troponin (Cardiac Troponin I and T) is _____ from the cytosolic pool of myocytes. (Text A)

2. It is _____ in a large number of tissues even in the skeletal muscle. (Text A)

3. _____ markers are widely used for monitoring cancer patients and screening certain tumors. (Text B)

4. Patients with plasmacytomas such as myeloma overproduce monoclonal _____, also known as M protein. (Text B)

5. The determination of several serum enzymes can help detecting tumor_____ in cancer patients. (Text B)

Ⅱ. Translate the following into Chinese.

Other hormones and enzymes: endocrine glandneoplasms overproduce corresponding hormones. Clues about cancer can be obtained by measuring specific hormones. For example, breast furuncle cells can secrete prolactin and estrogen. The determination of several serum enzymes can help detecting tumor metastases in cancer patients. For example, tumors that metastasize to the liver can cause the increase in serum alkaline phosphatase, gamma glutamyl transferase and transaminases.

Lesson 14　Enzyme Activity Assay
酶活性测定

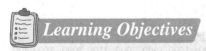 **Learning Objectives**

After studying this lesson, students are expected to be able to

1. master some medical words and terms concerning enzyme activity assay;

2. be familiar with the conditions and methods of enzyme activity assay;

3. know about the basic medical knowledge about enzyme activity assay.

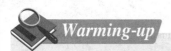

1. What are the factors on which enzyme rates depend?
2. What are the effects of pH?
3. What is continuous assay?

Text A   Conditions for Enzyme Activity Assay
酶活性测定条件

All enzymes need the right environments for effective function. Enzyme rates depend on solution conditions and substrate concentration. Conditions that denature the protein abolish enzyme activity, such as high temperatures, extreme pH levels or high salt concentrations, while raising substrate concentration ([S]) tends to increase activity when [S] is low.

Salt Concentration

Most enzymes cannot tolerate extremely high salt concentrations. The ions interfere with the weak ionic bonds of enzyme proteins. Typical enzymes are active in salt concentrations of 1-500 mM.

Effects of Temperature

All enzymes work within a range of temperature specific to the organism. Increase in temperature generally leads to increase in reaction rates. However, there is a limit to the increase because higher temperatures lead to a sharp decrease in reaction rates. This is due to the denaturation (alteration) of protein structure resulting from the breakdown of the weak ionic and hydrogen bonds that stabilize the three dimensional structure of the enzyme active site. The "optimum" temperature for human enzymes is usually between 35℃ and 40℃. The average temperature for humans is 37℃. Human enzymes start to denature quickly at temperatures above 40℃. Enzymes from thermophilic archaea found in the hot springs are stable up to 100℃. However, the idea of an "optimum" rate of an enzyme reaction is misleading, as the rate observed at any given temperature is the product of two rates, the reaction rate and the denaturation rate. If you were to use an assay measuring activity for one second, it would give high activity at high temperatures, however if you were to use an assay measuring product formation over an hour, it would give you low activity at these temperatures.

Effects of pH

Most enzymes are sensitive to pH and have specific ranges of activity. All have an optimum pH. The pH can stop enzyme activity by denaturing the three dimensional structure of the enzyme by breaking ionic, and hydrogen bonds. Most enzymes function between the pH of 6 and 8; however, pepsin in the stomach works best at the pH of 2 and trypsin at the pH of 8.

Substrate Saturation

Increasing the substrate concentration increases the rate of reaction (enzyme activity). However, enzyme saturation limits reaction rates. An enzyme is saturated when the active sites of all the molecules are occupied most of the time. At the saturation point, the reaction will not speed up, no matter how much

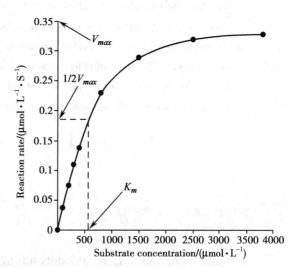

V_{max}: maximum reaction rate; K_m: Michaelis-Menten constant.

Figure 3-1　Saturation curve for an enzyme reaction showing the relationship between the substrate concentration (S) and rate (v)

additional substrate is added. To find the maximum speed of an enzymatic reaction, the substrate concentration is increased until a constant rate of product formation is seen. This is shown in the saturation curve (figure 3-1).

Level of crowding

The phenomenon of macromolecular crowding alters the properties of molecules in a solution when high concentrations of macromolecules such as proteins are present. The large amounts of macromolecules in a solution will alter the rates and equilibrium constants of enzyme reactions, through an effect called macromolecular crowding.

Text B   Enzyme Activity Assay
酶活性测定

Amounts of enzymes can either be expressed as molar amounts, as with any other chemical, or measured in terms of activity, in enzyme units. Enzyme assays are laboratory methods for measuring enzymatic activity. Enzyme activity is a measure of the quantity of active enzyme present and is thus dependent on conditions, which should be specified.

All enzyme assays measure either the consumption of substrate or production of product over time. Enzyme activity = moles of substrate converted per unit time = rate × reaction volume. The rate of a reaction is the concentration of substrate disappearing (or product produced) per unit time ($mol \cdot L^{-1} \cdot s^{-1}$). The SI unit is katal, 1 katal = 1mol / s, but this is an excessively large unit. A more practical and commonly used unit is enzyme unit (U), 1 U = 1 μmol / min. 1 U corresponds to 16. 67 nanokatals.

A large number of different methods of measuring the concentrations of substrates and products exist and many enzymes can be assayed in several different ways. Enzyme assays can be split into two groups according to their sampling method: continuous assays, where the assay gives a continuous reading of activity, and discontinuous assays, where samples are taken, the reaction stops and then the concentration of substrates or products is determined.

Continuous assay is most convenient in that it gives the rate of reaction with one assay and no further work is necessary. There are many different types of continuous assays. For example:

Spectrophotometric assays

In spectrophotometric assays, you follow the course of the reaction by measuring a change in how much light the assay solution absorbs. If this light is in the visible region you can actually see a change in the color of the assay, these are called colorimetric assays. The MTT (3-(4,5-Dimethylthiazol-2-yl)-2,5- diphenyltetrazolium bromide, a yellow tetrazole) assay, a redox assay using a tetrazolium dye as substrate is an example of a colorimetric assay.

UV light is often used, since the common coenzymes reduced nicotinamide adenine dinucleotide (NADH) and reduced nicotinamide adenine dinucleotide phosphate (NADPH) absorb UV light in their reduced forms, but do not in their oxidized forms. An oxidoreductase using NADH as a substrate could therefore be assayed by following the decrease in UV absorbance at a wavelength of 340 nm as it consumes the coenzyme.

Direct versus coupled assays

$$Glucose + ATP \xrightarrow{\ Hexokinase\ } glucose\text{-}6\text{-}phosphate + ADP$$

$$glucose\text{-}6\text{-}phosphate + NADP^{+} \xrightarrow{\ G\text{-}6\text{-}PDH\ } 6\text{-}Phosphoglucose\text{-}\gamma\text{-}Lactone + NADPH$$

Even when the enzyme reaction does not result in a change in the absorbance of light, it can still be possible to use a spectrophotometric assay for the enzyme by using a coupled assay. Here, the product of one reaction is used as the substrate of another, easily detectable reaction. For example, figure shows the coupled assay for the enzyme hexokinase, which can be assayed by coupling its production of glucose-6-phosphate to

NADPH production, using glucose-6-phosphate dehydrogenase (G-6-PDH).

New Words

enzyme /ˈenzaɪm/ n. ［生化］酶

substrate /ˈsʌbstreɪ/ n. ［生化］基质，基片，酶作用物（等于 substratum）

denature /diˈneɪtʃə/ vt. 改变本性，(使)变性，(使)改变

organism /ˈɔːrɡənɪzəm/ n. 有机体，生物体，微生物

stabilize /ˈsteɪbəlaɪz/ vt. 使安定，使坚固

optimum /ˈɑːptɪməm/ adj. 最佳的，最适宜的

thermophilic /ˌθɜːməuˈfilik/ adj. 嗜热的

archaea /ɑːˈkiə/ n. 古细菌，古生菌

misleading /ˌmɪsˈliːdɪŋ/ adj. 令人误解的，引入歧途的

pepsin /ˈpepsɪn/ n. 胃蛋白酶，助消化药

molecule /ˈmɑːlɪkjuːl/ n. ［化学］分子，微粒

formation /fɔːrˈmeɪʃn/ n. 形成，队形，编队，构造

macromolecular /ˌmækrəuməuˈlekjulə/ adj. ［化学］大分子的

property /ˈprɑːpərti/ n. 性质，性能，财产，所有权（复数 properties）

equilibrium /ˌiːkwɪˈlɪbriəm/ n. 平衡，均衡

molar /ˈmoulər/ adj. 磨碎的，臼齿的；［物理］质量上的；［化学］摩尔的

consumption /kənˈsʌmpʃn/ n. 消费，消耗

spectrophotometric /ˌspektrəufəuˈtɒmitrik/ adj. 分光光度计的，光谱光度测量的

redox /ridˈɑks/ n. ［化学］氧化还原反应

tetrazolium /ˌtetrəˈzəuliəm/ n. ［化学］四唑

colorimetric /kʌləriˈmetrik/ adj. 比色分析的

phosphate /ˈfɑːsfeɪt/ n. 磷酸盐，磷肥

glucose /ˈgluːkous/ n. 葡萄糖，葡糖（等于 dextrose）

hexokinase /ˌheksəuˈkaineis/ n. ［生化］己糖激酶

Phrases and Expressions

nicotinamide adenine dinucleotide   烟酰胺腺嘌呤二核苷酸，辅酶Ⅰ

nicotinamide adenine dinucleotide phosphate   烟酰胺腺嘌呤二核苷酸磷酸，辅酶Ⅱ

Notes

1. This is due to the denaturation (alteration) of protein structure resulting from the breakdown of the weak ionic and hydrogen bonds that stabilize the three dimensional structure of the enzyme active site.

这是由于稳定酶活性中心三维结构的弱离子键和氢键断裂，造成蛋白质结构变性（改变）所致。

2. Most enzymes function between the pH of 6 and 8; however, pepsin in the stomach works best at the pH of 2 and trypsin at the pH of 8.

多数酶在 pH 值为 6~8 时发挥催化作用，然而胃蛋白酶在 pH 值为 2 时催化作用最强，胰蛋白酶在 pH 值为 8 时催化作用最强。

3. At the saturation point, the reaction will not speed up, no matter how much additional substrate is added.

在饱和点，无论增加多少额外底物，反应速率都不会增加。

4. To find the maximum speed of an enzymatic reaction, the substrate concentration is increased until a constant rate of product formation is seen.

为了获得酶促反应的最大速率，会不断增加底物浓度，直到产物生成达到一个稳定的速率。

5. Amounts of enzymes can either be expressed as molar amounts, as with any other chemical, or meas-

ured in terms of activity, in enzyme units.

酶的量可以像任何其他化学物质一样用摩尔量来表示,或者用酶的活力,即酶单位来衡量。

6. Enzyme assays can be split into two groups according to their sampling method: continuous assays, where the assay gives a continuous reading of activity, and discontinuous assays, where samples are taken, the reaction stops and then the concentration of substrates or products is determined.

根据取样方法不同,酶测定方法可以分成两类:连续测定法与不连续测定法。连续测定法对酶的活性进行连续读数;不连续测定法是在反应终止后进行读取吸光度,再测定底物或产物的浓度。

7. Continuous assay is most convenient in that it gives the rate of reaction with one assay and no further work is necessary.

连续测定法最为便捷,只需一次测定法就可以得到反应速率,无需进一步的工作。

8. Even when the enzyme reaction does not result in a change in the absorbance of light, it can still be possible to use a spectrophotometric assay for the enzyme by using a coupled assay.

即使酶的反应没有导致光吸收的改变,仍然可以使用偶联法对酶进行分光光度测定。

Exercises

I. Fill in the blanks according to the texts.

1. Conditions that denature the protein abolish enzyme activity, such as high temperatures, extremes of pH levels or high salt concentrations, while raising substrate concentration ([S]) tends to_____ activity when [S] is low. (Text A)

2. Human enzymes start to_____ quickly at temperatures above 40℃. Enzymes from thermophilic archaea found in the hot springs are stable up to 100℃. (Text A)

3. The phenomenon of macromolecular crowding alters the properties of molecules in a solution when high concentrations of macromolecules such as proteins are_____. (Text A)

4. Amounts of enzymes can either be expressed as molar amounts, as with any other chemical, or measured in terms of activity, in_____ units. (Text B)

5. Enzyme assays can be split into two groups according to their sampling method: continuous assays, where the assay gives a continuous reading of activity, and_____ assays, where samples are taken, the reaction stops and then the concentration of substrates or products is determined. (Text B)

II. Translate the following into Chinese.

All enzyme assays measure either the consumption of substrate or production of product over time. Enzyme activity = moles of substrate converted per unit time = rate × reaction volume. The rate of a reaction is the concentration of substrate disappearing (or product produced) per unit time ($mol \cdot L^{-1} \cdot s^{-1}$). The SI unit is katal, 1 katal = 1mol/s, but this is an excessively large unit. A more practical and commonly used unit is enzyme unit (U), 1 U = 1 μmol/min. 1 U corresponds to 16.67 nanokatals.

Lesson 15 Point-of-care Testing
床旁检验

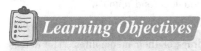 **Learning Objectives**

After studying this lesson, students are expected to be able to

1. master some key words and phrases;

2. be familiar with some medical terms about POCT;

3. understand the main idea of the whole texts.

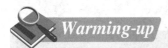

Warming-up

1. What is the definition of Point-of-care Testing?
2. What kinds of items does POCT include?
3. What does drug abuse mean?

Text A　Point-of-care Testing
床旁检验

Point-of-care testing (POCT) is defined as medical testing at or near the site of patient care. Other terminologies include Bedside Testing, Extra-Laboratory Testing and Disseminated Laboratory Testing. POCT includes blood glucose testing, blood gas and electrolytes analysis, rapid coagulation testing, rapid cardiac markers diagnostics, drugs of abuse screening, urine strips testing, pregnancy testing, fecal occult blood analysis, food pathogens screening, hemoglobin diagnostics, infectious disease testing and cholesterol screening.

POCT is accomplished through the use of transportable, portable and handheld instruments and test kits. Examples of POCT devices include Blood Glucose Meters, Urinalysis Test Strips, Pregnancy Test Kits, Coagulometers, HbA1C Analysers, Rapid Test Kits for Infectious Disease Markers, Bilirubinometers, Blood Gas Analysers, Electrolyte Analysers, Lipid Analysers, Cardiac Marker Test Kits, and so on. Many point-of-care test systems are realized as easy-to-use membrane-based test strips, often enclosed by a plastic test cassette. This concept often is realized in test systems for detecting pathogens. Very recently such test systems for rheumatology diagnostics have been developed, too. These tests require only a single drop of whole blood, urine or saliva, and they can be performed and interpreted by any general physician within minutes. Cheaper, smaller, faster, and smarter POCT devices have promoted the use of POCT approaches by making it cost-effective for many diseases, such as diabetes, carpal tunnel syndrome (CTS) and acute coronary syndrome.

The driving notion behind POCT is to bring the test conveniently and immediately to the patients. Potential operational benefits of POCT are more rapid decision making and triage, reduce operating times, reduce high-dependency, postoperative care time, reduce emergency room time, reduce the number of outpatient clinic visits, reduce the number of hospital beds required, ensure optimal use of professional time. This increases the likelihood that the patient, physician, and care team will receive the results quicker, which allows for immediate clinical management decisions to be made. POCT has become established worldwide and finds vital roles in public health.

Text B　Screening Test of Drug Abuse
药物滥用筛查试验

Drug abuse refers to a maladaptive pattern of use of a drug that is not considered dependent. Some of the drugs most often associated with this term include alcohol, amphetamines, barbiturates, benzodiazepines (particularly temazepam, nimetazepam, and flunitrazepam), cocaine, methaqualone and opioids.

A drug test is a technical analysis of biological specimen — for example urine, hair, blood, sweat, oral fluid or saliva to determine the presence or absence of specified parent drugs or their metabolites. The detection windows depend upon multiple factors, namely, drug class, amount and frequency of use, metabolic rate, body mass, age, overall health and urine pH. For ease of use, the detection times of metabolites have been incorporated into each parent drug. For example, heroin and cocaine can only be detected for a few hours after use, but their metabolites can be detected for several days in urine. In this type of situation, we will report the (longer) detection times of the metabolites.

One Step Tests for drugs of abuse are lateral flow, one-step, qualitative, competitive inhibition immunoassays. One-Step drug of abuse (DOA) tests are based on the principle of the highly specific immunochemical reactions of antigens and antibodies. One-step drug of abuse (DOA) rapid Screening tests employ unique monoclonal antibodies to selectively identify specific drugs of abuse and the corresponding metabolites in urine samples with a high degree of sensitivity and specificity.

At present, we have 10 drug of abuse test devices (test strip or test cassette), which test Amphetamine (AMP), Barbiturates (BAR), Benzodiazepine (BZO), Cocaine (COC), Methamphetamine (MAMP), Methadone (MTD), Opiates (OPI), Phencyclidine (PCP), Tricyclic (TCA) and Marijuana (THC) respectively. At the same time, DOA test panels are widely used for urine sample screening.

For all our DOA screening test devices, the cut off concentration for specific drug of abuse (DOA) and its metabolites has been developed at the concentration standard set by NIDA (the National Institute on Drug Abuse) for the qualitative detection of corresponding drug in human urine specimens.

New Words

analysis /əˈnæləsɪs/ *n.* 分析,解析

abuse /əˈbjuːs/ *n.* 滥用

pregnancy /ˈpregnənsi/ *n.* 怀孕

rheumatology /ˌruːməˈtɒlədʒɪ/ *n.* 风湿病学

triage/ˈtriːɑːʒ/ *n.* 伤员验伤分类,分类

urine /ˈjʊrɪn/ *n.* 尿,小便

metabolite /mɛˈtæbəlaɪt/ *n.* [生化]代谢物

detection/dɪˈtekʃn/ *n.* 检查

specific /spəˈsɪfɪk/ *adj.* 特定的,具有特效的

reaction /rɪˈækʃn/ *n.* 反应

monoclonal /ˌmɑnoˈklonəl/ *adj.* 单细胞繁殖的

sample /ˈsæmpl/ *n.* 样本

qualitative/ˈkwɑːlɪteɪtɪv/ *adj.* 定性的

Phrases and Expressions

extra-laboratory testing	检验科外的检验
blood glucose testing	血糖检测
carpal tunnel syndrome (CTS)	腕管综合征
acute coronary syndrome	急性冠脉综合征
associate with ...	与……联系在一起,相关
be based on ...	根据……,以……为基础
competitive inhibition immunoassay	竞争性免疫抑制试验
NIDA (the national institute on drug abuse)	国家药物滥用研究所
cut off concentration	浓度界值

Notes

1. POCT includes blood glucose testing, blood gas and electrolytes analysis, rapid coagulation testing, rapid cardiac markers diagnostics, drugs of abuse screening, urine strips testing, pregnancy testing, fecal occult blood analysis, food pathogens screening, hemoglobin diagnostics, infectious disease testing and cholesterol screening.

床旁检验包括:血糖检测、血气和电解质分析、快速凝血测验、快速心脏标记物诊断、药物滥用筛查、尿试纸条检测、妊娠检测、粪便隐血分析、食物病原体筛查、血红蛋白检测、传染病筛查和胆固醇检测等。

2. Examples of POCT devices include Blood Glucose Meters, Urinalysis Test Strips, Pregnancy Test Kits, Coagulometers, HbA1C Analysers, Rapid Test Kits for Infectious Disease Markers, Bilirubinometers, Blood Gas Analysers, Electrolyte Analysers, Lipid Analysers, Cardiac Marker Test Kits, and so on.

床旁检验设备包括:血糖仪、尿检试纸、妊娠检测试剂盒、凝血计、HbA1C 分析仪、传染病标志物快速检测试剂盒、胆红素检测仪、血气分析仪、电解质分析仪、血脂分析仪、心脏标志物检测试剂盒等。

3. Cheaper, smaller, faster, and smarter POCT devices have promoted the use of POCT approaches by making it cost-effective for many diseases, such as diabetes, carpal tunnel syndrome (CTS) and acute coronary syndrome.

廉价、更小、更快、更智能的 POCT 装置在许多疾病显现出很高的性价比,如糖尿病、腕管综合征(CTS)和急性冠状动脉综合征,从而促进了它的应用。

4. The driving notion behind POCT is to bring the test conveniently and immediately to the patient.

促进 POCT 发展的观念是给病人方便和立即检验。

5. This increases the likelihood that the patient, physician, and care team will receive the results quicker, which allows for immediate clinical management decisions to be made.

这样可使病人、医生和护理人员更快地获得结果,并立刻做出临床处理方案。

6. Some of the drugs most often associated with this term include alcohol, amphetamines, barbiturates, benzodiazepines (particularly temazepam, nimetazepam, and flunitrazepam), cocaine, methaqualone and opioids.

通常与这一术语最相关的一些药物包括乙醇、安非他命、巴比妥药物、苯二氮䓬类药物(特别是替马西泮、尼美西泮和氟硝西泮)、可卡因、甲喹酮和阿片类药物。

7. A drug test is a technical analysis of a biological specimen — for example urine, hair, blood, sweat, oral fluid or saliva to determine the presence or absence of specified parent drugs or their metabolites.

药物测试是对生物样本的技术分析,如尿液、毛发、血液、汗液或唾液,以确定是否存在指定的母体药物或其代谢物。

8. The detection windows depend upon multiple factors, namely, drug class, amount and frequency of use, metabolic rate, body mass, age, overall health and urine pH.

检测窗口期取决于多方面因素——药物类别、使用量及使用频率,代谢率、体重、年龄、总体健康状况以及尿液 pH 值。

9. One Step Tests for drugs of abuse are lateral flow, one-step, qualitative, competitive inhibition immunoassays.

药物滥用的一步检测法是利用层析进行一步定性竞争性免疫抑制实验。

10. For all our DOA screening test devices, the cut off concentration for specific drug of abuse (DOA) and its metabolites has been developed at the concentration standard set by NIDA (the National Institute on Drug Abuse) for the qualitative detection of corresponding drug in human urinespecimens.

为了定量检测病人尿液标本中相应药物,所有药物滥用筛查检测设备中特定的药物及其代谢物的参考浓度界值已按照 NIDA(国家药物滥用研究所)设定的浓度标准开发。

Exercises

Ⅰ. Fill in the blanks according to the texts.

1. POCT is accomplished through the use of transportable, ＿＿＿＿＿＿＿ and handheld instruments and test kits. (Text A)

2. These tests require only a single drop of whole ＿＿＿＿＿＿＿, urine or saliva, and they can be performed and interpreted by any general physician within minutes. (Text A)

3. One Step Tests for drugs of abuse are lateral flow, one-step, ＿＿＿＿＿＿＿, competitive inhibition immunoassays. (Text B)

4. One-step drug of abuse (DOA) rapid Screening tests employ unique monoclonal antibodies to selec-

tively identify specific drugs of abuse and the corresponding metabolites in urine samples with a high degree of
_____ and specificity. (Text B)

5. At the same time, DOA test panels are widely used for urine _____ screening. (Text B)

Ⅱ. Translate the following into Chinese.

Point-of-care testing (POCT) is defined as medical testing at or near the site of patient care. Other terminologies include Bedside Testing, Extra-Laboratory Testing and Disseminated Laboratory Testing. POCT includes blood glucose testing, blood gas and electrolytes analysis, rapid coagulation testing, rapid cardiac markers diagnostics, drugs of abuse screening, urine strips testing, pregnancy testing, fecal occult blood analysis, food pathogens screening, hemoglobin diagnostics, infectious disease testing and cholesterol screening.

Lesson 16 Flow Cytometry Analysis
流式细胞仪分析

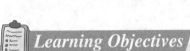
Learning Objectives

After studying this lesson, students are expected to be able to

1. master the basic knowledge of flow cytometry;

2. be familiar with some medical words and terms about flow cytometry analysis;

3. know about the principle and components of flow cytometer.

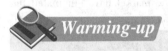
Warming-up

1. Have you ever heard about flow cytometry?

2. What is flow cytometry used for?

3. What is the principle of flow cytometer?

Text A Application of Flow Cytometry Analysis in Medicine
流式细胞仪分析在医学中的应用

Flow cytometry (FCM) is a laser based biophysical technology to analyze the characteristics of cells or particles. It can count and sort cells, detect biomarker and monitor protein engineering, by suspending cells in a stream of fluid and passing them by an electronic detection apparatus. This technology allows simultaneous multi-parameter analysis of single cells. It has applied to a number of fields, including molecular biology, pathology, immunology, plant biology and marine biology. It is widely used in health research and in treatment for a variety of tasks, (especially in transplantation, hematology, tumor immunology and chemotherapy, prenatal diagnosis, genetics and sperm sorting for sex preselection).

Flow cytometry analysis is most often clinically used to help diagnosis and monitoring of leukemia and lymphoma patients, providing the counts of helper-T lymphocytes needed to monitor the course and treatment of HIV infection, the evaluation of peripheral blood hematopoietic stem cell grafts, and many other diseases. Flow cytometry is quite sensitive; it can detect rare cell types and residual levels of disease. It usually chooses blood, body fluids, or bone marrow as specimens. In most cases, no special preparation is required. If bone marrow aspiration is necessary or a biopsy is required from a solid tumor, the patient should be appropriately prepared for these procedures. However, the flow cytometry itself does not require patients for any additional preparation.

The physician will select a specimen based on the type of cancer the patient may be diagnosed with. In the case of lymphoma, the specimen may be collected by means of fine needle aspiration, and then tissue specimen is isolated into single cells. Leukemia analysis requires blood sample from patient. The patient's blood sample will be separated, and the red blood cells will be removed by a simple lysis step. Each sample particle will pass one or more beams of light from the flow cytometer. Light scattering or fluorescence emission (supposing the particle is labeled by a fluorochrome) can provide information about the particle's properties. Fluorescence measurements taken at different wavelengths can provide quantitative and qualitative data of fluorescently labeled cell surface receptors or intracellular molecules such as DNA and cytokines. The specificity of detection is controlled by filters, which transmit other wavelengths while shielding certain wavelengths. The physician uses this information to determine the specific type of leukemia, such as myelogenous or lymphocytic, which in turn, helps to determine the type of treatment that will be best suited to the patient.

Text B Principle and Components of Flow Cytometer
流式细胞仪的原理与组成

The underlying principle of flow cytometry is that a cell suspension is focused into a single cell stream which passes through a light source (typically a laser beam). The scattered and emitted fluorescent light (if the cells are labeled by a fluorochrome) is subsequently measured by using a range of detectors and these measurements are used to generate multi-parameter data sets that describe the physical characteristics of the cells and their fluorescent properties. The size and granularity of cells can be identified on the basis of their forward and side light scatter characteristics (FSc and SSc respectively). FSC correlates with the cell volume and SSC depends on the inner complexity of the particle (i. e. , shape of the nucleus, the amount and type of cytoplasmic granules or the membrane roughness). Some flow cytometers on the market have eliminated the need for fluorescence and use only light scatter for measurement. Other flow cytometers form images of each cell's fluorescence, scattered light, and transmitted light.

A flow cytometer has five main components:

1. A flow cell— liquid stream (sheath fluid). Focus cells into the centre of a narrow stream of liquid called sheath fluid and only single cells can pass through the illuminating beam of light in the flow chamber.

2. A measuring system — commonly used ones are measurement of impedance (or conductivity) and optical systems lamps (mercury, xenon); high-power water-cooled lasers (argon, krypton, dye laser); low-power air-cooled lasers (argon 488 nm), red-HeNe (633 nm), green-HeNe, HeCd (UV); diode lasers (blue, green, red, violet) resulting in light signals.

3. A detector and Analogue-to-Digital Conversion (ADC) system— which generates FSC (forward scatter) and SSC (side scatter) as well as fluorescence signals from light into electrical signals that can be processed by a computer.

4. An amplification system—linear or logarithmic.

5. A computer for analyses of the signals.

The process of collecting data about samples by using the flow cytometer is called "acquisition". This acquisition is done by a computer physically connected to the flow cytometer, and the software which handles the digital interface of the cytometer. Modern flow cytometer can achieve real-time detection. It can analyze thousands of particles per second and is able to actively isolate particles having specified properties.

The data generated by flow-cytometers can be plotted in a single dimension, to produce a histogram, or in two-dimensional dot plots or even in three dimensions. The regions on these plots can be sequentially separated, based on fluorescence intensity, by creating a series of subset extractions, termed "gates." Specific gating protocols exist for diagnostic and clinical purposes especially in relation to hematology.

New Words

laser /ˈleɪzər/ *n.* 激光

biophysical /ˌbaɪəʊˈfɪzɪkəl/ *adj.* 生物物理学的

suspend /səˈspend/ *vt. & vi.* 延缓,使暂停,悬浮

apparatus /ˌæpəˈrætəs/ *n.* 装置,设备,仪器,器官

marine /məˈriːn/ *n.* 海运业

chemotherapy /ˌkiːmoʊˈθerəpi/ *n.* [临床]化学疗法

lymphoma /lɪmˈfoʊmə/ *n.* [肿瘤]淋巴瘤

sensitive /ˈsensətɪv/ *adj.* 敏感的,灵敏的

biopsy /ˈbaɪɑːpsi/ *n.* 活组织检查

fluorescence /fləˈresns/ *n.* 荧光,荧光性

shield /ʃiːld/ *vi.* 防御,起保护作用

myelogenous /ˌmaɪəˈlɔdʒənəs/ *adj.* 骨髓性的

granularity /ˌgrænjuˈlærɪti/ *n.* 间隔尺寸

mercury /ˈmɜːrkjəri/ *n.* [化学]汞,水银

xenon /ˈzenɑːn/ *n.* [化学]氙

argon /ˈɑːrgɑːn/ *n.* [化学]氩

krypton /ˈkrɪptɑːn/ *n.* [化学]氪

logarithmic /ˌlɔːgəˈrɪðmɪk/ *adj.* 对数的

acquisition /ˌækwɪˈzɪʃn/ *n.* 获得物,获得

dimension /daɪˈmenʃn/ *n.* 方面,维,尺寸

histogram /ˈhɪstəgræm/ *n.* [统计]直方图,柱状图

Phrases and Expressions

protein engineering	蛋白质工程
sheath fluid	鞘液
cell suspension	细胞悬液
analogue-to-digital conversion(ADC)	模数转换
forward scatter	前向散射
side scatter	侧向散射

Notes

1. It is widely used in health research and in treatment for a variety of tasks,(especially in transplantation, hematology, tumor immunology and chemotherapy, prenatal diagnosis, genetics and sperm sorting for sex preselection).

它被广泛应用在医学研究和各种治疗任务(尤其是在移植、血液学、肿瘤免疫学和化疗、产前诊断、遗传和性别预选的精子分类)中。

2. The physician will select a specimen based on the type of cancer the patient may be diagnosed with.

医生依据病人拟诊断的癌症类型选择标本。

3. The physician uses this information to determine the specific type of leukemia, such as myelogenous or lymphocytic, which in turn, helps to determine the type of treatment that will be best suited to the patient.

医生用该信息确定白血病的特定类型,诸如髓细胞性白血病或淋巴细胞白血病;确定了白血病类型后,又有助于确定最适合病人的治疗方案。

4. The scattered and emitted fluorescent light (if the cells are labeled by a fluorochrome) is subsequently measured by using a range of detectors and these measurements are used to generate multi-parameter data sets that describe the physical characteristics of the cells and their fluorescent properties.

随后使用一系列探测器进行测量散射和发射的荧光(如果细胞是荧光标记的),这些测量被用来生成描述细胞物理特性和荧光特性的多参数数据集。

5. Focus cells into the centre of a narrow stream of liquid called sheath fluid and only single cells can pass through the illuminating beam of light in the flow chamber.

聚焦细胞进入被称为鞘液的狭窄液体流的中心,并且只有单个细胞可以通过流动室的照明光束。

6. The data generated by flow-cytometers can be plotted in a single dimension, to produce a histogram, or in two-dimensional dot plots or even in three dimensions.

流式细胞仪产生的数据能绘制成单参数直方图或双参数点图,甚至三维立体图。

Exercises

Ⅰ. Fill in the blanks according to the texts.

1. It can count and sort cells, detect＿＿＿＿＿＿ and monitor protein engineering, by suspending cells in a stream of fluid and passing them by an electronic detection apparatus. (Text A)

2. Flow cytometry is quite＿＿＿＿＿＿; it can detect rare cell types and residual levels of disease. (Text A)

3. The underlying principle of flow cytometry is that a cell ＿＿＿＿＿＿ is focused into a single cell stream which passes through a light source (typically a laser beam). (Text B)

4. The process of collecting data about samples by using the flow cytometer is called "＿＿＿＿＿＿". (Text B)

5. It can analyze thousands of particles per second and is able to actively isolate particles having specified ＿＿＿＿＿＿. (Text B)

Ⅱ. Translate the following into Chinese.

A measuring system— commonly used are measurement of impedance (or conductivity) and optical systems: lamps (mercury, xenon); high-power water-cooled lasers (argon, krypton, dye laser); low-power air-cooled lasers (argon 488 nm), red-HeNe (633 nm), green-HeNe, HeCd (UV); diode lasers (blue, green, red, violet) resulting in light signals.

Lesson 17 Viral Epidemiology and HIV Tests
病毒流行病学与 HIV 检测

 Learning Objectives

After studying this lesson, students are expected to be able to

1. master some medical words and terms about viral epidemiology and HIV tests;

2. be familiar with the structure and replication cycle of viruses, and the incubation periods for viral diseases;

3. know about the procedure of ELISA and Western blot, and the differences between them.

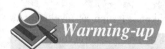 *Warming-up*

1. What parts do virus particles consist of? And what are the steps of viral replication cycle?

2. What are the incubation periods for viral diseases?

3. What are the two tests combined for the diagnosis of HIV infection in the United States?

Text A Viral Epidemiology
病毒流行病学

A virus is a small infectious agent that can replicate only inside the living cells of organisms. Virus particles consist of two (or three) parts: the genetic material made from either DNA or RNA, which are long molecules that carry genetic information; the protein coat, which protects these genes (and the envelope of lipids, which surrounds the protein coat when they are outside a cell). The shapes of viruses range from simple helical and icosahedral forms to more complex structures. The average virus is about one-hundredth the size of the average bacterium. Most viruses are too small to be seen directly with a light microscope.

For a virus to replicate it must infect a living cell. All viruses employ a common set of steps in their replication cycle. These steps are attachment, penetration, uncoating, replication, assembly, maturation, and release.

Transmission of viruses can be vertical, that is from mother to child, or horizontal, which means from person to person. Examples of vertical transmission include hepatitis B virus and human immunodeficiency virus (HIV) where the baby is born already infected with the virus. Horizontal transmission is the most common mechanism of spread of viruses in populations. Transmission can occur when: body fluids are exchanged during sexual activity, e. g., HIV; blood is exchanged by contaminated transfusion or needle sharing, e. g., hepatitis C; exchange of saliva by mouth, e. g., Epstein-Barr virus; contaminated food or water is ingested, e. g., norovirus; aerosols containing virions are inhaled, e. g., influenza virus; and insect vectors such as mosquitoes penetrate the skin of a host, e. g., dengue. The rate or speed of transmission of viral infections depends on factors including population density, the number of susceptible individuals, the quality of healthcare and the weather. Most viral infections of humans and of other animals have incubation periods during which the infection causes no signs or symptoms. Incubation periods for viral diseases range from a few days to weeks but are known for most infections.

Examples of common human diseases caused by viruses include the common cold, influenza, chickenpox and cold sores. Many serious diseases, such as Ebola, AIDS, avian influenza, SARS and COVID-19, are also caused by viruses. The relative ability of viruses to cause disease is described in terms of virulence.

Viral epidemiology is the branch of medical science that deals with the transmission and control of virus infections in humans. Epidemiology is used to break the chain of infection in populations during outbreaks of viral diseases. Control measures are based on knowledge of how the virus is transmitted. It is important to find the source, or sources, of the outbreak and to identify the virus.

Text B HIV Tests
HIV 检测

HIV tests are used to detect the presence of the human immunodeficiency virus (HIV), the virus that causes AIDS (acquired immunodeficiency syndrome), in serum, saliva, or urine. Such tests may detect antibodies, antigens or RNA.

Tests used for the diagnosis of HIV infection in a particular person require a high degree of both sensitivity and specificity. In the United States, this is achieved using an algorithm combining two tests for HIV antibodies. If antibodies are detected by an initial test based on the ELISA method, then a second test using the Western blot procedure determines the size of the antigens in the test kit binding to the antibodies. The combination of these two methods is highly accurate.

In an ELISA test, a person's serum is diluted 400-fold and applied to a plate to which HIV antigens have been attached. If antibodies to HIV are present in the serum, they may bind to these HIV antigens. The plate is then washed to remove all other components of the serum. A specially prepared "secondary antibody" — an antibody that binds to human antibodies — is then applied to the plate, followed by another wash. This secondary antibody is chemically linked in advance to an enzyme. Thus the plate will contain enzyme in proportion to the amount of secondary antibody bound to the plate. A substrate for the enzyme is applied, and catalysis by the enzyme leads to a change in color or fluorescence. ELISA results are reported as a number; the most controversial aspect of this test is determining the "cut-off" point between a positive and negative result.

Like the ELISA procedure, the western blot is an antibody detection test. However, unlike the ELISA method, the viral proteins are separated first and immobilized. In subsequent steps, the binding of serum antibodies to specific HIV proteins is visualized.

Specifically, cells that may be HIV-infected are opened and the proteins within are placed into a slab of gel, to which an electrical current is applied. Different proteins will move with different velocities in this field, depending on their size, while their electrical charge is leveled by a surfactant called sodium lauryl sulfate. Some commercially prepared Western blot test kits contain the HIV proteins already on a cellulose acetate strip. Once the proteins are well-separated, they are transferred to a membrane and the procedure continues, which is similar to an ELISA: the person's diluted serum is applied to the membrane and antibodies in the serum may attach to some of the HIV proteins. Antibodies that do not attach are washed away, and enzyme-linked antibodies with the capability to attach to the person's antibodies determine to which HIV proteins the person has antibodies.

The HIV proteins used in western blotting can be produced by recombinant DNA uisng a technique called recombinant immunoblot assay (RIBA).

New Words

replicate /ˈreplɪkeɪt/ *v.* 复制,折叠

helical /ˈhelɪkl/ *adj.* 螺旋形的

icosahedral /ˌaɪkəʊsəˈhedrəl/ *adj.* [数] 二十面体的

penetration /ˌpenəˈtreɪʃn/ *n.* 穿入,侵入,渗透

uncoating /ˌʌnˈkəʊtiŋ/ *n.* 病毒脱壳

maturation /ˌmætʃuˈreɪʃn/ *n.* 成熟,化脓

norovirus /ˈnɔːrəʊvaɪrəs/ *n.* 诺瓦克病毒

aerosol /ˈerəsɒl/ *n.* [物化] 气溶胶,气雾剂

virion /ˈvaɪərɪˌɑn/ *n.* [病毒] 病毒粒子,病毒体

inhale /ɪnˈheɪl/ *vt.* 吸入

mosquito /məˈskiːtəʊ/ *n.* 蚊子

dengue /ˈdeŋgi/ *n.* 登革热

incubation /ˌɪŋkjuˈbeɪʃn/ *n.* [病毒] [医] 潜伏,孵化

symptom /ˈsɪmptəm/ *n.* [临床] 症状,征兆

sore /sɔːr/ *n.* 疡,疮

virulence /ˈvɪrələns/ *n.* 毒力,毒性,恶意(等于 virulency)

algorithm /ˈælgərɪðəm/ *n.* [计] [数] 算法,运算法则

surfactant /sɜːrˈfæktənt/ *n.* 表面活性剂

Phrases and Expressions

influenza virus	流感病毒
cold sores	唇疱疹,感冒疮
avian influenza	禽流感
SARS (severe acute respiratory syndromes)	严重急性呼吸综合征
COVID-19	新型冠状病毒肺炎
initial test	初筛试验

western blot	免疫印迹
test kit	试剂盒
recombinant immunoblot assay (RIBA)	重组免疫印迹试验

Notes

1. Virus particles consist of two (or three) parts: the genetic material made from either DNA or RNA, which are long molecules that carry genetic information; the protein coat, which protects these genes (and the envelope of lipids, which surrounds the protein coat when they are outside a cell).

病毒颗粒由两(三)部分组成:遗传物质、蛋白衣壳(和脂质包膜)。遗传物质为 DNA 或 RNA,这些长链分子携带遗传信息;蛋白衣壳保护这些遗传物质;当病毒在宿主细胞外时,脂质包膜包绕在蛋白衣壳外。

2. The average virus is about one-hundredth the size of the average bacterium. Most viruses are too small to be seen directly with a light microscope.

普通病毒约为普通细菌大小的百分之一。大多数病毒太小以致光学显微镜不能直接观察。

3. Transmission can occur when: body fluids are exchanged during sexual activity, e. g., HIV; blood is exchanged by contaminated transfusion or needle sharing, e. g., hepatitis C; exchange of saliva by mouth, e. g., Epstein-Barr virus; contaminated food or water is ingested, e. g., norovirus; aerosols containing virions are inhaled, e. g., influenza virus; and insect vectors such as mosquitoes penetrate the skin of a host, e. g., dengue.

下列途径能够传播病毒:性行为时体液交换,如人类免疫缺陷病毒;受污染的输血过程或共用针头时血液交换,如丙型肝炎;口腔唾液交换,如 EB 病毒;摄入污染的食物或水,如诺瓦克病毒;吸入含有病毒体的气溶胶,如流感病毒;昆虫媒介如蚊子叮咬宿主的皮肤(吸血),例如登革热。

4. The rate or speed of transmission of viral infections depends on factors including population density, the number of susceptible individuals, the quality of healthcare and the weather.

病毒感染的传播速率或速度取决于以下因素,包括人口密度、易感个体的数量,卫生保健的质量和气候。

5. In an ELISA test, a person's serum is diluted 400-fold and applied to a plate to which HIV antigens have been attached.

酶联免疫吸附试验中,将受检者的血清标本稀释 400 倍,而后与包被在固相反应板上的 HIV 抗原进行反应。

6. A specially prepared "secondary antibody" — an antibody that binds to human antibodies — is then applied to the plate, followed by another wash.

然后,将专门制备的"第二抗体"——即一种结合人抗体的抗体,加入反应板中(反应),随后又一次洗涤。

7. ELISA results are reported as a number; the most controversial aspect of this test is determining the "cut-off" point between a positive and negative result.

酶联免疫吸附试验结果报告为一个值;该试验最有争议的方面是决定一个阳性和阴性结果之间的分界点。

8. Specifically, cells that may be HIV-infected are opened and the proteins within are placed into a slab of gel, to which an electrical current is applied.

特别的方法,将可能受 HIV 感染的细胞破碎,(提取的)细胞内蛋白质加样到凝胶平板,再给它施加电流。

9. Antibodies that do not attach are washed away, and enzyme-linked antibodies with the capability to attach to the person's antibodies determine to which HIV proteins the person has antibodies.

未吸附的抗体被洗脱,能与人抗体结合的酶联抗体确定人具有的抗体所针对的 HIV 蛋白质种类。

Exercises

Ⅰ. Fill in the blanks according to the texts.

1. A virus is a small infectiousagent that can replicate only inside the ＿＿＿＿＿＿ cells of organisms. (Text A)

2. The rate or speed of transmission of viral infections depends on factors that including population density, the number of ＿＿＿＿＿＿ individuals, the quality of healthcare and the weather. (Text A)

3. Control measures are used that are based on knowledge of how the virus is ＿＿＿＿＿＿. It is important to find the source, or sources, of the outbreak and to identify the virus. (Text A)

4. HIV tests are used to detect the presence of HIV, the virus that causes AIDS, in serum, saliva, or urine. Such tests may detect ＿＿＿＿＿＿, antigens or RNA. (Text B)

5. A ＿＿＿＿＿＿ for the enzyme is applied, and catalysis by the enzyme leads to a change in color or fluorescence. (Text B)

Ⅱ. Translate the following into Chinese.

HIV infection leads to a progressive reduction in the number of T cells expressing CD4. Counting the CD4 cells in a blood sample by using monoclonal antibody technology and flow cytometry indicates the stage of infection. CD4 cells count test measures the number of T cells expressing CD4. Results are usually expressed in the number of cells per microliter (or cubic millimeter, mm^3) of blood.

Lesson 18 Antibiotic Susceptibility Testing Methods
抗生素药物敏感试验方法

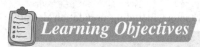

Learning Objectives

After studying this lesson, students are expected to be able to

1. master some medical words and terms about antibiotic susceptibility test;

2. be familiar with the process of antibiotic susceptibility test;

3. know about the methods of measuring antibiotic susceptibility testing results.

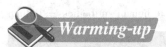

Warming-up

1. What is MIC?

2. What does a lower MIC indicate?

3. What is the zone of inhibition in K-B testing?

Text A Minimum Inhibitory Concentration
最小抑菌浓度

In microbiology, the minimum inhibitory concentration (MIC) is the lowest concentration of an antimicrobial agent, or other substance, that will inhibit the visible growth of a microorganism after overnight incubation. MICs are important in diagnostic laboratories to confirm resistance of microorganisms to an antimicrobial agent and also to monitor the activity of new antimicrobial agents. A lower MIC is an indication of a better antimicrobial agent. A MIC is generally regarded as the most basic laboratory measurement of the activity of an antimicrobial agent against an organism. Clinically, MICs are used not only to determine the amount of antibiotic that the patient will receive but also the type of antibiotic used, which in turn lowers the chance for microbial resistance to specific antimicrobial agents. Currently, there are a few web-based, freely accessible MIC databases.

Once the MIC is calculated, it can be compared to established values for a given bacterium and antibiotic: e. g. , a MIC>0. 06 μg/mL may be interpreted as a penicillin-resistant *Streptococcus pneumoniae*. Such information may be useful to the clinician, who can change the empirical treatment to a more custom-tailored treatment that is directed only at the causative bacterium.

Text B   Kirby-Bauer Disc Diffusion Method
纸片扩散法

Antibiotic susceptibility or antibiotic sensitivity is the susceptibility of bacteria to antibiotics. Because susceptibility can vary even within a species (with some strains being more resistant than others), antibiotic susceptibility testing (AST) is usually carried out to determine which antibiotic will be most successful in treating a bacterial infection in vivo.

The disc diffusion test is most widely used among the antibiotic susceptibility testing methods. Kirby-Bauer antibiotic testing (K-B testing or disc diffusion antibiotic sensitivity testing) is a test which uses antibiotic-impregnated wafers to test whether particular bacteria are susceptible to specific antibiotics (figure 3-2). A known quantity of bacteria is grown on Mueller-Hinton agar plates (4 mm thickness plate) in the presence of thin wafers containing relevant antibiotics. If the bacteria are susceptible to a particular antibiotic, an area of clearing surrounds the wafer where bacteria are not capable of growing (called a zone of inhibition).

In Kirby-Bauer testing, white wafers containing antibiotics are placed on a plate of bacteria. Circles

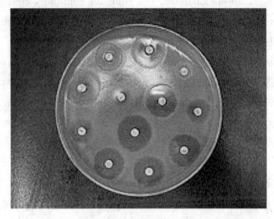

Figure 3-2　Kirby-Bauer Disc Diffusion Method

of poor bacterial growth surrounding some wafers indicate susceptibility to the antibiotic. Zones of inhibition are measured to the nearest whole millimeter using sliding calipers, ruler or template prepared for this purpose which is held on the back of inverted petri plate. Use of a single disk for each antibiotic with careful standardization of the test conditions permits the report of susceptible or resistant for a microorganism by comparing the size of the inhibition zone against the standard size of the same drug.

The size of the inhibition zone along with the rate of antibiotic diffusion is used to estimate the bacteria's sensitivity to that particular antibiotic. In general, larger zones correlate with smaller MIC of antibiotic for that bacterium. This information can be used to choose appropriate antibiotics to combat a particular infection.

New Words

antimicrobial /ˌæntimaɪˈkrobiəl/ *n.* 抗菌剂,杀菌剂

resistance /rɪˈzɪstəns/ *n.* 耐药性

indication /ˌɪndɪˈkeɪʃn/ *n.* 指示,指出

measurement /ˈmeʒərmənt/ *n.* 测量,度量,尺寸

accessible /əkˈsesəbl/ *adj.* 易接近的,可进入的,可理解的

wafer /ˈweɪfər/ *n.* 圆片,晶片,薄片

combat /ˈkɑːmbæt/ *v.* 反对,与……战斗

interpret /ɪnˈtɜːrprət/ *v.* 解释,理解

笔记

137

empirical /ɪmˈpɪrɪkl/ *adj.* 凭经验的

custom-tailored /ˌkʌstəmˈteɪlərd/ *adj.* 定制的，量体裁衣的

inverted /ɪnˈvɜːtɪd/ *adj.* 倒转的，反向的

Phrases and Expressions

Kirby-Bauer antibiotic testing	K-B 药物敏感性试验
antibiotic-impregnated wafers	抗生素浸渍片
sliding calipers	游标卡尺
zone of inhibition	抑菌圈
petri plate	培养皿
streptococcus pneumoniae	肺炎链球菌
in vivo	在活的有机体内
Mueller-Hinton agar plates	水解酪蛋白培养基琼脂平板

Notes

1. In microbiology, the minimum inhibitory concentration (MIC) is the lowest concentration of an antimicrobial agent, or other substance, that will inhibit the visible growth of a microorganism after overnight incubation.

在微生物学中，最低抑菌浓度(MIC)是指抗菌药物(或其他物质)能够抑制过夜培养的微生物可见生长的最低浓度。

2. Kirby-Bauer antibiotic testing (K-B testing or disc diffusion antibiotic sensitivity testing) is a test which uses antibiotic-impregnated wafers to test whether particular bacteria are susceptible to specific antibiotics.

K-B 药物敏感试验(K-B 法或纸片扩散法药物敏感试验)是用抗生素浸渍纸片检测特定细菌是否对特定抗生素敏感的试验。

3. Clinically, MICs are used not only to determine the amount of antibiotic that the patient will receive but also the type of antibiotic used, which in turn lowers the opportunity for microbial resistance to specific antimicrobial agents.

临床上，MICs 不仅用来确定病人接受抗生素的用量，还用来确定病人使用抗生素的类型，由此降低微生物对特定抗菌药物产生耐药性的概率。

4. In general, larger zones correlate with smaller MIC of antibiotic for that bacterium.

总的来说，抑菌圈区域越大，代表抗生素对此种细菌的 MIC 越小。

5. Circles of poor bacterial growth surrounding some wafers indicate susceptibility to the antibiotic.

纸药片周围细菌生长不良的环形区域代表细菌对此抗生素敏感。

Exercises

Ⅰ. Fill in the blanks according to the texts.

1. MICs are important in diagnostic laboratories to confirm _____ of microorganisms to an antimicrobial agent and also to monitor the activity of new antimicrobial agents. (Text A)

2. Kirby-Bauer antibiotic testing (KB testing or disc diffusion antibiotic sensitivity testing) is a test which uses antibiotic-impregnated wafers to test whether particular bacteria are_____ to specific antibiotics. (Text B)

3. In general, larger zones _____ with smaller MIC of antibiotic for that bacterium. (Text B)

4. The disk _____ test is used most widely among the antibiotic susceptibility testing methods. (Text B)

5. Zones of inhibition are measured to the nearest whole _____ using sliding calipers，ruler or template prepared for this purpose which is held on the back of inverted petri plate. （Text B）

Ⅱ. Translate the following into Chinese.

Antibiotic susceptibility or antibiotic sensitivity is the susceptibility of bacteria to antibiotics. Because susceptibility can vary even within a species（with some strains being more resistant than others），antibiotic susceptibility testing（AST）is usually carried out to determine which antibiotic will be most successful in treating a bacterial infection in vivo.

Lesson 19   Polymerase Chain Reaction Technology
聚合酶链反应技术

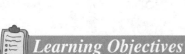
Learning Objectives

After studying this lesson，students are expected to be able to
1. master the chemical composition and structure of DNA；
2. be familiar with the genetic base-pair sequence；
3. know about the PCR reaction；
4. perform the steps in PCR.

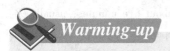
Warming-up

1. What are the four types of chemical bases in the genetic code?
2. What is the polymerase chain reaction?

Text A   Central Dogma of Molecular Biology
分子生物学中心法则

One of the most exciting developments in genetics is the initiation of the Human Genome Project. It is designed to provide a complete genetic map outlining the locations and functions of about 40,000 genes that are found in human cells.

To understand genes and their biological functions in heredity，it is necessary to understand the chemical composition and structure of DNA. The complete DNA molecule is often called the blueprint of life，because it carries all the instructions for the growth and functions of organisms，in the form of genes. This fundamental molecule is called a double helix. The two sides of the DNA ladder are made up of alternate sugar and phosphate molecules，linking to a chain. The rungs or steps of DNA are made from a combination of four different chemical bases. Two of these，adenine and guanine，are known aspurines，and the other two，cytosine and thymine，are pyrimidines. The four letters of the genetic code — A, G, C and T，refer to these bases. In this genetic code，A combines with T and C with G，forming base pairs. Specific sequences of these base pairs make up the genes.

Genetic information is copied during the process of DNA duplication，which is started by proteins in the cells. To produce same genetic information during cell mitosis，the DNA hydrogen bonds are broken，splitting the DNA in half lengthwise. This process begins a few hours before the beginning of cell mitosis. Once it is completed，each half of the DNA ladder is capable of forming a new DNA molecule with the same genetic code.

Genes usually express their functional effects through the production of proteins. Cells contain hundreds of different proteins and complex molecules that make up many solid body tissues and control most biological processes. It is the genetic base-pair sequence in DNA that determines the amino acids sequence which forms particular proteins.

Since the sites of protein production lie outside the cell nucleus, coded messages pass from the DNA in the nucleus to the cytoplasm. This transfer of messages is achieved by RNA or ribonucleic acid, especially by messenger RNA or mRNA. This messenger RNA molecule is used to produce a relevant amino acid sequence through translation process. To form the protein, other RNA molecules are linked to the amino-acids together in a sequence.

Text B Polymerase Chain Reaction
聚合酶链反应

DNA can be amplified by using a procedure called the polymerase chain reaction (PCR) in the laboratory. Because it can amplify extremely small amounts of DNA, PCR is often used to test the presence of specific DNA sequences.

To perform the PCR reaction, the tube containing the solution is placed into a machine called a DNA thermal cycler. Thermal cyclers are basically programmable heating blocks. They usually contain a thick aluminum block with holes. Under programmable computer control, the block can be quickly cooled or heated to specific temperatures. Changing the temperature of the block and the reaction mixture can control each cycle in a PCR reaction.

The first step in PCR is to heat the mixture to a high temperature for about five minutes, usually 94-95℃. The hydrogen bonds are broken at these temperatures, and the DNA separates into single strand. This process is called denaturation.

In the second step, the PCR mixture is cooled to a lower temperature, usually between about 50℃ and 65℃. This allows the primers to anneal to their specific complementary sequences in the template DNA. The temperature for this step needs to be low enough to allow the primers to bind, but no cooler. A lower annealing temperature might allow the primers to bind to regions in the template DNA that are not perfect complements. It may lead to the amplification of non-specific sequences. The annealing step usually takes about fifteen to thirty seconds, which is very short.

In the third step, the reaction is heated again, usually to about 72℃, the temperature at which the DNA polymerase is most active. Most enzymes are destroyed at 72℃. To solve this problem, scientists purified DNA polymerases from microorganisms that live in hot springs or other places. These organisms' enzymes are most active at high temperatures. The most commonly used enzyme for PCR is called Taq DNA polymerase.

During each duplication cycle, the number of the target sequence molecules doubles, because the products and templates of one round all become the templates for the next round. In theory, after n rounds of duplication, 2^n copies of the target sequence are produced. After thirty cycles, PCR can produce 2^{30} or more than ten billion copies of a single target DNA sequence.

New Words

outline/ˈaʊtlaɪn/ *n.* 轮廓,大纲,概要,略图 *vt.* 概述,略述,描画……轮廓

heredity /həˈredəti/ *n.* 遗传,遗传性

fundamental /ˌfʌndəˈmentl/ *adj.* 基本的,根本的

rung /rʌŋ/ *n.* 阶梯

adenine /ˈædənɪn/ *n.* [生化] 腺嘌呤

guanine /ˈɡwɑnin/ *n.* [生化] 鸟嘌呤

purine /ˈpjuriːn/ *n.* [有化] 嘌呤

cytosine /ˈsaɪtoˌsin/ *n.* ［生化］胞嘧啶

thymine /ˈθaɪmɪn/ *n.* ［生化］胸腺嘧啶

pyrimidine /paɪˈrɪməˌdin/ *n.* ［生化］嘧啶

sequence /ˈsiːkwəns/ *n.* ［数］［计］序列，顺序，续发事件

duplication /ˌduːplɪˈkeɪʃn/ *n.* 复制

split /splɪt/ *v.* 分离

lengthwise /ˈlɛŋθˌwaɪz/ *adv.* 纵长地

amplify /ˈæmplɪfaɪ/ *v.* 扩大

perform /pərˈfɔːrm/ *v.* 执行

programmable /ˈprouɡræməbl/ *adj.* ［计］可编程的，可设计的

denaturation /diˌnetʃəˈreʃən/ *n.* 变性

primer /ˈpraɪmər/ *n.* 引物

anneal /əˈniːl/ *v.* 使退火

template /ˈtemplət/ *n.* 模板

purify /ˈpjʊrɪfaɪ/ *v.* 净化

Phrases and Expressions

double helix	双螺旋
genetic code	遗传密码
base pair	碱基对
cell mitosis	细胞分裂
hydrogen bond	氢键
messenger RNA	信使 RNA
thermal cycler	热循环仪
Taq DNA polymerase	Taq DNA 聚合酶

Notes

1. The two sides of the DNA ladder are made up of alternate sugar and phosphate molecules, linking to a chain.

DNA 螺旋梯的两侧是由交替的糖和磷酸盐分子组成，连接成骨架。

2. To produce same genetic information during cell mitosis, the DNA hydrogen bonds are broken, splitting the DNA in half lengthwise.

为了在细胞有丝分裂过程中产生相同的遗传信息，DNA 氢键断裂，将 DNA 纵向分裂成两半。

3. Once it is completed, each half of the DNA ladder is capable of forming a new DNA molecule with the same genetic code.

一旦完成，DNA 螺旋梯的每条链都能够形成具有相同遗传密码的新的 DNA 分子。

4. Since the sites of protein production lie outside the cell nucleus, coded messages pass from the DNA in the nucleus to the cytoplasm.

由于蛋白质产生的部位位于细胞核之外，编码信息从细胞核中的 DNA 传递到细胞质。

5. DNA can be amplified by using a procedure called the polymerase chain reaction (PCR) in the laboratory.

DNA 可以用实验室中称为聚合酶链反应(PCR)的方法扩增。

6. To perform the PCR reaction, the tube containing the solution is placed into a machine called a DNA thermal cycler.

为了进行 PCR 反应，将含有溶液的试管放入一台称为 DNA 热循环仪的仪器中。

7. Changing the temperature of the block and the reaction mixture can control each cycle in a PCR reac-

tion.

改变铝板和反应混合物的温度可以控制 PCR 反应的每次循环。

8. During each duplication cycle, the number of the target sequence molecules doubles, because the products and templates of one round all become the templates for the next round.

在每个复制周期中,靶序列的分子数加倍,因为一轮复制的产物和模板都成为下一轮的模板。

Exercises

Ⅰ. Fill in the blanks according to the texts.

1. It is designed to provide a complete genetic map_____ the locations and functions of about 40,000 genes that are found in human cells. (Text A)

2. This_____ molecule is called a double helix. (Text A)

3. It is the genetic base-pair sequence in DNA that_____ the amino acids sequence which forms particular proteins. (Text A)

4. Under_____ computer control, the block can be quickly cooled or heated to specific temperatures. (Text B)

5. _____, after n rounds of duplication, 2^n copies of the target sequence are produced. (Text B)

Ⅱ. Translate the following into Chinese.

Genes usually express their functional effects through the production of proteins. Cells contain hundreds of different proteins and complex molecules that make up many solid body tissues and control most biological processes. It is the genetic base-pair sequence in DNA that determines the amino acids sequence which forms particular proteins.

Lesson 20 Biochip Technology
生物芯片技术

Learning Objectives

After studying this lesson, students are expected to be able to

1. master the principle of DNA microarray and protein microarray;

2. be familiar with the preparation methods of DNA microarray and protein microarray;

3. know about the clinical application prospects of biochips technology.

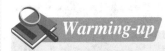 Warming-up

1. What is the principle of DNA hybridization technique?

2. What methods could be used for labeling nucleic acids?

3. What is the principle of specific binding of antibody and antigen?

Text A DNA Microarray
DNA 芯片

DNA microarray (or DNA chip) is part of the process of microarray profiling, which is also known as gene microarray. A DNA microarray is a collection of microscopic DNA spots attached to a solid surface. In standard microarrays, the probes are synthesized and then attached via surface engineering to a solid surface by a covalent bond to a chemical matrix. The solid surface can be glass or a silicon chip, in which case they are colloquially known as an Affy chip when an Affymetrix chip is used. Other microarray platforms, such as Illumina, use microscopic beads, instead of the large solid support. Alternatively, microarrays can be constructed by the direct synthesis of oligonucleotide probes on solid surfaces.

Scientists use DNA microarrays to measure the expression level of large numbers of genes simultaneously or to genotype multiple regions of a genome. Each DNA spot contains picomoles (10^{-12} moles) of a specific DNA sequence, known as probes (or reporters). These can be a short section of a gene or other DNA elements that are used to hybridize a cDNA or cRNA sample (called target) under high-stringency conditions.

The core principle behind microarrays is hybridization between two DNA strands, the property of complementary nucleic acid sequences to specifically pair with each other by forming hydrogen bonds between complementary nucleotide base pairs. A high number of complementary base pairs in a nucleotide sequence mean tighter non-covalent bonding between the two strands. After washing off of non-specific bonding sequences, only strongly paired strands will remain hybridized. Probe-target hybridization is usually detected and quantified by detection of fluorophore-labeled, silver-labeled or chemiluminescence-labeled targets to determine relative abundance of nucleic acid sequences in the target. So fluorescently labeled target sequences that bind to a probe sequence generate a signal that depends on the strength of the hybridization determined by the number of paired bases, the hybridization conditions (such as temperature) and washing after hybridization. Total strength of the signal, from a spot (feature), depends upon the amount of target sample binding to the probes present on that spot.

Microarrays use relative quantization in which the intensity of a feature is compared to the intensity of the same feature under a different condition, and the identity of the feature is known by its position.

Text B   Protein Microarray
蛋白质芯片

A protein microarray (or protein chip), provides an approach to identify protein-protein interactions, the substrates of protein kinases, transcription factor protein-activation or the targets of biologically active small molecules. The array is a piece of glass on which different molecules of protein or specific DNA binding sequences (as capture probes for the proteins) have been affixed at separate locations in an ordered manner thus forming a microscopic array.

The most common protein microarray is the antibody microarray, where antibodies are spotted onto the protein chip and are used as capture molecules to detect proteins from cell lysate solutions. Antibodies have several problems including the fact that there are no antibodies for most proteins and also problems with specificity in some commercial antibody preparations. Nevertheless, antibodies still represent the most effective protein capture agent for microarrays.

Antibodies are the most widely used capture molecules for the preparation of microarrays. However, antigens are used in applications where antibodies are detected in serum. Recently, nucleic acids, receptors and enzymes have been used as capture molecules, which allows a vast variety of experiments to be conducted on protein-protein interactions and all other protein binding substrates. More recently there has been a push towards other types of capture molecules which are more similar in their nature such as peptides or aptamers.

Protein chips differ from analytical arrays, which are composed of full-length functional proteins or protein domains. They are used to study the biochemical activities of the entire proteome in a single experiment.

New Words

biochip /ˈbaɪɒˌtʃɪp/ *n.* [生物] 生物芯片

microarray /ˌmaikrəuəˈrei/ *n.* 微阵列, 微阵列芯片

synthesize /ˈsɪnθəsaɪz/ *vt.* 合成

via /ˈvaɪə/ *prep.* 通过

silicon /ˈsɪlɪkən/ *n.* ［化学］硅,硅元素

covalent /ˌkoʊˈveɪlənt/ *adj.* 共价的

Illumina /ɪˈljuːmɪnə/ *n.* 依诺米那(公司名)

beads /biːdz/ *n.* 磁珠

alternatively /ɔːlˈtɜːrnətɪvli/ *adv.* 要不,或者

oligonucleotide /ˌɔligəʊˈnjuːkliəutaid/ *n.* ［生化］寡核苷酸

picomole /ˈpaikəuməul/ *n.* 皮摩尔,微微摩尔

hybridize /ˈhaɪbrɪdaɪz/ *v.* 杂交

stringency /ˈstrɪndʒənsi/ *n.* 严格

complementary /ˌkɑːmplɪˈmentri/ *adj.* 互补的

fluorophore /ˈfluərəˌfɔːr/ *n.* ［化学］荧光团

silver /ˈsɪlvər/ *n.* 银

kinase /ˈkɪnneɪz/ *n.* ［生化］激酶,致活酶

transcription /trænˈskrɪpʃn/ *n.* 转录

affix /əˈfɪks/ *vt.* 粘上,署名 n. ［语］词缀,附加物

microscopic /ˌmaɪkrəˈskɑːpɪk/ *adj.* 微观的

lysate /ˈlaiseit/ *n.* 溶菌产物,溶解产物

receptor /rɪˈseptər/ *n.* ［生化］受体,接受器,感觉器官

aptamer /ˈæpteɪmər/ *n.* 适体,适配体

domain /douˈmeɪn/ *n.* 结构域

Phrases and Expressions

microarray profiling	微阵列谱
surface engineering	表面工程
protein-protein interaction	蛋白质-蛋白质相互作用

Notes

1. In standard microarrays, the probes are synthesized and then attached via surface engineering to a solid surface by a covalent bond to a chemical matrix.

在标准芯片中,探针被合成后,通过以共价键与化学基质结合这样的表面工程吸附到一个固体表面。

2. The solid surface can be glass or a silicon chip, in which case they are colloquially known as an Affy chip when an Affymetrix chip is used.

固体表面可以是玻璃或一种硅芯片,当使用 Affymetrix 芯片时,他们通俗被称为 Affy 芯片。

3. The core principle behind microarrays is hybridization between two DNA strands, the property of complementary nucleic acid sequences to specifically pair with each other by forming hydrogen bonds between complementary nucleotide base pairs.

基因芯片的核心原理是两条 DNA 链之间的杂交,即互补核酸序列通过互补核苷酸碱基对之间形成氢键彼此特异配对的特性。

4. Probe-target hybridization is usually detected and quantified by detection of fluorophore-labeled, silver-labeled or chemiluminescence-labeled targets to determine relative abundance of nucleic acid sequences in the target.

检测与定量探针-靶向目标之间的杂交,通常是通过检测荧光标记的、银标记的或化学发光标记的

靶向物,来决定靶向目标中核酸序列的相对多少。

5. So fluorescently labeled target sequences that bind to a probe sequence generate a signal that depends on the strength of the hybridization determined by the number of paired bases, the hybridization conditions (such as temperature) and washing after hybridization.

所以荧光标记的靶标序列与探针结合产生的信号强度依赖于杂交配对碱基数,杂交条件(例如温度)以及杂交后的洗脱情况。

6. Total strength of the signal, from a spot (feature), depends upon the amount of target sample binding to the probes present on that spot. Microarrays use relative quantization in which the intensity of a feature is compared to the intensity of the same feature under a different condition and the identity of the feature is known by its position.

源于一个点(特性)的信号总强度,取决于该点探针所结合的靶向样品的数量。基因芯片使用相对量化,指的是一个特征的强度与不同条件下同一特征的强度的比值,而这一特征的一致性根据它的位置得知。

7. A protein microarray (or protein chip), provides an approach to identify protein-protein interactions, the substrates of protein kinases, transcription factor protein-activation or the targets of biologically active small molecules.

蛋白质微阵列(也称蛋白质芯片),可以用来鉴定蛋白质-蛋白质的相互作用、鉴定蛋白激酶的底物、鉴定活化蛋白质的转录因子或鉴定生物活性小分子的靶标。

8. The array is a piece of glass on which different molecules of protein or specific DNA binding sequences (as capture probes for the proteins) have been affixed at separate locations in an ordered manner thus forming a microscopic array.

在一块玻璃上面,将不同蛋白质分子或者特异性 DNA 序列(作为蛋白质捕获探针),按照有序方式分别黏附在不同的位置,形成微阵列。

9. The most common protein microarray is the antibody microarray, where antibodies are spotted onto the protein chip and are used as capture molecules to detect proteins from cell lysate solutions.

最常见的蛋白质微阵列是抗体微阵列。在抗体微阵列上,抗体固化在蛋白芯片上用作捕获分子,检测细胞裂解液中蛋白质。

10. More recently there has been a push towards other types of capture molecules which are more similar in their nature such as peptides oraptamers.

最近,更倾向于使用其他类型的捕获分子。这些捕获分子更接近于它们的天然状态,比如多肽或适配体。

Exercises

Ⅰ. Fill in the blanks according to the texts.

1. DNA microarray (or DNA chip) is part of the process of microarray profiling, which is also known as _____ microarray. (Text A)

2. The core principle behind microarrays is _____ between two DNA strands, the property of complementary nucleic acid sequences to specifically pair with each other by forming hydrogen bonds between complementary nucleotide base pairs. (Text A)

3. Total strength of the signal, from a spot (feature), depends upon the _____ of target sample binding to the probes present on that spot. (Text A)

4. A protein microarray (or protein chip), provides an approach to identify protein-protein interactions, the _____ of protein kinases, transcription factor protein-activation or the targets of biologically active small molecules. (Text B)

5. Antibodies are the most widely used capture molecules for the preparation of microarrays. However,

_____ are used in applications where antibodies are detected in serum. (Text B)

Ⅱ. Translate the following into Chinese.

Protein chips differ from analytical arrays, which are composed of full-length functional proteins or protein domains. They are used to study the biochemical activities of the entire proteome in a single experiment.

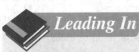

Chapter Ⅳ　Laboratory Techniques in Pathology
病理学检验技术

 Leading In

Through the study of this chapter, you will learn some common pathological laboratory techniques, as well as some basic vocabularies and expressions related to them. After studying this chapter, you will master some relevant medical terms and the glass-slides-making technique, be familiar with the process of making glass slides and biological staining and cytopathological laboratory techniques, and understand the general ideas of the texts and learning purposes of pathological laboratory techniques. Besides, you should be able to describe the process of tissue embedding and tissue blocks making in English, choose proper cytopathological laboratory techniques to make diagnoses, and determine the different parts and status of cells according to HE Staining and Giemsa Staining.

Lesson 1　Pathological Laboratory Techniques
病理学检验技术

Learning Objectives

After studying this lesson, students are expected to be able to

1. master the basic techniques of making glass slides;
2. be familiar with the process of making glass slides;
3. know about the purposes of studying pathologicallaboratory techniques;
4. describe the process of embedding the tissue and making tissue blocks in English.

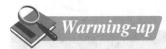 **Warming-up**

1. What is the basic pathological techniques?
2. How do we make glass slides?

Text A　Making Glass Slides
病理制片技术

Pathology is the study of diseases by scientific methods, particularly the structural and functional changes in tissues and organs. "As is our pathology, so is our medicine" said William Osler, a famous American physician and medical historian.

The development of pathology promotes the progress of pathological technology — Making Glass Slides. Gross observation with the naked eye and morphological observation at the level of optical microscope are the most traditional and basic techniques in pathological research and learning. With the development of molecular biology and the establishment of corresponding molecular pathology techniques, some new advanced techniques of making glass slides have been applied to the study of pathology and the pathological diagnosis of diseases.

Basic pathological techniques of making glass slides include tissue fixation, paraffin section, hematoxylin-eosin staining and common special staining techniques. In addition, it includes a brief overview of ancillary techniques that pathologists sometimes use (e. g. , electron microscopy).

In the past 30 years, the development of immunology, cell biology, molecular biology, cytogenetics and the application of techniques, such as immunohistochemistry, flow cytometry, image analysis and molecular biology have greatly promoted the development of traditional pathological techniques of making glass slides.

In particular, the interdisciplinary development has led to the emergence of many new branches of pathology, such as immunopathology, molecular pathology, genetic pathology and quantitative pathology, which have led to the research of diseases from the organ, tissue, cell and subcellular to the molecular level. Obviously, the techniques of making glass slides are very important, so that we can make the morphological observation more objective, repetitive and comparable.

This article aims to help students understand the process of making glass slides, from harvesting tissues to generating glass slides, producing a pathology report.

Text B Process of Making Glass Slides
病理制片过程

The process of making glass slides suitable for clinical diagnosis and histopathological analysis involves a number of steps performed in the laboratory: trimming, tissue processing, embedding, microtoming and staining.

Trimming

The first step of trimming is fixing tissues collected during the necropsy with formalin, the freshly dissected tissues are fixed with 10% formalin for 24-48 hours at room temperature. Then the formalin-fixed tissues are further cut up in order to fit into embedding cassettes.

The tissues from the same area of the organ should be trimmed in the same way and all gross lesions must be identified and included in the cassette.

Tissue Processing

In order to make paraffin wax firm, intact, and in the correct orientation for sectioning, cassettes are placed in a machine that allows the tissues to undergo a series of steps which include tissue dehydration, clearing and impregnation with paraffin wax.

Embedding

Tissue embedding is a tissue preparation technique. During embedding, tissue samples are embedded in embedding material, such as wax. A trained technician places the paraffin wax-infiltrated tissues into a metal mould, and adds additional wax into it, then moves the metal to the cooling stage, which is chilled to produce tissue blocks. When the paraffin block is transparent, removed it completely, the block is ready to be sliced. The paraffin tissue block can be stored at room temperature for years.

Microtoming

Rotary microtome is a machine for cutting a wax block into sections. Thin sections (4-6 μm) are cut using this device. First, setting the micro knife on the knife holder, and then putting the embedded tissue on the specimen holder. The operation of the microtome is based upon the rotary action of a hand wheel, a technician may start with a large thickness (15-25 μm) and go to the sections (4-6 μm). The thin wax sections

148

are floated in a water to stretch for several minutes and then carefully pick up with a clean slide. The glass slides are placed in an oven to melt off the wax, so the tissue section is ready for further experiment.

Histochemical Staining

In order to diagnose disease based on the tissues on the glass slides under the microscope, histochemical staining is needed. All the tissues are transparent before staining, so it is difficult to see the cellular structures under the microscope.

Haematoxylin and eosin (H&E) stain is the most commonlyused stain method. The haematoxylin binds to the nuclei of the cells, making them blue and the eosin binds to the cytoplasm, making it pink. After staining, mounting with a coverslip and final checking, the glass slides are transported to the pathologist.

New Words

ancillary /ˈænsəleri/ *adj.* 辅助的，副的，从属的

fixation /fɪkˈseɪʃn/ *n.* 固定，定位，定影

embed /ɪmˈbed/ *v.* ［医］植入，埋藏

cytogenetics /ˌsaɪtodʒəˈnɛtɪks/ *n.* 细胞遗传学

immunohistochemistry /ˈɪmjʊnəʊˌhɪstəʊˈkemɪstrɪ/ *n.* 免疫组织化学

multidisciplinary /ˌmʌltiˈdɪsəpləneri/ *adj.* 有关各种学问的

trimming /ˈtrɪmɪŋ/ *n.* 整理，装饰品，配料，修剪下来的东西

formalin /ˈfɔrməlɪn/ *n.* ［药］福尔马林

orientation /ˌɔːriənˈteɪʃn/ *n.* 方向，定向，适应，情况介绍

impregnation /ˌimpregˈneiʃən/ *n.* 注入，受精，怀孕，受胎

section /ˈsekʃn/ *n.* 截面，节段，型材 *v.* 把……切成片，把……作成截面

Phrases and Expressions

optical microscope	光学显微镜
molecular pathology	分子病理学
pathological diagnosis	病理学诊断
paraffin section	石蜡切片
gross lesion	肉眼损害
formalin-fixed	福尔马林固定
paraffin wax	固体石蜡
metal mould	金属铸模
specimen holder	标本夹，样品夹，试样架
melt off	熔化掉

Notes

1. Pathology is the study of diseases by scientific methods, particularly the structural and functional changes in tissues and organs. "As is our pathology, so is our medicine" said William Osler, a famous American physician and medical historian.

病理学是用科学的方法研究疾病，尤其是研究组织和器官在结构、功能上的变化。美国著名医生和医学史专家 William Osler 说："病理学为医学之本"。

2. Basic pathological techniques of making glass slides include tissue fixation, paraffin section, hematoxylin-eosin staining and common special staining techniques.

病理制片基本技术包括组织固定、石蜡切片、苏木精-伊红染色和常见的特殊染色技术。

3. In the past 30 years, the development of immunology, cell biology, molecular biology, cytogenetics and the application of techniques, such as immunohistochemistry, flow cytometry, image analysis and molecu-

lar biology have greatly promoted the development of traditional pathological techniques of making glass slides.

近30年来,免疫学、细胞生物学、分子生物学、细胞遗传学的发展以及免疫组织化学、流式细胞术、图像分析、分子生物学等技术的应用,极大地促进了传统病理制片技术的发展。

4. In particular, the interdisciplinary development has led to the emergence of many new branches of pathology, such as immunopathology, molecular pathology, genetic pathology and quantitative pathology, which have led to the research of diseases from the organ, tissue, cell and subcellular level to the molecular level.

特别是跨学科的发展,使免疫病理学、分子病理学、遗传病理学和定量病理学等许多新的病理学分支应运而生,并导致从器官、组织、细胞和亚细胞水平对疾病的研究达到了分子水平。

5. The process of making glass slides suitable for clinical diagnosis and histopathological analysis involves a number of steps performed in the laboratory: trimming, embedding, microtoming and staining.

在病理实验室中,制作适合临床诊断和组织病理学分析的玻片过程涉及多个步骤:修剪、包埋、切片和染色。

6. The tissues from the same area of the organ should be trimmed in the same way and all gross lesions must be identified and included in the cassette.

相同区域的组织病灶应以相同的方法修整,保证大体标本的病灶不被遗漏。

7. In order to make paraffin wax firm, intact, and in the correct orientation for sectioning, cassettes are placed in a machine that allows the tissues to undergo a series of steps which include tissue dehydration, clearing and impregnation with paraffin wax.

为了使石蜡块中的组织固定完整、病灶定位准确,将组织盒放置在脱水机中,组织经历一系列处理,包括组织脱水、透明和浸蜡。

8. A trained technician places the paraffin wax-infiltrated tissues into a metal mould, and adds additional wax into it, then moves the metal to the cooling stage, which is chilled to produce tissue blocks.

专业技术人员将石蜡渗过的组织放置到金属模具中,向其中注满石蜡,然后将金属模具移动到冷却系统。当石蜡块冷却至透明后,移开,制成组织蜡块。

9. Rotary microtome is a machine for cutting a wax block into sections. Thin sections (4-6 μm) are cut using this device.

组织切片机是将蜡块切割成薄切片(4~6μm)的机器。

10. Haematoxylin and eosin (H&E) stain is the most commonly used stain method. The haematoxylin binds to the nuclei of the cells, making them blue and the eosin binds to the cytoplasm, making it pink.

苏木精-伊红(H&E)染色是最常用的染色方法。苏木精可与细胞核结合,把它们染成蓝色,而伊红结合到细胞质中,将其染成粉红色。

Exercises

I. Fill in the blanks according to the texts.

1. Pathology is the study of diseases by scientific methods, particularly the structural and _____ changes in tissues and organs. (Text A)

2. Gross observation with the naked eye and morphological observation at the level of optical _____ are the most traditional and basic techniques in pathological research and learning. (Text A)

3. The first step of _____ is fixing tissues collected during the necropsy with formalin, the freshly dissected tissues are fixed with 10% formalin for 24-48 hours at room temperature. (Text B)

4. When the paraffin block is _____, removed it completely, the block is ready to be sliced. (Text B)

5. After staining, mounting with a _____ and final checking, the glass slides are transported to the pathologist. (Text B)

II. Translate the following into Chinese.

In order to diagnose disease based on the tissues on the glass slides under the microscope, histochemical staining is needed. All the tissues are transparent before staining, so it is difficult to make out the cellular structures under the microscope.

Lesson 2   Cytopathological Laboratory Techniques
细胞病理学检验技术

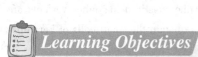

After studying this lesson, students are expected to be able to

1. master some key words and phrases;
2. be familiar with some medical terms aboutcytopathological techniques;

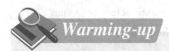

1. What is cytopathology?
2. What is Pap staining used for?

Text A   Cytopathological Test
细胞病理学检验

Cytopathology is a branch of pathology that studies and diagnoses diseases on the cellular level. Cytopathological tests are sometimes called smear tests because the samples may be smeared across a glass microscope slide for subsequent staining and microscopic examination. However, cytology samples may be prepared in other ways, including cytocentrifugation. Different types of smear tests may also be used for cancer diagnoses. In this sense, it is termed a cytological smear. Cytopathology is generally used on samples of free cells or tissue fragments, in contrast to histopathology, which studies whole tissues.

A common application of cytopathology is the Pap smear (also called Papanicolaou test, Pap test or cervical smear), which is used as a screening tool to detect precancerous cervical lesions and prevent cervical cancer. In taking a Pap smear, a speculum is used to open the vaginal canal and allow the collection of cells from the outer opening of the cervix of the uterus and the endocervix. The cells are examined under a microscope to look for abnormalities. The test aims to detect potentially pre-cancerous changes, which are usually caused by sexually transmitted humanpapillomaviruses.

The test remains an effective, widely used method for early detection of cervical pre-cancer and cancer. The test may also detect infections and abnormalities in the endocervix and endometrium. Cytopathology is also commonly used to investigate thyroid lesions, diseases involving sterile body cavities (peritoneal, pleural and cerebrospinal) and a wide range of other body sites. It is usually used to aid in the diagnosis of cancer, but also helps in the diagnosis of certain infectious diseases and other inflammatory conditions.

Text B   Pap Stain
巴氏染色

Papanicolaou stain (also called Pap stain) is amultichromatic staining histological technique developed by George Papanikolaou, the father of cytopathology. Pap staining is used to differentiate cells in smear preparations of various bodily secretions; the specimens can be gynecological smears (Pap smears), sputum, brushings, washings, urine, cerebrospinal fluid, abdominal fluid, pleural fluid, synovial fluid, seminal fluid, fine needle aspiration material, tumor touch samples, or other materials containing cells.

Pap staining is a very reliable technique. The classic form of Pap stain involves five dyes in three solutions:

(1) A nuclear stain, haematoxylin, is used to stain cell nuclei. The unmordanted haematein may be responsible for the yellow color imparted to glycogen.

(2) First OG-6 counterstain (-6 denotes the concentration of phosphotungstic acid; other variants are OG-5 and OG-8). Orange G is used to stain keratin. Its original role was to stain the small cells of keratinizing squamous cell carcinoma present in sputum.

(3) Second EA (Eosin Azure) counterstain, comprising three dyes; the number denotes the proportion of the dyes, e. g. , EA-36, EA-50, EA-65.

Eosin Y stains the superficial epithelial squamous cells, nucleoli, cilia and red blood cells.

Light Green SF yellowish stains the cytoplasm of other cells, including non-keratinized squamous cells. This dye is now quite expensive and difficult to obtain, therefore some manufacturers are switching to Fast Green FCF. However it produces visually different results and is not considered satisfactory by some.

Bismarck brown Y stains nothing and in contemporary formulations it is often omitted.

When performed properly, the stained specimen should display hues from the entire spectrum: red, orange, yellow, green, blue, and violet. The chromatin patterns are well visible, the cells from borderline lesions are easier to interpret and the photomicrographs are better. The staining results in very transparent cells, so even thick specimens with overlapping cells can be interpreted.

On a well prepared specimen, the cell nuclei are crisp blue to black. Cells with high content of keratin are yellow, glycogen stains yellow as well. Superficial cells are orange to pink, and intermediate and parabasal cells are turquoise green to blue. Metaplastic cells often stain both green and pink at once.

New Words

diagnose /ˌdaɪəɡˈnoʊs/ *vt. & vi.* 诊断,断定,判断

cancer /ˈkænsər/ *n.* 癌症,恶性肿瘤

canal /kəˈnæl/ *n.* 管道

microscope /ˈmaɪkrəskoʊp/ *n.* 显微镜

sexually /ˈsekʃəli/ *adv.* 两性之间地

abnormality /ˌæbnɔːrˈmæləti/ *n.* 畸形,变态

cavity /ˈkævəti/ *n.* 腔,洞

haematein /ˌhɛməˈtiːn/ *n.* 氧化苏木精

lesion /ˈliːʒn/ *n.* 功能障碍

dye /daɪ/ *n.* 染色,染料

nuclei /ˈnjʊklɪˌai/ *n.* 核心,核子

Phrases and Expressions

smear tests	涂片检查,子宫抹片检查
cytological smear	细胞涂片
Pap smear	帕普涂片,巴氏涂片,宫颈涂片
cervical lesion	子宫颈病变
Papanicolaou stain	巴氏染色法
gynecological smear	妇科涂片
phosphotungstic acid	磷钨酸
Bismarck brown Y stains	俾斯麦棕 Y 染色剂

| superficial cell | 表层细胞 |
| parabasal cell | 副底层细胞 |

Notes

1. Cytopathological tests are sometimes called smear tests because the samples may be smeared across a glass microscope slide for subsequent staining and microscopic examination.

细胞病理学检查有时被称为涂片检查,因为样本可能被涂在玻璃载玻片上,用于后续染色和显微镜检查。

2. Cytopathology is generally used on samples of free cells or tissue fragments, in contrast to histopathology, which studies whole tissues.

相比之下,细胞病理学通常使用游离细胞或组织碎片为标本,组织病理学以完整组织为标本。

3. In taking a Pap smear, a speculum is used to open the vaginal canal and allow the collection of cells from the outer opening of the cervix of the uterus and the endocervix.

进行巴氏涂片检查时,使用窥器扩开阴道,从宫颈外口和宫颈内膜上收集细胞。

4. Cytopathology is also commonly used to investigate thyroid lesions, diseases involving sterile body cavities (peritoneal, pleural, and cerebrospinal), and a wide range of other body sites.

细胞病理学也常用于检查甲状腺病变、机体无菌腔隙(腹膜腔、胸膜腔和脑脊髓腔)以及其他广泛部位的相关疾病。

5. Pap staining is used to differentiate cells in smear preparations of various bodily secretions。

巴氏染色可用于鉴别各种机体分泌物涂片上的细胞。

6. A nuclear stain, haematoxylin, is used to stain cell nuclei. The unmordanted haematein may be responsible for the yellow color imparted to glycogen.

苏木精用于细胞核染色。未经媒染的苏木红可能与糖原被着色成黄色有关。

7. Eosin Y stains the superficial epithelial squamous cells, nucleoli, cilia and red blood cells.

伊红可使浅表鳞状细胞、核仁、纤毛和红细胞染色。

8. The chromatin patterns are well visible, the cells from borderline lesions are easier to interpret and the photomicrographs are better.

染色质形态易于见到,病变边缘部位的细胞在读片时更易于被解读,且显微照片拍摄效果更好。

9. On a well prepared specimen, the cell nuclei are crisp blue to black.

在一个制备良好的标本上,细胞核是清晰的蓝到黑。

Exercises

Ⅰ. Fill in the blanks according to the texts.

1. Cytopathology is a branch of pathology that studies and _____ diseases on the cellular level. (Text A)

2. The test remains an _____, widely used method for early detection of cervical pre-cancer and cancer. (Text A)

3. Pap staining is a very _____ technique. (Text B)

4. This dye is now quite _____ and difficult to obtain, therefore some manufacturers are switching to Fast Green FCF. However it produces visually different results and is not considered satisfactory by some. (Text B)

5. Metaplastic cells often stain both green and _____ at once. (Text B)

Ⅱ. Translate the following into Chinese.

Fine-needle Aspiration Cytology (FNAC or Needle aspiration biopsy) — A needle attached to a syringe is used to collect cells from lesions or masses in various body organs. FNAC can be performed under palpation guidance, the clinician can feel the lesion on a mass in superficial regions like the neck, thyroid or breast. FNAC may also be assisted by ultrasound for sampling of deep-seated lesions within the body that cannot be localized via palpation.

Lesson 3 Biological Staining
生物染色

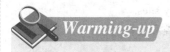

Learning Objectives

After studying this lesson, students are expected to be able to

1. master some key words and phrases;
2. be familiar with some medical terms about biological staining;
3. know about the main idea of the whole texts.

Warming-up

1. What is staining?
2. What is dyestuff?

Text A   Stain and Stainability of Biological Tissue
染色和生物组织的染色性

Staining is an auxiliary technique used in microscopy to enhance contrast in the microscopic image. Dye is a colored substance, also called a dyestuff, which imparts more or less permanent color to other materials. Compounds used for dyeing are generally organic compounds containing conjugated double bonds. The group producing the colour is the chromophore; othernoncoloured groups that influence or intensify the colour are called auxochromes.

Stains and dyes are frequently used in biology and medicine to highlight structures in biological tissues for viewing, often with the aid of different microscopes. Stains may be used to define and examine bulk tissues (e.g., muscle fibers or connective tissues), cell populations (e.g., different blood cells), or organelles within individual cells. In biochemistry it involves adding a class-specific (DNA, proteins, lipids, carbohydrates, etc.) dye to a substrate to qualify or quantify the presence of a specific compound. Staining and fluorescent tagging can serve similar purposes. Biological staining is also used to mark cells in flow cytometry, and to flag proteins or nucleic acids in gel electrophoresis.

Positive affinity for a specific stain may be designated by the suffix-philic. For example, tissues that can be stained by an azure dye may be referred to as azurophilic. This may also be used for more generalized staining properties, such as acidophilic for tissues easily stained by acidic stains (H&E stain is most representative), basophilic when staining in basic dyes and amphophilic when staining with either acid or basic dyes. In contrast, chromophobic tissues do not take up coloured dye readily.

An acidophile (or acidophil) is a term used byhistologists to describe a particular staining pattern of cells and tissues when using H&E stain. The most common dye of such kind is eosin, which stains acidophilic organisms red and is the source of the related term eosinophilic. Basophilic is a technical term used by histologists. It describes the microscopic appearance of cells and tissues after a histological section has been stained with a basic dye. The most common dye of the kind is haematoxylin.

Text B　HE Stain and Giemsa Stain
苏木精-伊红染色和吉姆萨染色

Hematoxylin and eosin（H&E）stain is a popular staining method in histology. The staining method involves application of hemalum, which is a complex formed from aluminium ions and oxidized haematoxylin. It stains nuclei of cells blue. The nuclear staining is followed by being counterstained with an aqueous or alcoholic solution of Eosin Y. The eosinophilic structures of cells appear in various shades of red, pink or orange. Eosin is a fluorescent red dye resulting from the action of bromine on fluorescein. It can be used to stain cytoplasm, collagen and muscle fibers for examination under the microscope. Structures that stain readily with eosin are termed eosinophilic. The eosinophilic are generally composed of intracellular or extracellular protein. The Lewy bodies and Mallory bodies are examples of eosinophilic structures. Most of the cytoplasm is eosinophilic. Red blood cells are stained intensely red.

Giemsa stain, named after Gustav Giemsa, an early German microbiologist, is used in cytogenetics and for the histopathological diagnosis of malaria and other parasites. Giemsa's solution is a mixture of methylene blue, eosin, and azure B. The stain is usually prepared from commercially available Giemsa powder.

Giemsa stain is a classic blood film stain for peripheral blood smears and bone marrow specimens. A thin film of the specimen on a microscope slide is fixed in pure methanol for 30 seconds, by immersing it or by putting a few drops of methanol on the slide. The slide is immersed to a freshly prepared 5% Giemsa stain solution for 20-30 minutes, then flushed with tap water and left to dry. A blood film or peripheral blood smear stained in such a way allows the various blood cells to be examined microscopically. Erythrocytes stain pink, platelets show a light pale pink, lymphocyte cytoplasm stains sky blue, monocyte cytoplasm stains pale blue, and leukocyte nuclear chromatin stains magenta.

Giemsa stain is specific for the phosphate groups of DNA and attaches itself to regions of DNA where there are high amounts of adenine-thymine bonding. It is used in Giemsa banding, commonly called G-banding, to stain chromosomes and often used to create an idiogram.

New Words

auxiliary /ɔːgˈzɪliəri/ *adj.* 辅助的,副的,附加的

permanent /ˈpɜːrmənənt/ *adj.* 永久的,永恒的,不变的

bulk /bʌlk/ *n.* 大块

histologist /hisˈtɔlədʒist/ *n.* ［解剖］组织学家,组织论学家

haematoxylin /ˌhiːməˈtɔksilin/ *n.* 苏木精

eosin /ˈiːəusin/ *n.* 曙红（鲜红色的染料）

alcoholic /ˌælkəˈhɑːlɪk/ *adj.* 酒精的,含酒精的

collagen /ˈkɑːlədʒən/ *n.* ［生化］胶原,胶原质

fiber /ˈfaɪbɚ/ *n.* 纤维,光纤（等于fibre）

malaria /məˈleəriə/ *n.* ［内科］疟疾,瘴气

available /əˈveɪləbl/ *adj.* 可获得的,可购得的,可找到的,有空的

immerse /ɪˈmɜːrs/ *vt.* 沉浸,使陷入

chromatin /ˈkrɒmətɪn/ *n.* 核染色质,核染质

Phrases and Expressions

organic compound	有机化合物
fluorescent tagging	荧光标记
histological section	组织切片
Mallory body	酒精小体,马洛里小体

Giemsa stain	吉姆萨染色
methylene blue	亚甲蓝
tap water	自来水
adenine-thymine bonding	腺嘌呤-胸腺嘧啶键合

Notes

1. Compounds used for dyeing are generally organic compounds containing conjugated double bonds.
用来染色的化合物通常是含有共轭双键的有机物。

2. Stains and dyes are frequently used in biology and medicine to highlight structures in biological tissues for viewing, often with the aid of different microscopes.
在生物学和医学中,染色剂和染料经常被用于突出生物组织的结构以供观察,通常需借助不同类别的显微镜。

3. In biochemistry it involves adding a class-specific (DNA, proteins, lipids, carbohydrates, etc.) dye to a substrate to qualify or quantify the presence of a specific compound.
生物化学中,它涉及在基质中加入特定类别的染料来限定或量化特定化合物(DNA、蛋白质、脂类、碳水化合物等)的存在。

4. An acidophile (or acidophil) is a term used byhistologists to describe a particular staining pattern of cells and tissues when using H&E stain.
嗜酸性一词,被组织学家用来描述苏木精和伊红(H&E)染色细胞和组织所显示的一种特殊染色模式。

5. The most common dye of such kind is eosin, which stains acidophilic organisms red and is the source of the related term eosinophilic.
这种染料最常见的是伊红,嗜酸性生物体被伊红染成红色,这就是相关术语嗜伊红的来源。

6. Hematoxylin and eosin (H&E) stain is a popular staining method in histology.
苏木精和伊红(H&E)染色,是一种常用的组织学染色方法。

7. The nuclear staining is followed by being counterstained with an aqueous or alcoholic solution of Eosin Y. The eosinophilic structures of cells appear in various shades of red, pink or orange.
核染色后,用含有伊红 Y 的水溶液或醇溶液复染,被伊红 Y 染色的成分,其嗜酸性结构呈现红色、粉红色或橘红色等不同的色彩。

8. Giemsa stain, named after Gustav Giemsa, an early German microbiologist, is used in cytogenetics and for the histopathological diagnosis of malaria and other parasites.
吉姆萨染色是以早期德国微生物学家古斯塔夫·吉姆萨的名字命名的,被用于细胞遗传学和疟疾及其他寄生虫的组织病理学诊断。

9. A blood film or peripheral blood smear stained in such a way allows the various blood cells to be examined microscopically.
血液涂片或外周血涂片,以这种方式染色便于各种血细胞的显微镜检查。

10. It is specific for the phosphate groups of DNA and attaches itself to regions of DNA where there are high amounts of adenine-thymine bonding.
它对 DNA 的磷酸基团有特异性,结合到腺嘌呤-胸腺嘧啶(A-T)键含量高的 DNA 区域。

Exercises

Ⅰ. Fill in the blanks according to the texts.

1. _____ affinity for a specific stain may be designated by the suffix-philic. (Text A)

2. Basophilic is a _____ term used by histologists. (Text A)

3. The staining method _____ application of hemalum, which is a complex formed from aluminiumions and oxidized haematoxylin. (Text B)

4. A thin film of the specimen on a microscope _____ is fixed in pure methanol for 30 seconds, by immersing it or by putting a few drops of methanol on the slide. (Text B)

5. Erythrocytes stain pink, platelets show a light _____ pink, lymphocyte cytoplasm stains sky blue, monocyte cytoplasm stains pale blue, and leukocyte nuclear chromatin stains magenta. (Text B)

Ⅱ. Translate the following into Chinese.

In vitro staining involves colouring cells or structures that are no longer living. Certain stains are often combined to reveal more details and features than a single stain alone. Combined with specific protocols for fixation and sample preparation, scientists and physicians can use these standard techniques as consistent, repeatable diagnostic tools. A counterstain is stain that makes cells or structures more visible, when not completely visible with the principal stain.

Chapter V

Extended Reading
拓展阅读

Leading In

Through the study of this chapter, you will learn vocabularies related to clinical laboratory professionals, medical terminologies, clinical test reports and imported medical laboratory instruments. You will be familiar with the educational history of clinical laboratory personnel, the construction of medical terminologies, the format of clinical test reports and the main button bars of the AU480. You will also know about the meaning of roots and affixes, the structure and routine operation of i1000SR and the operation flow of XN-550. Furthermore, you will have the ability to acquire the meaning of medical terms according to roots and affixes, read clinical test reports in English, identify the button bars and the symbols of display correctly, and perform some related operations.

Lesson 1   Professionals within the Clinical Laboratory
临床检验人员

Learning Objectives

After studying this lesson, students are expected to be able to
1. master some key words and phrases;
2. be familiar with the educational history of clinical laboratory personnel;
3. know about several kinds of clinical laboratory professionals.

Warming-up

1. How many disciplines do students in laboratory medicine mainly study?
2. What are the differences between CLS and CLT?

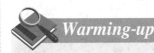

Text A   Clinical Laboratory Professionals
临床检验人员

Medical Laboratory Technology is a young profession started in the 1920s. Since then, most laboratory testings have been done by clinical laboratory professionals. Students in laboratory medicine mainly study four disciplines, namely, hematology, chemistry, microbiology and immunohematology.

Medical Laboratory Scientist

A medical laboratory scientist is a healthcare professional who performs chemical, hematological, immunologic, microscopic and bacteriological diagnostic analyses on body fluids such as blood, urine or sputum. Medical laboratory scientists work in clinical laboratories at hospitals, reference labs, and biotechnology labs.

Pathologist

A pathologist is a doctor who has specialized in pathology after receiving his or her medical degree. Pathology is the study of blood, fluid, and tissue samples, which allow doctors to make diagnoses of various illnesses by looking for specific factors lacking or present in these samples. In medical care, this professional is a very valuable part of the medical team, since many diseases are diagnosed or ruled out by microscopic and lab analysis of fluid or tissue samples.

Phlebotomist

Phlebotomists are people trained to draw blood from patients for clinical or medical testings. Phlebotomists collect blood primarily by performing venipunctures. Blood may be collected from infants by means of a heel stick. Some explain their work to patients and provide assistance when patients have adverse reactions after their blood is drawn.

Histotechnologist

A histotechnologist is a highly specialized person in the medical field and is important to the treatment of patients. They perform diagnostic tests on patients' tissue samples to examine the microscopic aspects of diseases. In addition to diagnosing diseases at the cellular level, they provide guidance on how to treat these diseases in a way that is specifically suitable to a patient's pathology.

Clinical Biochemist

A clinical biochemist is a lab-based medical professional, responsible for the analysis and explanation of results obtained through the diagnostic testing of physiological samples (both solid and fluid). They often work in research capacities, studying biological systems and organisms. This can include the study of living tissue, molecules, and genetic patterns. Typically, these professionals work in laboratories conducting experiments in order to analyze the results. Sometimes, clinical biochemists must work long hours to finish a particular project.

Biomedical Scientist

A biomedical scientist is ascientist trained in biology, particularly in the context of medicine. These scientists work to gain knowledge on the main principles of how the human body works and to find new ways to treat diseases by developing advanced diagnostic tools or new therapeutic strategies. The research of biomedical scientists is referred to as biomedical research. Biomedical scientists make research in a laboratory setting, using living organisms as models. These can include cultured human or animal cells, such as flies, fish, mice, and so on. They may also work with human tissue specimens to do experiments.

All of the above are laboratory professionals. Without these professionals, diagnosis and treatment would be more difficult, wasting more time and more money.

Text B   Education History of Clinical Laboratory Personnel
临床检验人员的教育历史

The clinical laboratory professional plays an important role in the diagnosis and treatment of a patient. The testing results can help to determine or rule out a putative diagnosis of disease, such as diabetes or other chronic illness. To prepare for this profession, the education is very serious. The education of clinical laboratory science is closely linked with pathology, but they are also different from each other. Clinical laboratory science has its own educational standards. However, pathology is its origin. Pathology is widely defined as the study of disease, including the cause, development and results of the disease process.

The education of clinical laboratory personnel evolved from on-the-job training to formal education programs. In the early days, the training was mainly in the hospital. Then, academic programs were developed in the university. In order to reflect the function of the laboratory profession, terminology appeared. The new term explains the responsibilities, career chances and the role of the laboratory personnel. There are two types of clinical laboratory professionals — clinical laboratory scientist (CLS) and clinical laboratory technician (CLT). CLS refers to a graduate with a baccalaureate degree and CLT refers to one with an associate degree. At present, both are used in most prints and documents.

There are various types of educational programs for clinical laboratory scientist. CLS programs have "3+1", "4+1", "2+2" or integrated program.

A "3+1" program often provides basic knowledge on science and meets general education requirements of a college or university. During the first 3 years in this program, students take courses. In the forth year, students spend 52 weeks at a hospital. By learning in the hospital, they get doctors' formal teaching and more practical experience.

In a "4+1" program, one must have a baccalaureate degree, such as biology. The program offers one year of training which includes lectures and practical experience about every discipline. In the end, students receive a post baccalaureate degree of this program.

In a "2+2" program, students need to take courses and have trainings during their first two years. Then, students need to make a formal application to continue the next 2 years' study. In the final 2 years, students take clinical laboratory science lectures and laboratory courses.

An integrated program is similar to the "2+2" program. However, students can take CLS courses in the first 3 years. In the forth year, students finish this program.

Clinical laboratory technician programs are usually offered in a community college or junior college. In the end, students receive an associate degree. They learn science and take general education courses in the first year and practice clinical techinques in the second year. When they graduate, they can take some national certification examinations.

New Words

professional /prə'feʃənl/ *adj.* 专业的,职业的 *n.* 专业人员

bacteriological /bækˌtɪrɪə'lɑːdʒɪkl/ *adj.* [微]细菌学的,细菌学上的

diagnostic /ˌdaɪəg'nɑːstɪk/ *adj.* 诊断的,特征的 *n.* 诊断法,诊断结论

biotechnology /ˌbaɪoʊtek'nɑːlədʒi/ *n.* [生物]生物技术,生物工艺学

pathologist /pə'θɑːlədʒɪst/ *n.* 病理学家

phlebotomist /fli'bɒtəmist/ *n.* 采血员,抽血者

venipuncture /'veniˌpʌŋktʃə/ *n.* 静脉穿刺(等于 venepuncture)

histotechnologist /ˌhistəˌtek'nɑːlədʒist/ *n.* 组织病理技术员

cellular /'seljələr/ *adj.* 细胞的,由细胞组成的

personnel /ˌpɜːrsə'nel/ *n.* 人员

putative /'pjuːtətɪv/ *adj.* 推定的,假定的

terminology /ˌtɜːrmɪ'nɑːlədʒi/ *n.* 术语,术语学,用词

certification /ˌsɜːrtɪfɪ'keɪʃn/ *n.* 证明,鉴定

Phrases and Expressions

draw blood	抽血
heel stick	足跟采血
adverse reaction	不良反应
baccalaureate degree	学士学位
associate degree	大专文凭

integrated program	综合课程
post baccalaureate degree	硕士学位
on the basis of . . .	根据……

Notes

1. A medical laboratory scientist is a healthcare professional who performs chemical, hematological, immunologic, microscopic and bacteriological diagnostic analyses on body fluids such as blood, urine or sputum.

医学检验科学家是医疗专业人士，对体液（例如血液、尿液或痰液等）进行化学、血液学、免疫学、显微镜学和细菌学诊断分析。

2. A pathologist is a doctor who has specialized in pathology after receiving his or her medical degree.

病理学家是在接受医学学位后专门从事病理学的医生。

3. Phlebotomists are people trained to draw blood from patients for clinical or medical testings.

采血员是指因临床或医学检测需要，经培训后为病人抽血的人。

4. Ahistotechnologist is a highly specialized person in the medical field and is important to the treatment of patients.

组织病理技术员是医学领域高度专业化的一类人，对病人的治疗非常重要。

5. A clinical biochemist is a lab-based medical professional, responsible for the analysis and explanation of results obtained through the diagnostic testing of physiological samples (both solid and fluid).

临床生化学家是基于实验室的医学专业人员，负责分析和解释通过对生理样品（固体和流体）的诊断性测试获得的结果。

6. A biomedical scientist is ascientist trained in biology, particularly in the context of medicine.

生物医学科学家是受过生物学培训的科学家，尤其是在医学背景下。

7. The education of clinical laboratory personnel evolved from on-the-job training to formal education programs.

临床检验人员的教育经历了从在职培训到正规教育的过程。

8. Clinical laboratory technician programs are usually offered in a community college or junior college.

临床检验技术员的学习课程是在社区学院或大专院校进行的。

Exercises

Ⅰ. Fill in the blanks according to the texts.

1. Students in laboratory medicine mainlystudy four _____, namely, hematology, chemistry, microbiology and immunohematology. (Text A)

2. In medical care, this professional is a very valuable part of the medical team, since many diseases are diagnosed or _____ by microscopic and lab analysis of fluid or tissue samples. (Text A)

3. They often work in _____, studying biological systems and organisms. (Text A)

4. The clinical laboratory professional plays an important role in the _____ and treatment of a patient. (Text B)

5. Clinical laboratory _____ programs are usually offered in a community college or junior college. (Text B)

Ⅱ. Translate the following into Chinese.

The clinical laboratory professional plays an important role in the diagnosis and treatment of a patient. The testing results can help to determine or eliminate a putative diagnosis of disease, such as diabetes or other chronic illness. To prepare for this profession, the education is very serious. The education of clinical laboratory science is closely linked with pathology, but they are also different from each other.

Lesson 2 Medical Terminology
医学术语

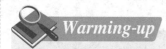

After studying this lesson, students are expected to be able to

1. master the construction of medical terminology;
2. be familiar with some common medical affixes and roots;
3. know about the classification of medical terminology;
4. get the meaning of a medical term with the help of the affix and root.

1. What is medical terminology?
2. Can you tell the construction of medical terms?

Text A Brief Introduction to Medical Terminology
医学术语简介

Medical terminology refers to the study of terms that are used in medicine only, and it is a branch of morphology which is concerned with the internal organization of words. As professionals of clinical laboratory, we know that many medical words are difficult to spell and pronounce. Studying the rules of lexical construction will help us learn medical words better and more easily.

Almost every medical term can be divided into two parts, the root and the affix, and the affix falls into two parts, i. e. , the prefix and the suffix. A prefix always comes at the beginning of a word, which relates to the meaning of a word. For example, atrophy and hypertrophy have common root and different prefix. Atrophy means "(of an organ or part of the body) to waste away, become smaller", while hypertrophy means "increase in the number or size of cells in a tissue". A suffix usually appears at the end of a word, most of which concern the property of a word, such as pediatrician and pediatric, surgeon and surgical, physician and physically. In addition to that, some suffixes also pertain to the meaning, like bacteremia and bacteriuria, leukemia and leukocyte, neurology and neurologist. A root is the base form of a word and can't be further analyzed without changing its meaning, which undertakes the main meaning of a word.

A root is usually combined with a prefix or a suffix by a combining vowel, and the vowel is usually "O". When coming up against medical terms, you should pay attention to prefix, root and suffix. If the first letter of a suffix is a vowel, the combining vowel should be deleted when the suffix is combined with other morphemes. For example, gastritis contains gastr- and -itis, and the first letter of the suffix is "i" which is a vowel, so gastritis is not gastroitis.

You can infer the meaning of a new word with the help of the root and affix, if you have acquired some relevant morphemes. For example, electrocardiogram consists of a prefix: electr-, a root: -cardi-, a suffix: -gram and two combining vowels "O". Reading a medical term from the suffix backward to the prefix, as to electrocardiogram, -gram refers to reading or recording, -cardi- pertains to the heart , and electr- means electrical. In accordance with the meaning of the suffix, the root and the prefix, you can conjecture the meaning of electrocardiogram: the electrical recording of the heart's cycle or activity.

Text B Classification of Medical Terminology
医学术语分类

In accordance to medical subject, medical terminology consists of the terms of foundation medicine and of clinical medicine. According to human body, medical terminology can be divided into more than 20 categories, such as the terms of digestive system, respiratory system, cardiovascular system, urinary system, nervous system, genital system, cell genetics, diagnostics, stomatognathic system. In addition to that, medical terminology also includes positional terms, color terms, shape terms and so forth. There are some common affixes of several medical categories listed below.

Digestive System

Affix	Chinese Meaning	Domination	Example
pharyngo-	咽	pharynx	pharyngectomy 咽切除术
jejuno-	空肠	jejunum	jejunostomy 空肠造口术
ileo-	回肠	ileum	ileorrhaphy 回肠缝合术
-pepsia	消化	pepsia	dyspepsia 消化不良
-gest-		digest	digestion 消化，领悟
ano-	肛门	anus	anoplasty 肛门成形术
cholecysto-	胆囊	cholecyst	cholecystostomy 胆囊造口术
appendio-	阑尾	appendix	appendicitis 阑尾炎，盲肠炎
sigmoido-	乙状结肠	sigmoid	sigmoidopexy 乙状结肠固定术
hepato-	肝	hepar（liver）	hepatobiliary 肝胆（管）的
colo-	结肠	colon	colopexy 结肠固定术
typhlo-	盲肠	typhlon	typhlocolitis 盲肠结肠炎
ceco-		cecum	cecocele 盲肠突出
entero-	肠	enteron	enterogastritis 肠胃炎
-duodeno-	十二指肠	duodenum	Duodenostomy 十二指肠切除术
esophago-	食管	esophagus	esophagology 食管病学
procto-	直肠，肛部	procto	proctodynia 肛部痛
recto-	直肠	rectum	rectorrhaphy 直肠缝术
gastro-	胃的，与胃有关的	gastric	gastrorrhagia 胃出血

Respiratory System

Affix	Chinese Meaning	Domination	Example
bronchio-	支气管	bronchus	Bronchiolitis 毛细支气管炎
pleuro-	胸膜	pleura	pleurorrhea 胸膜腔渗液
glotto-	声门	glottis	glottogram 声门图
pneumono-	肺的	pneumonic	pneumonopathy 肺脏疾病
pulmo-	肺的，肺病的	pulmonic	pulmonitis 肺炎
pulmono-	与肺有关的	pulmonology	pulmonohepatic 肺肝的
pneumato-	气体，呼吸	pneumatocele	pneumatometry 肺活量计
-spiro-	呼吸的	respiratory	spirography 呼吸运动记录器
-pnea	窒息，呼吸暂停	apnea	bradypnea 呼吸徐缓
tracheo-	气管	trachea	tracheoaerocele 气管气疝
rhino-	鼻尖	rhinarium	rhinoplastic 鼻整形术的
naso-	鼻（骨）	nose（nasal）	nasoscope 电光鼻镜
laryngo-	咽喉	laryngopharynx	laryngoptosis 喉下垂
-alveolo-	肺泡，齿槽	alveoli	interalveolar 牙槽间的

163

Cardiovascular System

Affix	Chinese Meaning	Domination	Example
sphygmo-	脉搏	sphygmus	sphygmogram 脉搏记录仪
arterio-	动脉	arteriole（artery）	arterio 动脉
phlebo-	静脉	phlebo	phleboid 静脉炎
veno-		vena（vein）	venosclerosis 静脉硬化
aorto-	主动脉	aorta	aortogastric 主动脉和胃的
angio-	血管（学）	angiography	angiopathy 血管病
vaso-	血管	vessel（vaso）	vasodepression 血管减压
ventriculo-	心室	ventricle	ventriculomyotomy 心室肌切开术
valvulo-	瓣膜	valve	valvoplasty 瓣膜成形术
-cuspid	尖瓣，瓣	cuspid	tricuspid 三尖瓣
cardio-	心脏（病）的	cardiac	cardiocentesis 心脏穿刺术
atrio-	心房	atrium	atriotomy 心房切开术
capillaro-	细血管	capillary	capillaropathy 毛细管病
capillari-			capillariasis 毛细线虫病
hemo-	出血	hemorrhage	hemochrome 血色素
hema-		haemorrhage	hematimeter 血细胞计数器
hemato-	血液（学）	hematology	hematocyanin 血蓝蛋白,血蓝质
sangui-	血,血液	sanguis	sanguiferous 带血的,含血的

New Words

atrophy /ˈætrəfi/ n. ［病理］萎缩

hypertrophy /haɪˈpɜːrtrəfi/ n. ［病理］肥大,肥厚,过度增大

pediatrician /ˌpidiəˈtrɪʃən/ n. 儿科医生（等于 paediatrician）

pediatric /ˌpiːdiˈætrɪk/ adj. 小儿科的

surgeon /ˈsɜːrdʒən/ n. 外科医生

physically /ˈfɪzɪkli/ adv. 身体上地

bacteremia /ˌbæktəˈrimiə/ n. ［内科］菌血症

bacteriuria /bækˌtiəriˈjuəriə/ n. ［泌尿］菌尿症,细菌尿

neurology /nʊˈrɑːlədʒi/ n. 神经病学,神经学

neurologist /nʊˈrɑːlədʒɪst/ n. 神经学家,神经科专业医师

gastritis /gæˈstraɪtɪs/ n. ［内科］胃炎

relevant /ˈreləvənt/ adj. 相关的

morpheme /ˈmɔːrfiːm/ n. ［语］词素

electrocardiogram /ɪˌlektroʊˈkɑːrdioʊgræm/ n. ［内科］心电图

conjecture /kənˈdʒektʃər/ vt. 推测,揣摩

Phrases and Expressions

refer to ...　　　　　　　　　指的是……

be concerned with ...　　　　涉及……,关心……

fall into ...	分成……
relate to ...	与……有关
take ... for example	以……为例
in addition to ...	除……之外(还有,也)
pertain to	关于
come up against ...	碰到……
consist of ...	由……组成
in accordance to ...	根据……

Notes

1. Medical terminology refers to the study of terms that are used in medicine only, and it is a branch of morphology which is concerned with the internal organization of words.

医学术语仅研究用于医学的术语,它是词法的一个分支。词法专门研究词的内部结构。

2. A root is the base form of a word and can't be further analyzed without changing its meaning, which undertakes the main meaning of a word.

词根是词的基本形式,在不改变词义的情况下就无法进一步分解,承载着词的主要意义。

Exercises

Ⅰ. Fill in the blanks according to the texts.

1. Almost every medical term can be divided into two parts, the root and the _____. (Text A)

2. A root is usually combined with a prefix or a suffix by a combining _____. (Text A)

3. If the first letter of a suffix is a vowel, the combining vowel should be _____. (Text A)

4. You can infer the meaning of a new word with the help of the root and the affix, if you have acquired some relevant _____. (Text A)

5. In accordance to medical subject, medical terminology consists of the terms of foundation medicine and the words of _____ medicine. (Text B)

Ⅱ. Translate the following into Chinese.

A root is usually combined with a prefix or a suffix by a combining vowel, and the vowel is usually "O". When coming up against medical terms, you should pay attention to prefix, root and suffix. If the first letter of a suffix is a vowel, the combining vowel should be deleted.

Lesson 3 Clinical Test Report
临床检验报告

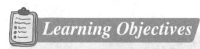 **Learning Objectives**

After studying this lesson, students are expected to be able to

1. master some key words and expressions related to clinical test reports;

2. be familiar with the format of clinical test reports;

3. read clinical test reports correctly.

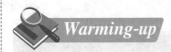

Warming-up

1. What is the main function of red blood cells in the blood?
2. How many types of hepatitis do you know?

Text A　Test Reports of Full Blood Count and Liver Function
血常规与肝功能检验报告

Full Blood Count Test Report

The Full Blood Count (FBC blood test), also known as the Full Blood Examination (FBE) or Complete Blood Count (CBC), provides important information about the numbers and development of cells in the blood: red blood cells that carry oxygen, white blood cells that fight infection and platelets that help blood to clot.

Abnormalities in any of these can tell us a lot about a range of important conditions including some nutritional factors, medications and, occasionally, exposure to toxic substances. Abnormalities in the FBE blood test can be caused by anemia, infections, some blood cancers such as leukemia and some inherited conditions.

Table 5-1 shows a full blood count test report.

Table 5-1　Full Blood Count Test Report

PATHOLOGY: Final Report

Req No:	P468620	P469129		
Date:	04/08/18	05/08/18		
Time:	15:45	05:40	Units	Ref Range

BLOOD COUNT

WCC	6.8	6.3	$\times 10^9$/L	4.0-11.0
Hb	132	126	g/L	115-160
Plat	372	336	$\times 10^9$/L	150-450
HCT	0.416	0.396	L/L	0.33-0.47
RCC	4.98	4.66	$\times 10^{12}$/L	3.8-5.2
MCV	83.5	85	fL	80-100
MCH	26.5	27	pg	27.0-33.0
MCHC	317	318	g/L	310-365
RDW	13.2	13.2	%	<16.5

White Cell Differential

Neuts	3.47	2.86	$\times 10^9$/L	1.8-7.7
Lymphs	2.31	2.39	$\times 10^9$/L	1.0-4.0
Mono	0.54	0.61	$\times 10^9$/L	0.2-1.0
Eos	0.39	0.43	$\times 10^9$/L	0.04-0.5
Baso	0.07	0.04	$\times 10^9$/L	<0.1
LeftShift	0.03	0.01	$\times 10^9$/L	
LeftShif %	0.4	0.2	%	<1.0

Liver Function Test Report

The Liver Function Tests (LFT) are a group of blood tests that measure some enzymes, proteins, and substances that are produced or excreted by the liver. The amount of these substances in the blood can be affected by liver injury.

There are many diseases, infections and lifestyle factors that can cause damage to the liver. A significant amount of liver damage may be present before symptoms appear, so pathology is key to early diagnosis and effective treatment.

Table 5-2 shows a liver function test report.

Table 5-2　Liver Function Test Report

CUMULATIVE SERUM BIOCHEMISTRY

Date			30/08/18
Time			00:00
Lab No			69218180
Sodium	136	mmol/L	137-147
Potass	3.5	mmol/L	3.5-5.0
Chloride	102	mmol/L	96-109
Bicarb	24	mmol/L	25-33
An. Gap	14	mmol/L	4-17
Gluc	4.5	mmol/L	3.0-7.7
Urea	3.0	mmol/L	2.0-7.0
Creat	55	μmol/L	40-110
eGFR	>90	mL/min	>59
Urate	0.21	mmol/L	0.14-0.35
T. Bili	6	μmol/L	2-20
Alk. P	51	U/L	30-115
GGT	19	U/L	0-45
ALT	15	U/L	0-45
AST	18	U/L	0-41
LD	162	U/L	80-250
Calcium	2.29	mmol/L	2.25-2.65
Corr. Ca	2.48	mmol/L	2.25-2.65
Phos	0.8	mmol/L	0.8-1.5
T. Prot	70	g/L	60-82
Alb	36	g/L	35-50
Glob	34	g/L	20-40
Chol	5.7	mmol/L	3.6-6.7
Trig	0.8	mmol/L	0.3-4.0

Text B　Test Reports of Rheumatoid Arthritis and Hepatitis
类风湿性关节炎与肝炎检验报告

Rheumatoid Arthritis Test Report

Rheumatoid arthritis, an autoimmune disorder, mainly affects your joints and occurs when your immune system mistakenly attacks your own body's tissues. Unlike the wear-and-tear damage of osteoarthritis, rheumatoid arthritis affects the lining of your joints, causing a painful swelling that can eventually result in bone erosion and joint deformity.

People with rheumatoid arthritis often have an elevated erythrocyte sedimentation rate (ESR, or sed rate) or C-reactive protein (CRP), which may indicate the presence of an inflammatory process in the body. Other common blood tests look for rheumatoid factors and anti-cyclic citrullinated peptide (anti-CCP) antibodies. Table 5-3 shows a test report of rheumatoid.

Table 5-3 Rheumatoid Arthritis Test Report

RHEUMATOID SEROLOGY

Rheumatoid Factor (RA latex)   <14 IU/mL   (0-14)

COMMENT

Result within normal limits.

Rheumatoid factor (RF) may be detected in up to 60% of patients with rheumatoid arthritis. However RF is also found in other disease states including autoimmune diseases, infective diseases and neoplasm. RF may also be detected in healthy individuals.

Anti-CCP antibody is a specific test for rheumatoid arthritis and has prognostic significance. Anti-CCP antibody testing is recommended in the diagnosis of rheumatoid arthritis.

Hepatitis Test Report

Hepatitis is an illness that inflames and damages your liver. It affects the liver's ability to do its job, which includes making proteins and clearing the blood of unwanted impurities. Hepatitis is usually, but not always, caused by an infection.

Hepatitis A infection is spread by direct contact with a person who has the illness, or by consuming food or water contaminated with the feces of an infected person.

Hepatitis B spreads through contact with the bodily fluids (such as blood, sweat, saliva or semen) of a person who has it. You can have hepatitis B without knowing it and may be a carrier.

Hepatitis C is usually transferred by blood, such as between intravenous drug users, or between a mother and her baby.

Infection with hepatitis A, B and C can be confirmed with blood tests.

Table 5-4 shows a test report of hepatitis.

Table 5-4 Hepatitis Test Report

HEPATITIS SEROLOGY

Hepatitis B surface antigen   (HBsAg): Negative
Hepatitis C IgG antibody   (HCVIgG): Negative

If contact with hepatitis is suspected, please repeat serology as indicated.
INCUBATION PERIOD (HEPATITIS A): 2-8 weeks
(HEPATITIS B): 1-6 months
(HEPATITIS C): 1-6 months

New Words

toxic /ˈtɑːksɪk/ adj. 有毒的，中毒的

excrete /ɪkˈskriːt/ vt. 排泄，分泌

osteoarthritis /ˌɑːstioʊɑːrˈθraɪtɪs/ n. ［外科］骨关节炎

lining /ˈlaɪnɪŋ/ n. (身体器官内壁的)膜

swell /swel/ v. 肿胀

erosion /ɪˈrəʊʒn/ *n.* 侵蚀

deformity /dɪˈfɔːrməti/ *n.* 畸形

Phrases and Expressions

blood count	血细胞计数
white cell differential	白细胞分类
rheumatoid arthritis	类风湿性关节炎
autoimmune disorder	自身免疫性疾病
erythrocyte sedimentation rate（ESR, or sed rate）	红细胞沉降率
C-reactive protein（CRP）	C 反应蛋白
rheumatoid factor	类风湿因子
surface antigen	表面抗原
IgG antibody	免疫球蛋白 G 抗体
incubation period	潜伏期

Notes

1. Red blood cells that carry oxygen, white blood cells that fight infection and platelets that help blood to clot.

携带氧气的红细胞、抗感染的白细胞和帮助血液凝固的血小板。

2. The Liver Function Tests（LFT）are a group of blood tests that measure some enzymes, proteins, and substances that are produced or excreted by the liver.

肝功能检验（LFT）是一组血液检验，测量某些酶、蛋白质和由肝脏代谢或排泄产生的物质。

3. People with rheumatoid arthritis often have an elevated erythrocyte sedimentation rate（ESR or sed rate）or C-reactive protein（CRP）, which may indicate the presence of an inflammatory process in the body.

类风湿性关节炎病人的红细胞沉降率（ESR 或 sed 率）或 C 反应蛋白（CRP）升高，这可能表明体内存在炎症过程。

4. Other common blood tests look for rheumatoid factors and anti-cyclic citrullinated peptide（anti-CCP）antibodies.

其他常见的血液检测项目查找类风湿因子和抗环瓜氨酸肽（anti-CCP）抗体。

5. Rheumatoid factor（RF）may be detected in up to 60% of patients with rheumatoid arthritis. However RF is also found in other disease states including autoimmune diseases, infective diseases and neoplasm. RF may also be detected in healthy individuals.

高达 60% 的类风湿性关节炎病人可检测到类风湿因子（RF）。然而，RF 也见于其他疾病状态，包括自身免疫性疾病、感染性疾病和肿瘤；也可能在健康个体中检测到 RF。

6. Anti-CCP antibody is a specific test for rheumatoid arthritis and has prognostic significance. Anti-CCP antibody testing is recommended in the diagnosis of rheumatoid arthritis.

抗 CCP 抗体是类风湿性关节炎的特异性检测方法，具有预后意义。抗 CCP 抗体检测被推荐用于类风湿性关节炎的诊断。

7. Hepatitis is an illness that inflames and damages your liver. It affects the liver's ability to do its job, which includes making proteins and clearing the blood of unwanted impurities.

肝炎是一种炎症性疾病，可以损伤肝脏。它影响肝脏正常合成蛋白质和清除血液中多余杂质的功能。

8. Hepatitis A infection is spread by direct contact with a person who has the illness, or by consuming food or water contaminated with the feces of an infected person.

甲型肝炎通过与该病病人直接接触，或食用被感染者粪便污染的食物或水传播。

9. Hepatitis B spreads through contact with the bodily fluids（such as blood, sweat, saliva or semen）of a person who has it. You can have hepatitis B without knowing it and may be a carrier.

乙型肝炎通过接触感染者的体液（如血液、汗水、唾液或精液）传播。你可能在不知情的情况下感染了乙型肝炎，而且可能是携带者。

10. Hepatitis C is usually transferred by blood, such as between intravenous drug users, or between a mother and her baby.

丙型肝炎通常通过血液传播,例如在静脉药瘾者之间,或在母亲和胎儿之间。

Exercises

Ⅰ. Fill in the blanks according to the texts.

1. _____ help blood to clot. (Text A)

2. Abnormalities in the FBE blood test can be caused by _____, infections, some blood cancers such as leukemia and some inherited conditions. (Text A)

3. The Liver Function Tests (LFT) are a group of blood tests that measure some _____, proteins, and substances that are produced or excreted by the liver. (Text A)

4. Other common blood tests look for _____ factor and anti-cyclic citrullinated peptide (anti-CCP) antibodies. (Text B)

5. _____ is an illness that inflames and damages your liver. (Text B)

Ⅱ. Translate the following into Chinese.

Rheumatoid arthritis, an autoimmune disorder, mainly affects your joints and occurs when your immune system mistakenly attacks your own body's tissues. Unlike the wear-and-tear damage of osteoarthritis, rheumatoid arthritis affects the lining of your joints, causing a painful swelling that can eventually result in bone erosion and joint deformity.

Lesson 4   Index of Imported Medical Laboratory Instruments
进口医学检验设备索引

Learning Objectives

After studying this lesson, students are expected to be able to

1. master some key words and expressions related to imported medical laboratory instrument;

2. be familiar with the main button bars of AU480;

3. know about the structure of i1000SR and the operation procedure of i1000SR and Sysmex XN-550;

4. read the symbols on the LCD of BD Phoenix™ 100 correctly.

Warming-up

1. What kind of imported medical laboratory instruments do you know?

2. Do you know the routine operation of them?

Text A   Instruments for Biochemical and Immunological Reaction Test
生化和免疫检验设备

Biochemical Test Instrument

The AU480 chemistry analyzer is the ideal primary chemistry analyzer for low- to mid-volume hospitals and laboratories, or dedicated specialty chemistry or STAT analyzer for larger laboratories. With throughput of up to 400 photometric tests per hour, increased onboard testing, reduced sample volume and easy operation, the AU480 delivers efficiency for laboratories around the world (figure 5-1).

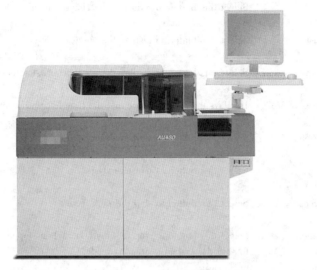

Figure 5-1 AU480 Chemistry Analyzer

The following chart shows the graphical user interface of the AU480 (figure 5-2).

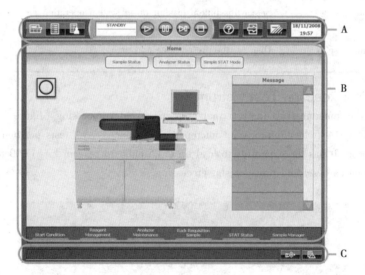

A. Functional Control Area; B. Menu Area; C. Alarm Area.

Figure 5-2 Graphical User Interface

All of the Start Up Procedures can be accessed byHome > Jump button as opposed to the User Menu and Menu options (figure 5-3).

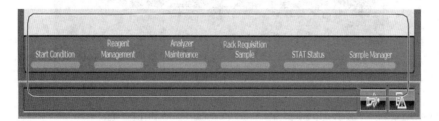

Figure 5-3 Jump Button Overview

Table 5-5 shows shows main button bars of the AU480.

Table 5-5 Main Button Bars

Button	Item	Actions
Home (icon)	Home	Select this button to return to the Home screen.
Menu List (icon)	Menu List	Select this button to display the Menu list screen.
User menu (icon)	User menu	Select this button to display the user menu list screen set by the user.
STOP	Mode Display area	Displays the present mode and the time left until completion of the operation.
Measure Start (icon)	Measure Start	Select this button to start analysis.
Pause (icon)	Pause	Select this button to pause analysis.
Feeder Stop (icon)	Feeder Stop	Select this button to stop the rack feeder.
Stop/Standby (icon)	Stop/Standby	Select this button to stop the analysis. When stopped, this button can be used to shift the system to standby mode.
Online Help (icon)	Online Help	Select this button to display online operational help.
Logout (icon)	Logout	Select this button to log out the user.
End (icon)	End	Select this button to shut down system operation and switch off the auxiliary power supply (End Process).
2007/07/23 10:22	Time Display area	Displays the present date and time.

Immunological Reaction Test Instrument

An i1000SR is an immunoassay analyzer that performs sample processing (figure 5-4, figure 5-5). It processes up to 100 CMIA (chemiluminescent microparticle immunoassay) tests per hour when using a one step 11 STAT protocol. It has the capability to load up to 25 onboard reagent kits (100 tests) in a temperature-controlled reagent carousel and provides stat processing.

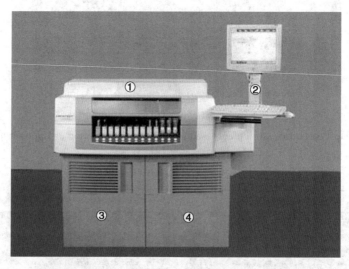

Figure 5-4 i1000SR Processing Module (Front View)

①Processing center cover: Provides access to the components that perform assay processing activities; ②SCC articulated arm: Provides access to the SCC monitor, keyboard, and mouse; ③Supply and waste center door: Provides access to the bulk storage and waste storage area; ④Card cage and SCC center door: Provides access to the card cage and SCC components.

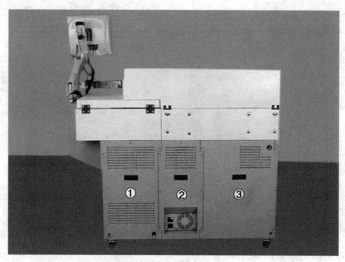

Figure 5-5　i1000SR Processing Module (Rear View)

①SCC rear panel：Provides access to the SCC CPU back panel connectors；②Card cage rear panel：Provides access to the card cage backplane and power supply；③Fluidics rear panel：Provides access to the fluidics components.

The following chart shows a routine operation of i1000SR.

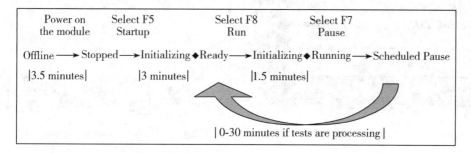

Text B　Instruments for Microbiological and Clinical Test
微生物和临床检验设备

Microbiological Test Instrument

The BD Phoenix™ Automated Microbiology System is intended for the rapid identification (ID) and antimicrobial susceptibility testing (AST) of clinically significant bacteria (figure 5-6). The Phoenix system provides rapid results for most aerobic and facultative anaerobic Gram-positive bacteria as well as most aerobic and facultative anaerobic Gram-negative bacteria of human origin. The Phoenix system is also intended for the rapid identification of yeast and yeast-like organisms.

The overall layout of the instrument is shown in figure 5-7.

The keypad and LCD display are located on the front of the instrument, at the top right. The keypad is used to enter commands to the instrument. The LCD display presents setup and status information, as well as the keypad definitions that allow you to perform routine operations. See figure 5-8.

The Main Status screen has three areas：the top region presents system status information；the middle region presents station status information；and the bottom region displays the current soft key definitions. See figure 5-9.

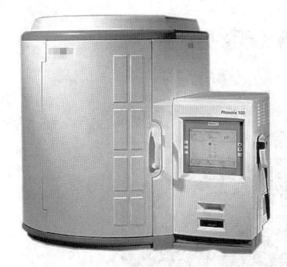

Figure 5-6   BD Phoenix 100 Instrument

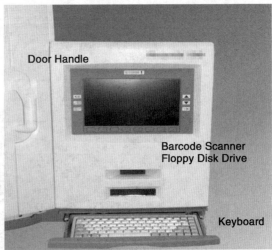

Figure 5-7   Phoenix Instrument Layout

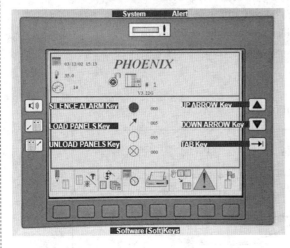

Figure 5-8   Keypad and LCD Display

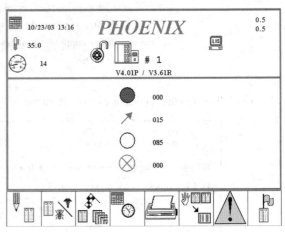

Figure 5-9   Main Status Screen (with Optional LIS Indicator)

Clinical Test Instrument

Sysmex introduced its first blood counter in 1963. It was the first company to use fluorescent flow cytometry and cell counting methods to reliably detect abnormal samples and reduce false positive results. Using a diode laser bench, fluorescent flow cytometry provides the sensitivity needed for measuring and differentiating cell types in whole blood and body fluid samples.

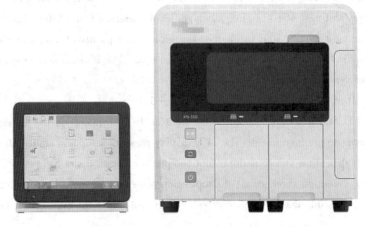

Figure 5-10   Automated Hematology Analyzer XN-550

The XN-550 features an automated sampler and improves workflow productivity with its Rerun and Reflex functionality, and continuous loading feature (figure 5-10). This model also has an integrated IPU and is operated via a compact LCD color touch screen. XN-550 incorporates the proven Sysmex technologies of fluorescence flow cytometry and cyanide-free SLS method for determining hemoglobin.

The flow chart below shows the sequence of operation of the instrument. The typical flow is shown in gray.

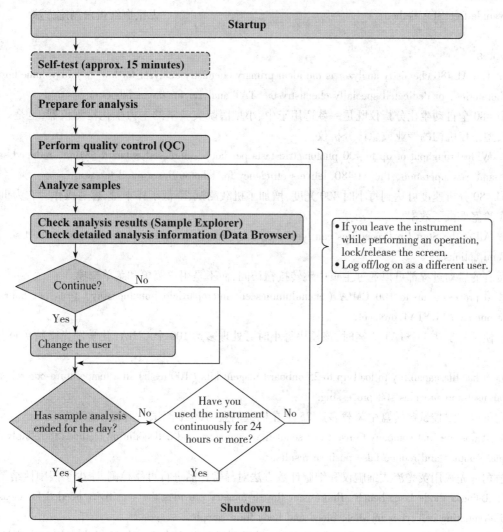

New Words

photometric /ˌfəʊtəʊˈmetrik/ *adj.* 测光的

protocol /ˈprəʊtəkɑːl/ *n.* 草案

carousel /ˌkærəˈsel/ *n.* 行李传送带

backplane /ˈbækˌpleɪn/ *n.* 背板

aerobic /eˈrəʊbɪk/ *adj.* 需氧的

anaerobic /ˌænəˈrəʊbɪk/ *adj.* 厌氧的

integrated /ˈɪntɪɡreɪtɪd/ *adj.* 集成的

compact /kəmˈpækt/ *adj.* 小巧的

incorporate /ɪnˈkɔːrpəreɪt/ *vt.* 包含

Phrases and Expressions

STAT analyzer　　　　　　　　　　　　　急诊分析仪

Graphical User Interface	图形用户界面
CMIA (chemiluminescent microparticle immunoassay)	化学发光微粒免疫分析测定
Gram-positive bacteria	革兰氏阳性菌
Gram-negative bacteria	革兰氏阴性菌
fluorescent flow cytometry	荧光流式细胞术
diode laser	半导体激光器
cyanide-free SLS method	无氰血红蛋白测定方法

Notes

1. The AU480 chemistry analyzer is the ideal primary chemistry analyzer for low- to mid-volume hospitals and laboratories, or dedicated specialty chemistry or STAT analyzer for larger laboratories.

AU480 全自动生化分析仪既是一款适用于中、小型医院实验室的主力生化检测仪器,也是一款适用于大型医疗机构的专业或急诊分析仪。

2. With throughput of up to 400 photometric tests per hour, increased onboard testing, reduced sample volume and easy operation, the AU480 delivers efficiency for laboratories around the world.

AU480 分析速度可达到每小时 400 光度,增加了机载测试,降低了样本量,容易操作。它为世界各地的实验室提供了效率。

3. All of the Start Up Procedures can be accessed by Home >Jump button as opposed to the User Menu and Menu options.

所有的启动过程都可以通过主页中跳转按钮访问,而不是用户菜单和菜单选项。

4. It processes up to 100 CMIA (chemiluminescent microparticle immunoassay) tests per hour when using a one step 11 STAT protocol.

在使用一步法 11 STAT 方案时,该模块每小时可处理多达 100 个 CMIA(化学发光微粒免疫分析)测试。

5. It has the capability to load up to 25 onboard reagent kits (100 tests) in a temperature-controlled reagent carousel and provides stat processing.

它可以在温控试剂转盘中装载多达 25 个在机试剂盒(100 个测试),并提供急诊检测。

6. It was the first company to use fluorescent flow cytometry and cell counting methods to reliably detect abnormal samples and reduce false positive results.

公司率先采用荧光流式细胞仪和细胞计数方法对异常样品进行可靠检测,减少了假阳性结果。

7. Using a diode laser bench, fluorescent flow cytometry provides the sensitivity needed for measuring and differentiating cell types in whole blood and body fluid samples.

使用半导体激光工作台,荧光流式细胞仪提供了测量和鉴别全血和体液样本中细胞类型所需的灵敏度。

8. The XN-550 features an automated sampler and improves workflow productivity with its Rerun and Reflex functionality, and continuous loading feature.

XN-550 具有自动采样功能,可以通过自动复检功能以及连续加载功能来提高工作流效率。

9. This model also has an integrated IPU and is operated via a compact LCD color touch screen.

这个型号还集成了 IPU 操作软件,通过小巧的 LCD 彩色触摸屏操作。

10. XN-550 incorporates the proven Sysmex technologies of fluorescence flow cytometry and cyanide-free SLS method for determining hemoglobin.

XN-550 包含了已经成熟的希森美康技术,如荧光流式细胞术和无氰 SLS 血红蛋白测定的方法。

Exercises

Ⅰ. Fill in the blanks according to the texts.

1. The AU480 is the ideal primary _____ analyzer for low- to mid-volume hospitals and la-

boratories. （Text A）

2. An i1000SR is an _____ analyzer that performs sample processing. （Text A）

3. The BD Phoenix™ Automated Microbiology System is mainly applicable to clinical microbiological laboratory for _____ type identification and drug sensitive test. （Text B）

4. Sysmex introduced its first _____ in 1963. （Text B）

5. The model of Sysmex hematology analyzer introduced in the text is _____. （Text B）

Ⅱ. Translate the following into Chinese.

The BD Phoenix™ Automated Microbiology System is intended for the rapid identification （ID） and antimicrobial susceptibility testing （AST） of clinically significant bacteria. The Phoenix system provides rapid results for most aerobic and facultative anaerobic Gram-positive bacteria as well as most aerobic and facultative anaerobic Gram-negative bacteria of human origin. The Phoenix system is also intended for the rapid identification of yeast and yeast-like organisms.

Lesson 4 Scan and Practice

笔记

Chapter Ⅰ　Medical Laboratory Science

Lesson 1　Laboratory Medicine

Ⅰ. Fill in the blanks according to the texts.

1. laboratory medicine　2. clinical pathology　3. clinical laboratory tests　4. assessment　5. Emergency Department

Ⅱ. Translate the following into Chinese.

在很多国家,主要有两种实验室来处理大多数医学标本。医院实验室附属于某一所医院,进行针对病人的检验。多数医疗决策是基于实验室检验。而私立实验室(或社区实验室)接受并分析来自全科医生、保险公司、临床研究机构和其他健康诊所的标本。

Lesson 2　Basic Clinical Laboratory Medicine

Ⅰ. Fill in the blanks according to the texts.

1. high-volume　2. urine　3. bleeding　4. hemoglobin　5. Parasitic

Ⅱ. Translate the following into Chinese.

红细胞,俗称红血球,在骨髓中产生,成熟后释放到血液中。红细胞中含有血红蛋白,即一种可以将氧气输送至全身的蛋白质。

Lesson 3　Clinical Laboratory Hematology

Ⅰ. Fill in the blanks according to the texts.

1. plasma　2. basophils　3. Anemia　4. leukemia　5. B lymphocytes

Ⅱ. Translate the following into Chinese.

血液的主要功能是把营养物质和氧气运输(送)到全身的组织和器官,并将代谢废物排出体外。同时,血液(白细胞)具有免疫防御功能,能帮助人体抵抗细菌、病毒、真菌和寄生虫等其他异物的侵袭。此外,血液(血小板)还具有凝血功能;当人体出血时,它可以发挥凝血和止血的作用。

Lesson 4　Clinical Laboratory Biochemistry

Ⅰ. Fill in the blanks according to the texts.

1. body fluids　2. basic metabolic panel(BMP)　3. meets　4. liver function　5. ALT

Ⅱ. Translate the following into Chinese.

肝功能检查包括总蛋白、白蛋白、总胆红素、直接胆红素、谷丙转氨酶、谷草转氨酶等。它们反映了肝细胞的合成、生物转化和损伤状态。虽然谷丙转氨酶分布广泛,但血浆中谷丙转氨酶活性的显著增加通常表明肝脏受损。因此,谷丙转氨酶常被用于鉴别由炎症或坏死引起的肝损伤。

Lesson 5　Clinical Laboratory Immunology

Ⅰ. Fill in the blanks according to the texts.

1. immunopathology　2. molecules　3. antibody　4. agglutination　5. immunolabeling

Ⅱ. Translate the following into Chinese.

免疫学检验技术是一门研究免疫学技术及其在医学检验领域应用的学科。以抗原与抗体间的特异结合反应为基础的各种免疫学技术的出现,使得我们可以用其检测临床标本中相应抗原或抗体的存在与数量,从而用于疾病的诊断和治疗。

Lesson 6 Clinical Laboratory Microbiology

Ⅰ. Fill in the blanks according to the texts.

1. viruses 2. Microbiological 3. motility 4. diffusion 5. lowest

Ⅱ. Translate the following into Chinese.

革兰氏染色,也称为革兰氏染色法,是一种用于鉴别细菌的染色方法。根据细胞壁的物理特性,革兰氏染色将细菌分为两大种类(革兰氏阳性和革兰氏阴性)。它的名字来源于丹麦细菌学家 Hans Christian Gram,他首次发明使用了这种技术。革兰氏染色常用于初步鉴定细菌的第一个步骤。

Lesson 7 Clinical Laboratory Molecular Biology

Ⅰ. Fill in the blanks according to the texts.

1. Activation 2. genetic diseases 3. quantitatively 4. chip techniques 5. DNA

Ⅱ. Translate the following into Chinese.

第一代测序技术,双脱氧末端终止法,是由 Sanger 等人发明的。这种方法的优点是读取序列准确,适合重复序列测序;其缺点是每次只能检测单一序列。

Chapter Ⅱ Basic Skills in the Laboratory

Lesson 1 Laboratory Safety—Everyone is Responsible

Ⅰ. Fill in the blanks according to the texts.

1. dangerous 2. occupational 3. pathogens 4. infectious 5. in which

Ⅱ. Translate the following into Chinese.

如果工作场所没有适当预警或操作程序,细菌、病毒和其他微生物在一些暴露条件下有致病的风险。普遍性预防能明显防止接触血液或其他潜在的传染性物质而引发感染。

Lesson 2 Asepsis

Ⅰ. Fill in the blanks according to the texts.

1. microorganisms 2. implementation 3. High-pressure 4. resistant 5. plateau

Ⅱ. Translate the following into Chinese.

现在很多医院都在使用更先进的预真空蒸汽灭菌器,其原理是灭菌器内的空气被吸干,使其处于真空状态,然后中央燃气供应商将蒸汽直接送到消毒室。

Lesson 3 Laboratory Purified Water and Solution Concentration

Ⅰ. Fill in the blanks according to the texts.

1. compound 2. solvent 3. processed 4. dissolve 5. concentration

Ⅱ. Translate the following into Chinese.

水质的技术标准已由一系列专业组织制定,包括美国国家临床实验室标准委员会 NCCLS,即现在的美国临床和实验标准化协会 CLSI。ISO 3696(1987)和 NCCLS(1988)根据水的纯度将水分为 1~3 级或 Ⅰ~Ⅲ类。

Lesson 4 Chemical and Diagnostic Reagents

Ⅰ. Fill in the blanks according to the texts.

1. Reagent-grade 2. standard 3. moles 4. diagnostic 5. controlled

Ⅱ. Translate the following into Chinese.

标准溶液常用来标定其他物质的浓度,如滴定法中的溶液。在分析化学中,标准溶液用标准物质配制,如基准物质。基准物质通常是一种易于称重的试剂,它的高纯度使得其重量能真实地代表所含物质的摩尔数。基准物质被用于校正其他相关工作标准。

Lesson 5 Work Flow for Clinical Specimen Collection

Ⅰ. Fill in the blanks according to the texts.

1. urine 2. transport 3. venipuncture 4. a heel stick 5. tourniquet

Ⅱ. Translate the following into Chinese.

将下列医疗用品摆放在紧挨着抽血椅的桌子上:安全针和真空采血套管、试管、止血带、手套、酒精棉签、绷带、棉花或纱布以及胶带。锐器容器应该始终置于伸手可及的位置。试管应按照采血顺序排列:红头试管、蓝头试管、血清分离试管(SST)、绿头试管、紫头试管、黄头试管和灰头试管。要让病人说出姓名以确认书写内容。

Lesson 6 Collection of Blood Plasma and Serum

Ⅰ. Fill in the blanks according to the texts.

1. Blood plasma 2. vacuum 3. coagulation function 4. fibrinogen 5. interface

Ⅱ. Translate the following into Chinese.

那么如何从血液中分离血清呢?如果用商用真空管,研究者可以使用红色帽的不含添加剂的管。收集全血后,让血液在室温下不受干扰凝固。这通常需要 15~30min。以 1 000~2 000×g 的离心力,离心 10min 分离血块。在实验室检测中,我们可以用这种血清做生化、免疫学和血清学检查。

Lesson 7 Microscopy and Microscope Slide

Ⅰ. Fill in the blanks according to the texts.

1. electron 2. microscopy 3. cover slip 4. surface tension 5. tissue cultures

Ⅱ. Translate the following into Chinese.

复合光学显微镜的有效功率或放大倍数是其目镜和物镜放大倍数的乘积。标准目镜的放大倍数包括×2、×5 和×10。标准物镜的放大倍数范围从×5 到×100。目镜和物镜的最大标准放大倍数分别是×10 和×100,因此,最终放大倍数是 1000×。

Lesson 8 Centrifugation and Electrophoresis Technology

Ⅰ. Fill in the blanks according to the texts.

1. Decantation 2. sedimentation 3. supernatant 4. cataphoresis 5. matrix

Ⅱ. Translate the following into Chinese.

离心机遵循沉淀原理进行工作,也就是向心加速度致使密度较高的物质沿着径向(试管底部)分离出来。基于同样的原理,密度较轻的物质将倾向移动到(试管)顶部。

Lesson 9 Absorption Spectroscopy

Ⅰ. Fill in the blanks according to the texts.

1. Spectroscopy 2. Beer-Lambert 3. coefficient 4. spectrophotometer 5. emitted

Ⅱ. Translate the following into Chinese.

分光光度法用于样本的定性和定量分析。最大光吸收波段的波长给出分子或离子的结构信息,且光吸收程度与吸光物种的量成比例。使用比尔-朗伯定律可以使吸收光谱与所给物质的含量在数量上相关联。

Lesson 10 Electrochemical Analysis

Ⅰ. Fill in the blanks according to the texts.

1. electrochemical 2. Electroanalytical 3. reference 4. fluoride-selective 5. ion-selective

Ⅱ. Translate the following into Chinese.

每个半电池都有一个特殊电压。每个半电池材质选择的不同将产生不同的电势差。每个反应都是离子的不同氧化态之间进行的平衡反应,当达到平衡时,电池将不再提供电压。

Lesson 11 Validation of Laboratory

Ⅰ. Fill in the blanks according to the texts.

1. validate 2. optical systems 3. precision 4. bias 5. false-negative

Ⅱ. Translate the following into Chinese.

检验项目的有效性是一个检验项目给一种疾病或状态作出正确诊断的能力。申请特定检验项目的临床医生在解读有效性低的检验结果时必须牢记这一点。有效性由两个标准判断。

Lesson 12 Laboratory Automation Technology

Ⅰ. Fill in the blanks according to the texts.

1. optimizing 2. integrated 3. unique 4. repetitive 5. direct

Ⅱ. Translate the following into Chinese.

一些分析仪需要将标本转移至标本杯。然而,为了保护实验室工作人员的健康和安全,促使许多制造商开发分析仪,采用封闭管取样,防止操作者直接接触标本。样品可以单独处理、分批处理或连续处理。

Lesson 13 Quality Assurance

Ⅰ. Fill in the blanks according to the texts.

1. specimen 2. External 3. proficiency 4. refers to 5. agency

Ⅱ. Translate the following into Chinese.

质量评价程序是一个保证操作高标准、在需要之处提高标准的管理过程。戴明循环的计划(P)、执行(D)、检查(C)和处理(A)最好地阐明了这个概念。如果循环的四个环节的任何一个出现滞后,则质量下降。在计划质量评价程序时,重要的是努力地在每一个环节去预防、发现和纠正误差。

Chapter Ⅲ Clinical Laboratory Techniques

Lesson 1 Complete Blood Count

Ⅰ. Fill in the blanks according to the texts.

1. evaluates 2. automated 3. diluted 4. aspirate 5. precise

Ⅱ. Translate the following into Chinese.

全血细胞计数检测红细胞(RBC)总数及其相关指标,包括平均红细胞体积(MCV)、血红蛋白浓度以及血细胞比容。血红蛋白浓度是由平均红细胞血红蛋白(MCH)与平均红细胞血红蛋白浓度(MCHC)测得。血细胞比容是红细胞的平均比容。

Lesson 2 Urine and Stool Examination

Ⅰ. Fill in the blanks according to the texts.

1. glucose 2. epithelial 3. kidney 4. microbiological 5. diet

Ⅱ. Translate the following into Chinese.

实验室粪便检验包括显微镜学检查、化学检验和微生物学检验。粪便检验对粪便的颜色、稠度、重量(体积)、形状、气味和黏液进行检验;还检验粪便的潜血、脂肪、肌肉纤维、胆汁、白细胞,以及被称为还原物质的糖类。粪便的pH值也可以被检测。粪便培养旨在发现是否有细菌引起感染。

Lesson 3　Vaginal Discharge and Semen Examination

Ⅰ. Fill in the blanks according to the texts.

1. vaginal smear　2. secretions　3. sperms　4. fertility　5. based on

Ⅱ. Translate the following into Chinese.

真菌性阴道炎常有白色奶酪块状物质排出。滴虫性阴道炎导致阴道分泌物呈黄绿色,泡沫状,并伴有难闻的气味。细菌性阴道炎通常产生的阴道分泌物薄且为乳白色,具有强烈的鱼腥味。

Lesson 4　Cerebrospinal Fluid and Sputum Examination

Ⅰ. Fill in the blanks according to the texts.

1. plasma　2. clarity　3. excreted　4. pus　5. positive

Ⅱ. Translate the following into Chinese.

颜色和透明度是脑脊液的重要诊断特征。出现稻草色、粉红色、黄色或琥珀色,表明胆红素、血红蛋白、红细胞或蛋白质的存在。浊度表示细胞的数量增加,目测有助于区分蛛网膜下腔出血与穿刺伤渗血。穿刺伤渗血在收集脑脊液时,液体常常逐渐变为澄清,澄清液体中或有血丝,或有凝固的样本。

Lesson 5　White Blood Cell

Ⅰ. Fill in the blanks according to the texts.

1. leukocytosis　2. Granulocytes　3. monocytes　4. Neutrophils　5. viral

Ⅱ. Translate the following into Chinese.

淋巴细胞是脊椎动物免疫系统中的一种白细胞。其名称源于它们是淋巴中发现的主要细胞类型。淋巴细胞包括三大类:T淋巴细胞(在细胞介导的细胞毒性适应性免疫中发挥作用)、B淋巴细胞(在体液、抗体介导的适应性免疫中发挥作用)和自然杀伤细胞(其在细胞介导的细胞毒性固有免疫中发挥作用)。

Lesson 6　Related Tests of Blood Coagulation

Ⅰ. Fill in the blanks according to the texts.

1. thrombocytes　2. hemostasis　3. extrinsic　4. intrinsic　5. thromboembolism

Ⅱ. Translate the following into Chinese.

血小板浓度降低称为血小板减少症,可由生成减少或者破坏增加导致。相反,如果血小板计数过高,会形成血凝块(血栓形成),血栓会阻塞血管,导致脑卒中、心肌梗死、肺栓塞或身体其他部位的血管堵塞,如胳膊或腿的末梢血管。

Lesson 7　Blood Group System and Cross-matching

Ⅰ. Fill in the blanks according to the texts.

1. named after　2. transfusion　3. hemolytic　4. compatibility　5. prior to

Ⅱ. Translate the following into Chinese.

国际输血协会目前确认了30种主要的血型系统(包括 ABO 和 Rh 系统)。因此,除了 ABO 抗原和恒河猴抗原,许多其他的抗原也表达在红细胞膜表面。例如,一个人可以是 AB RhD 阳性,同时 M 和 N 抗原阳性(MNS 系统),K 抗原阳性(Kell 系统),以及 Le^a 或 Le^b 抗原阳性(Lewis 系统)。

Lesson 8　Electrolytes in Body Fluids

Ⅰ. Fill in the blanks according to the texts.

1. cations　2. neurons　3. imbalance　4. except for　5. ion-selective electrode

Ⅱ. Translate the following into Chinese.

通过口服或在紧急状态时,静脉内给予含电解质的物质维持电解质平衡。电解质平衡通过激素调节,多余的电解质通常由肾脏排出。人体内的激素如抗利尿素、醛固酮和甲状旁腺素调节电解质平衡。严重的电解质紊乱,如脱水或水分过多,可导致心脏和神经系统并发症,如果不迅速纠正,将导致医疗紧急情况。

Lesson 9　Arterial Blood Gas Analysis

Ⅰ. Fill in the blanks according to the texts.

1. therapist　2. femoral　3. coagulation　4. acidosis　5. acid-base

Ⅱ. Translate the following into Chinese.

CaO_2 是血浆溶解氧和血红蛋白化学结合氧之和,通过公式计算:$CaO_2 = (PO_2 \times 0.003) + (SaO_2 \times 1.34 \times Hgb)$(公式中血红蛋白浓度以 g/d 表示)。

SaO_2 或 O_2 sats,表示氧饱和度,测量血红蛋白结合氧量占血液中氧量的百分比。

Lesson 10　Blood Lipids and Lipoproteins

Ⅰ. Fill in the blanks according to the texts.

1. biochemistry　2. glycerol　3. soluble　4. cholesterol　5. coronary

Ⅱ. Translate the following into Chinese.

血脂或脂质,是总胆固醇(TC)、高密度胆固醇酯(HDL-C)、低密度胆固醇酯(LDL-C)和甘油三酯的总称。广义上的血脂可能还包括极低密度胆固醇酯。血脂常用来确定高脂血症(各种胆固醇和甘油三酯水平的紊乱),其中许多是公认的心血管疾病、胰腺炎的危险因素。

Lesson 11　Diagnostic Tests of Endocrine

Ⅰ. Fill in the blanks according to the texts.

1. bloodstream　2. insulin　3. bioassays　4. glucose　5. diagnostic

Ⅱ. Translate the following into Chinese.

明显升高的游离甲状腺素(T_4)水平支持甲状腺功能亢进症的临床诊断结果,而明显降低的游离 T_4 水平加上典型的临床表现,可以诊断为甲状腺功能减退症。测量游离 T_4 水平以及其他甲状腺检查,结合临床发表现,可以鉴别甲状腺功能亢进和甲状腺功能减退。游离 T_4 因不受 T_4 结合蛋白水平的影响,故优于总 T_4。

Lesson 12　Liver and Renal Function Tests

Ⅰ. Fill in the blanks according to the texts.

1. state　2. responsible　3. elevated　4. controlling　5. adequate

Ⅱ. Translate the following into Chinese.

肾小球滤过率是单位时间内从肾小球毛细血管滤过到鲍氏囊中的液量。GFR 可以通过测量血液中任何稳定水平的化学物质来计算,这些物质能被肾脏自由过滤,但不能再被肾脏吸收或分泌。因此,测量所得出的速率就是尿液中物质的量,其源自可计算的血液量。GFR 通常记录为单位体积/时间,如毫升/分钟(mL/min)。

Lesson 13　Cardiac and Tumor Markers

Ⅰ. Fill in the blanks according to the texts.

1. released　2. distributed　3. tumour　4. immunoglobulin　5. metastases

Ⅱ. Translate the following into Chinese.

其他激素和酶:内分泌腺肿瘤过度分泌相应的激素。通过测定特殊的激素,可获得有关癌症的线索。例如,乳腺瘤细胞可以分泌催乳素和雌激素。多种血清酶的测定有助于发现癌症病人的肿瘤转移。例如:转移到肝脏的肿瘤引起血清碱性磷酸酶、γ谷氨酰转肽酶和转氨酶升高。

Lesson 14　Enzyme Activity Assay

Ⅰ. Fill in the blanks according to the texts.

1. increase　2. denature　3. present　4. enzyme　5. discontinuous

Ⅱ. Translate the following into Chinese.

酶是通过产物的生成量或底物的减少量来测定的。酶活性＝单位时间底物转化摩尔数＝反应速率×反应体积。反应速率是每单位时间内底物消耗的浓度（或产生的产物）（mol·L^{-1}·s^{-1}）。SI 单位是 katal，1 katal ＝ 1mol/s，但这个单位太大了。一个更加实际和常用的值为 1 酶单位（U）＝ 1 μmol/min。1 U 相当于 16.67 nkatals。

Lesson 15　Point-of-care Testing

Ⅰ. Fill in the blanks according to the texts.

1. portable　2. blood　3. qualitative　4. sensitivity　5. sample

Ⅱ. Translate the following into Chinese.

床旁检验（POCT）被定义为病人护理地点或附近的医学检验。其他术语包括床边检验、实验室外检验和传播实验室检验。床旁检验包括：血糖检测、血气和电解质分析、快速凝血检测、快速心脏标记物诊断、药物滥用筛查、尿试纸条检测、妊娠检测、粪便隐血分析、食物病原体筛查、血红蛋白检测、传染病筛查和胆固醇检测等。

Lesson 16　Flow Cytometry Analysis

Ⅰ. Fill in the blanks according to the texts.

1. biomarker　2. sensitive　3. suspension　4. acquisition　5. properties

Ⅱ. Translate the following into Chinese.

测量系统——常用电阻抗（或电导率）和光学系统测量：灯（汞灯、氙灯）；大功率水冷激光器（氩、氪、染料激光器）；低功耗风冷激光器（氩 488nm），红色氦氖（633nm），绿色氦氖，氦镉（紫外线）；二极管激光器（蓝、绿、红、紫）产生光信号。

Lesson 17　Viral Epidemiology and HIV Tests

Ⅰ. Fill in the blanks according to the texts.

1. living　2. susceptible　3. transmitted　4. antibodies　5. substrate

Ⅱ. Translate the following into Chinese.

人类免疫缺陷病毒的感染导致表达 CD4 的 T 细胞（即 CD4$^+$ T 细胞）数量逐步减少。通过单克隆抗体技术和流式细胞术计数血样中的 CD4 细胞可表明感染的阶段。CD4 细胞计数试验测量 CD4$^+$ T 细胞的数量。结果通常以每微升（或立方毫米，mm^3）血液中含有的细胞数量来表示。

Lesson 18　Antibiotic Susceptibility Testing Methods

Ⅰ. Fill in the blanks according to the texts.

1. resistance　2. susceptible　3. correlate　4. diffusion　5. millimeter

Ⅱ. Translate the following into Chinese.

抗生素药物敏感试验是检测细菌对抗生素敏感程度的实验。因为抗生素药物敏感程度是变化的，甚至在同一菌种中也是不同的（有的菌株耐药性就高于其他的菌株），因此抗生素药物敏感试验是用来确定哪种抗生素将是治疗体内细菌性感染的最佳选择。

Lesson 19　Polymerase Chain Reaction Technology

Ⅰ. Fill in the blanks according to the texts.

1. outlining　2. fundamental　3.　determines　4. programmable　5. In theory

Ⅱ. Translate the following into Chinese.

基因通常通过蛋白质的产生来表达其功能效应。细胞含有数百种不同的蛋白质和复合分子，它们构成了很多的固体组织，并控制其大多数的生物学过程。正是 DNA 中的遗传碱基对序列决定了组成特定蛋白质的氨基酸排列顺序。

Lesson 20　Biochip Technology

Ⅰ. Fill in the blanks according to the texts.

1. gene　2. hybridization　3. amount　4. substrates　5. antigens

Ⅱ. Translate the following into Chinese.

蛋白质芯片与由全长蛋白质或结构域构成的分析阵列不同。它们可以在单独的实验中进行完整蛋白质组的生化活性研究。

Chapter Ⅳ　Laboratory Techniques in Pathology

Lesson 1　Pathological Laboratory Techniques

Ⅰ. Fill in the blanks according to the texts.

1. functional　2. microscope　3. trimming　4. transparent　5. coverslip

Ⅱ. Translate the following into Chinese.

为了在显微镜下对玻片上的组织进行诊断,需要进行组织化学染色。由于在染色前,所有组织都是透明的,因此很难在显微镜下分辨细胞的结构。

Lesson 2　Cytopathological Laboratory Techniques

Ⅰ. Fill in the blanks according to the texts.

1. diagnoses　2. effective　3. reliable　4. expensive　5. pink

Ⅱ. Translate the following into Chinese.

细针穿刺细胞学(FNAC 或穿刺针穿刺活检)——针附在注射器上,用于收集各种身体器官病变或肿块的细胞。FNAC 可以在触诊指导下进行,临床医生可以在颈部、甲状腺或乳房等浅表区域的肿块上感觉到病变组织或病变位置。超声还可以辅助 FNAC 对体内无法通过触诊定位的深部病变进行取样。

Lesson 3　Biological Staining

Ⅰ. Fill in the blanks according to the texts.

1. positive　2. technical　3. involves　4. slide　5. pale

Ⅱ. Translate the following into Chinese.

体外染色包括给不再存活的细胞或结构染色。某些染色剂经常被结合起来,以揭示比单一染色剂更多的细节和特征。结合固定和样品制备的具体方案,科学家和医生可以使用这些标准技术作为一致的、可重复的诊断工具。当主染色剂不完全可见时,复染液可使细胞或结构更明显的染色。

Chapter Ⅴ　Extended Reading

Lesson 1　Professionals within the Clinical Laboratory

Ⅰ. Fill in the blanks according to the texts.

1. disciplines　2. ruled out　3. research capacities　4. diagnosis　5. technician

Ⅱ. Translate the following into Chinese.

临床检验人员在病人的诊断和治疗中起着重要的作用。检验结果有助于确定或排除疾病的假定诊断,例如糖尿病或其他慢性疾病。为了从事这个职业,教育是非常严谨的。临床检验科学教育与病理学密切相关,但也各不相同。

Lesson 2　Medical Terminology

Ⅰ. Fill in the blanks according to the texts.

1. affix   2. vowel   3. deleted   4. morphemes   5. clinical

II. Translate the following into Chinese.

词根通常通过连接元音与前缀或后缀组合在一起使用,连接元音通常是字母"O"。当遇到医学术语时,应该注意前缀、词根和后缀。如果后缀的第一个字母是元音,那么可以去掉连接元音。

Lesson 3   Clinical Test Report

I. Fill in the blanks according to the texts.

1. Platelets   2. anemia   3. enzymes   4. rheumatoid   5. Hepatitis

II. Translate the following into Chinese.

类风湿性关节炎是一种自身免疫性疾病,主要影响关节组织,当免疫系统错误地攻击自身组织时就会发生。与骨关节炎的磨损和撕裂损伤不同,类风湿性关节炎影响关节腔内壁,引起肿痛,最终导致骨侵蚀和关节畸形。

Lesson 4   Index of Imported Medical Laboratory Instruments

I. Fill in the blanks according to the texts.

1. chemistry   2. immunoassay   3. bacteria   4. blood counter   5. XN-550

II. Translate the following into Chinese.

BD Phoenix™ 全自动微生物分析系统可用于临床重要细菌的快速鉴定(ID)和药敏测试(AST)。全自动微生物分析系统能够为来自人源性的大部分需氧和兼性厌氧的革兰氏阳性细菌及革兰氏阴性细菌提供快速的结果。此系统也可以用于酵母菌以及似酵母菌的快速鉴定。

Appendix Ⅱ Glossary 词汇表

A

a sharps container 锐器容器(2-5)

abnormality /ˌæbnɔːrˈmæləti/ n. 畸形,变态(4-2)

abscess /ˈæbses/ n. 脓疮(3-4)

absorbance /əbˈsɔːrbəns/ n. ［物化］吸光度,吸收率(2-9)

absorption coefficient 吸收系数(2-9)

absorptivity /ˌæbsɔrpˈtɪvɪti/ n. 吸收率,吸收能力,吸收性(2-9)

abuse /əˈbjuːs/ n. 滥用(3-15)

acceleration /əkˌseləˈreɪʃn/ n. 加速度(2-8)

access /ˈækses/ n. 通道,进入,机会 v. 接近,使用,访问(2-1)

accessible /əkˈsesəbl/ adj. 易接近的,可进入的,可理解的(3-18)

accreditation /əˌkredɪˈteɪʃn/ n. 认证,鉴定合格,委派(2-13)

accreditation body 认证机构,认可机构(2-13)

accumulation /əˌkjuːmjəˈleɪʃn/ n. 积聚,累积,堆积物(2-2)

accurate /ˈækjərət/ adj. 精确的(3-12)

acetaminophen /əˌsiːtəˈmɪnəfen/ n. 对乙酰氨基酚(3-12)

acid-base balance 酸碱平衡(3-9)

acidosis /ˌæsɪˈdosɪs/ n. ［内科］酸中毒,酸毒症(3-9)

acquired /əˈkwaɪrd/ adj. ［医］后天的,已获得的(1-5)

acquired (or adaptive) immune response 获得性(或适应性)免疫应答(1-5)

acquisition /ˌækwɪˈzɪʃn/ n. 获得物,获得(3-16)

acute coronary syndrome 急性冠脉综合征(3-15)

additive /ˈædətɪv/ n. 添加物,添加剂(2-5)

address /əˈdres/ v. 演说,从事,提出(2-1)

adenine /ˈædənɪn/ n. ［生化］腺嘌呤(3-19)

adenine-thymine bonding 腺嘌呤-胸腺嘧啶键合(4-3)

adipose /ˈædɪˈpous/ adj. 脂肪的(3-10)

administration /ədˌmɪnɪˈstreɪʃn/ n. 管理,行政(2-1)

adrenal /ædˈrinl/ n. 肾上腺(3-11)

advanced stage 晚期(3-4)

adverse reaction 不良反应(5-1)

aerobic /eˈroubɪk/ adj. 需氧的(5-4)

aerosol /ˈerəsɑːl/ n. ［物化］气溶胶,气雾剂(3-17)

affix /əˈfɪks/ vt. 粘上,署名 n. ［语］词缀,附加物(3-20)

aforementioned /əˈfɔːrmenʃənd/ adj. 上述的,前面提及的(3-10)

agar /ˈeɪgɑːr/ n. 琼脂(1-6)

agglutination /əˌgluːtənˈeʃən/ n. 凝集(反应),胶合(1-5)

agranulocyte /eiˈgrænjuləusait/ n. ［组织］无颗粒白细胞(3-5)

AIDS (acquired immunodeficiency syndrome) 艾滋病(获得性免疫缺陷综合征)(1-5)

alanine aminotransferase (ALAT) 丙氨酸转氨酶(3-12)

ALT (alanine transaminase) 谷丙转氨酶(1-4)

alcoholic /ˌælkəˈhɑːlɪk/ adj. 酒精的,含酒精的(4-3)

aldosterone /ælˈdɑstəˌron/ n. ［生化］醛固酮,醛甾酮(3-8)

algorithm /ˈælgərɪðəm/ n. ［计］［数］算法,运算法则(3-17)

alkaline phosphatase(ALP) 碱性磷酸酶(2-12)

alkalosis /ˌælkəˈlosɪs/ n. 碱毒症(3-9)

allergy /ˈælərdʒi/ n. 过敏反应,过敏症,反感,厌恶(1-5)

allowable error limits 误差允许范围(2-9)

alpha fetoprotein (AFP)甲胎蛋白(3-13)

alternatively /ɔːlˈtɜːrnətɪvli/ adv. 要不,或者(3-20)

alveoli /ælˈviəlaɪ/ n. 肺泡(alveous 的复数)(3-4)

ambient /ˈæmbɪənt/ adj. 周围的,外界的(3-8)

ambulatory /ˈæmbjələtɔːri/ adj. 流动的,走动的(2-12)

American Chemical Society (ACS)美国化学学会(2-4)

American Society for Testing and Materials (ASTM)美国试验与材料学会(2-4)

amino acid 氨基酸(2-8)

amniotic /ˌæmniˈotɪk/ adj. ［昆］羊膜的(2-1)

ampere /æmˈpɪr/ n. 安培(计算电流强度的标准单位)(2-10)

amplification /ˌæmplɪfɪˈkeɪʃn/ n. ［电子］扩增(1-7)

amplify /ˈæmplɪfaɪ/ v. 扩大(3-19)

anaerobic /ˌænəˈroubɪk/ adj. 厌氧的(5-4)

analogue-to-digital conversion (ADC)模数转换(3-16)

analysis /əˈnæləsɪs/ n. 分析,解析(3-15)

analyte /ˈænəlait/ n. ［分化］分析物,被分析物(2-9)

analyze /ˈænəlaɪz/ v. 分析(2-3)

analyzer /ˈænəˌlaɪzə/ n. ［计］分析仪,分析者(2-5)

anatomic /ˌænəˈtɑmɪk/ adj. 组织的,解剖(学)的(等于 anatomical)(1-1)

ancillary /ˈænsəleri/ adj. 辅助的,副的,从属的(4-1)

anemia /əˈniːmiə/ n. 贫血(1-3)

anemic /əniːmɪk/ adj. 贫血的(3-1)

anion /ˈænaɪən/ n. [化学]阴离子,负离子(3-8)

anneal /əˈniːl/ v. 使退火(3-19)

anonymous /əˈnɑːnɪməs/ adj. 匿名的,无名的(2-13)

antibiotic /ˌæntibaɪˈɑːtɪk/ n. 抗生素 adj. 抗菌的(1-6)

antibiotic susceptibility testing(AST)抗生素药物敏感性试验
(1-6)

antibiotic-impregnated wafers 抗生素浸渍片(3-18)

antibody /ˈæntɪbɒːdɪ/ n. [免疫]抗体(1-5)

anticipated/ænˈtɪsəˌpetɪd/ adj. 预期的,期望的(2-1)

anticoagulant /ˌæntɪkoʊˈægjələnt/ n. (助剂)抗凝剂 adj. 抗凝
血的(3-6)

antidiuretic hormone 抗利尿激素(3-8)

antigen /ˈæntɪdʒən/ n. [免疫]抗原(1-5)

antimicrobial /ˌæntimaɪˈkrobiəl/ n. 抗菌剂,杀菌剂(3-18)

antiphospholipid /ˈæntɪfɒsfə(ʊ)ˈlɪpɪd/ n. [医]抗磷脂(3-6)

antiseptic /ˌænti'septɪk/ n. 抗菌剂(2-5)

apoprotein /ˌæpəˈprəutiːn/ n. [生化]载脂蛋白(3-10)

apparatus /ˌæpəˈrætəs/ n. 装置,设备,仪器,器官(3-16)

approve /əˈpruːv/ v. 批准,核准,赞成(2-4)

aptamer /ˈæpteɪmər/ n. 适体,适配体(3-20)

aqueous /ˈeɪkwɪəs/ adj. 水的,水般的(2-3)

archaea /ɑːˈkiə/ n. 古细菌,古生菌(3-14)

archaeology /ˌɑːrkiˈɑːlədʒi/ n. 考古学(1-7)

argon /ˈɑːrgɑːn/ n. [化学]氩(3-16)

arousal /əˈrauzl/ n. 唤起,觉醒(3-3)

arterial /ɑːrˈtɪriəl/ adj. [解剖]动脉的,干线的(2-1)

as a result of ... 作为……的结果(3-5)

asepsis /æˈsɛpsɪs/ n. 无菌,无菌操作(2-2)

aspartate aminotransferase(ASAT)天冬氨酸转氨酶(3-12)

aspartate transaminase(AST)谷草转氨酶(1-4)

aspirate /ˈæspərət/ v. 抽吸(3-1)

assay /əˈseɪ/ n. 化验,试验(1-2)

associate degree 大专文凭(5-1)

associate with ... 与……联系在一起,相关(3-15)

Association of Caribbean States(ACS)加勒比国家联盟(2-4)

assumed /əˈsuːmd/ adj. 假定的,假装的(3-7)

assurance /əˈʃurəns/ n. 保证,担保(2-11)

atomic absorption spectroscopy 原子吸收光谱法(2-9)

atomic emission spectroscopy 原子发射光谱法(2-9)

atrophy /ˈætrəfi/ n. [病理]萎缩(5-2)

atypical /ˌeɪˈtɪpɪkl/ adj. 非典型的,不合规则的(3-7)

autoantibody /ˌɔtoˈæntɪˌbɑdi/ n. [免疫]自身抗体,自体抗原
(1-5)

autoclave /ˈɔːtoʊkleɪv/ n. 高压灭菌器,高压锅 v. 用高压锅

烹饪(2-2)

autoclave sterilization 高压灭菌器消毒(2-2)

autoclaving /ˌɔːtəuˈkleiviŋ/ n. [医]高压灭菌法,高压蒸气
养护(2-3)

autoimmune /ˌɔːtoʊɪˈmjuːn/ adj. 自身免疫的(1-1)

autoimmune disorder 自身免疫性疾病(5-3)

autoimmunity /ˌɔːtəuɪˈmjuːnəti/ n. [免疫]自身免疫(性)
(1-5)

automated clinical and analytical testing 自动化临床检验和分
析检验(2-12)

automated hematology analyzers 自动血液分析仪(3-1)

auxiliary /ɔːgˈzɪliəri/ adj. 辅助的,副的,附加的(4-3)

available /əˈveɪləbl/ adj. 可获得的,可购得的,可找到的,有
空的(4-3)

avian influenza 禽流感(3-17)

axis /ˈæksɪs/ n. 轴(2-8)

B

baccalaureate degree 学士学位(5-1)

backplane /ˈbækˌplein/ n. 背板(5-4)

bacteremia /ˌbæktəˈrimiə/ n. [内科]菌血症(5-2)

bacteria /bækˈtɪrɪə/ n. [微]细菌(1-6)

bacteriological /bækˌtɪrɪəˈlɑːdʒɪkl/ adj. [微]细菌学的,细菌
学上的(5-1)

bacteriuria /bækˌtiəriˈjuəriə/ n. [泌尿]菌尿症,细菌尿
(5-2)

base pair 碱基对(3-19)

basic metabolic panel(BMP)基础代谢功能检查试验组合
(1-4)

basophil /ˈbeisəfil/ n. 嗜碱性粒细胞(1-2)

be based on ... 根据……,以……为基础(3-15)

be characterized as ... 被描述为……(3-5)

be composed of ... 由……组成(2-6)

be concerned with ... 涉及……,关心……(5-2)

be detected with ... 被检测到……(3-6)

be devised to ... 被设计来……(3-6)

be involved in ... 包括在……中(3-5)

be separated from ... 从……分离出来(2-6)

beads /biːdz/ n. 磁珠(3-20)

beverage /ˈbevəridʒ/ n. 饮料(3-11)

bias /ˈbaɪəs/ n. 偏倚,偏差(2-11)

bicarbonate /ˌbaɪˈkɑːrbənət/ n. 碳酸氢盐,重碳酸盐(3-9)

bile acids 胆汁酸(3-10)

biliary ducts 胆管(3-12)

bilirubin /ˌbɪlɪˈruːbɪn/ n. [生化]胆红素(1-4)

bioassay /ˌbaɪɒˈse/ n. [生物]生物测定,生物鉴定,活体检
定(3-11)

biochemistry /ˌbaɪoʊˈkemɪstri/ n. 生物化学(1-1)

biochip /ˈbaɪoˌtʃɪp/ n. ［生物］生物芯片(3-20)

biological hazard 生物危害(2-1)

biomarker /ˈbaɪɒmɑːkər/ n. 生物标志物(1-7)

biomolecule /ˌbaɪoʊˈmɒlɪkjuːl/ n. 生物分子(1-7)

biophysical /ˌbaɪoʊˈfɪzɪkəl/ adj. 生物物理学的(3-16)

biopsy /ˈbaɪɑːpsi/ 活组织检查(3-16)

biotechnology /ˌbaɪoʊtekˈnɑːlədʒi/ n. ［生物］生物技术,生物工艺学(5-1)

biotransformation /ˌbaɪoˌtrænsfərˈmeʃən/ n. ［环境］生物转化(1-4)

bipolar /ˌbaɪˈpoʊlər/ adj. 有两极的,双极的(3-10)

Bismarck brown Y stains 俾斯麦棕 Y 染色剂(4-2)

bleach /bliːtʃ/ n. 漂白剂(2-5)

blood borne pathogen 经血液传播的病原体(2-1)

blood clot 血凝块,血块(3-6)

blood count 血细胞计数(5-3)

blood film 血涂片(3-1)

blood glucose testing 血糖检测(3-15)

blood urea nitrogen 血尿素氮(2-12)

bone marrow 骨髓(3-5)

borne /bɔːrn/ v. 忍受,负荷(2-1)

bound /baʊnd/ adj. 有义务的 v. 束缚,限制 n. 界限,范围(3-9)

brachial artery 肱动脉,臂动脉(3-9)

bronchi /ˈbrɒnkai/ n. 细支气管(bronchus 的复数)(3-4)

bronchiectasis /ˌbrɒŋkɪˈektəsɪs/ n. ［内科］支气管扩张(3-4)

bubble /ˈbʌbl/ n. 气泡,泡沫 v. 沸腾,冒泡(3-9)

buffer /ˈbʌfər/ n. 缓冲器 v. 缓冲(2-4)

buffered solution 缓冲液(2-8)

buffy /ˈbʌfi/ adj. 淡黄色的(3-5)

bulk /bʌlk/ n. 大块(4-3)

by the same token 出于同样原因(2-8)

C

calculate /ˈkælkjuleɪt/ v. 计算,预测,打算(3-9)

calibrate /ˈkælɪbreɪt/ v. 校准(2-4)

calibration /ˌkælɪˈbreɪʃn/ n. 校准(2-9)

calibration curve 校准曲线(2-9)

calibration standard 校准标准(2-9)

calibrator /ˈkæliˌbreɪtə/ n. ［仪］校准器,口径测量器(等于 calibrater)(2-4)

canal /kəˈnæl/ n. 管道(4-2)

cancer /ˈkænsər/ n. 癌症,恶性肿瘤(4-2)

capillary /ˈkæpəleri/ n. 毛细管,毛细血管 adj. 毛细管的,毛状的(2-5)

capillary tubing 毛细管(2-10)

carbohydrate /ˌkɑːrboʊˈhaɪdreɪt/ n. ［有化］碳水化合物,糖类(1-3)

carbonate /ˈkɑːrbənət/ n. 碳酸盐(3-8)

carboxylic acid 羧酸(3-10)

cardiac /ˈkɑːrdiæk/ n. 强心剂,强胃剂 adj. 心脏的,心脏病的(2-2)

cardiovascular /ˌkɑːrdioʊˈvæskjələr/ adj. ［解剖］心血管的(3-10)

carousel /ˌkærəˈsel/ n. 行李传送带(5-4)

carpal tunnel syndrome（CTS）腕管综合征(3-15)

cast /kæst/ n. 管型(3-2)

catabolism /kəˈtæbəlɪzəm/ n. ［生化］分解代谢(3-12)

catalyst /ˈkætəlɪst/ n. ［物化］催化剂,刺激因素(2-4)

cataphoresis /ˌkætəfəˈriːsɪs/ n. ［化学］电泳,阳离子电泳,电透法(2-8)

categorize /ˈkætəɡəraɪz/ v. 将……分类(3-1)

catheter /ˈkæθətər/ n. ［医］导管,导尿管,尿液管(2-2)

cation /ˈkætaɪən/ n. ［化学］阳离子,正离子(3-8)

cavity /ˈkævəti/ n. 腔,洞(4-2)

cell mitosis 细胞分裂(3-19)

cell suspension 细胞悬液(3-16)

cellular /ˈseljələr/ adj. 细胞的,由细胞组成的(5-1)

cellulose acetate 醋酸纤维素(2-8)

centers for disease control and prevention（CDC）疾病预防控制中心(2-1)

central dogma 中心法则(1-7)

centrifugal force 离心力(2-8)

centrifugation /senˌtrifjuˈgeiʃən/ n. 离心法,离心过滤(3-5)

centrifuge /ˈsentrɪfjuːdʒ/ v. 用离心机分离(2-5)

centripetal /senˈtrɪpɪtl/ adj. 向心的(2-8)

cerebrospinal /ˌsɛrəbroˈspaɪnl/ adj. ［解剖］脑脊髓的(1-2)

cerebrospinal fluid 脑脊液(3-4)

certification /ˌsɜːrtɪfɪˈkeɪʃn/ n. 证明,鉴定(5-1)

certified /ˈsɜ˞təˌfaɪd/ adj. 被证明的,具有证明文件的(3-7)

cervical lesion 子宫颈病变(4-2)

chamber /ˈtʃeɪmbər/ n.（身体或器官内的）室,腔(3-1)

charge /tʃɑːrdʒ/ n. 电荷(2-8)

cheese /tʃiːz/ n. ［食品］乳酪,干酪(3-3)

chemical gas sterilization 化学气体灭菌(2-2)

Chemical Hygiene Plan（CHP）化学卫生计划(2-1)

chemiluminescence /ˌkɛməˌlʊːməˈnɛsəns/ n. 化学发光,化合光(1-5)

chemotherapy /ˌkiːmoʊˈθerəpi/ n. ［临床］化学疗法(3-16)

chip /tʃɪp/ n. 芯片,碎片(3-8)

chlamydia /kləˈmɪdiə/ n. 衣原体(3-3)

cholestasis /ˌkɒləˈstasɪs/ n. 胆汁阻塞,胆汁淤积(3-12)

cholestatic /ˌkəʊləˈstætɪk/ adj. 胆汁郁积的(3-12)

cholesterol /kəˈlestərɔːl/ n. ［生化］胆固醇(3-2)

choline /ˈkolin/ n. ［生化］胆碱(3-10)

chromatin /ˈkrəomətɪn/ n. 核染色质,核染质(4-3)

chromosome /ˈkrəoməsəom/ n. ［遗］［细胞］［染料］染色体 (1-7)

chylomicrons /ˌkaɪləoˈmaɪkrɔns/ n. ［生化］乳糜微粒(3-10)

circulate /ˈsɜːrkjəleɪt/ v. 循环(3-1)

cirrhosis /səˈrəosɪs/ n. ［内科］硬化,肝硬化（复数 cirrho-ses）(3-12)

citrate /ˈsɪtret/ n. 柠檬酸盐(2-6)

Clinical and Laboratory Standards Institute（CLSI）美国临床与实验室标准化研究所(2-3)

clinical blood cell number and morphological analysis 临床血细胞数量与形态分析检测(1-1)

Clinical Cellular and Molecular Genetics Laboratory 临床细胞分子遗传学检验室(1-1)

Clinical Chemistry Laboratory 临床化学检验室(1-1)

Clinical Hematology and Body Fluids Laboratory 临床血液与体液检验室(1-1)

clinical hemorrhage and thrombosis analysis 临床出血与血栓分析检测(1-1)

Clinical Immunology Laboratory 临床免疫检验室(1-1)

Clinical Microbiology Laboratory 临床微生物检验室(1-1)

closeness /ˈkləosnəs/ n. 接近,严密(2-11)

clot /klɑːt/ n. 凝块,黏团（尤指血块）v.（使）凝结成块,覆以黏性物质(3-1)

clotting /ˈklɔtɪŋ/ n. 凝血,结块(1-2)

clue cell 线索细胞(3-3)

CMIA（chemiluminescent microparticle immunoassay）化学发光微粒免疫分析测定(5-4)

coagulation /kəoˌægjuˈleɪʃn/ n. 凝固,凝结,凝结物(3-6)

coagulation factor 凝血因子(3-6)

cold sores 唇疱疹,感冒疮(3-17)

collagen /ˈkɑːlədʒən/ n. ［生化］胶原,胶原质(4-3)

colleague /ˈkɑːliːɡ/ n. 同事,同僚(2-13)

colloquially /kəˈləokwɪəli/ adv. 口语地,用通俗语(2-4)

coloration /ˌkʌləˈreɪʃn/ n. 着色(3-2)

colorimetric /kʌləriˈmetrik/ adj. 比色分析的(3-14)

combat /ˈkɑːmbæt/ v. 反对,与……战斗(3-18)

combinatorial /kəmˌbaɪnəˈtɔːrɪəl/ adj. 组合的(2-12)

combinatorial chemistry 组合化学(2-12)

come up against... 碰到……(5-2)

commitment /kəˈmɪtmənt/ n. 承诺,保证(2-13)

compact /kəmˈpækt/ adj. 小巧的(5-4)

compatibility testing 兼容性测试(3-7)

competitive /kəmˈpetətɪv/ adj. 竞争的(2-12)

competitive inhibition immunoassay 竞争性免疫抑制试验 (3-15)

complain /kəmˈpleɪn/ v. 抱怨(2-12)

complement /ˈkɑːmpləmənt/ n. 补体,补充物(1-5)

complement fixation test 补体结合实验(1-5)

complementary /ˌkɑːmplɪˈmentri/ adj. 互补的(3-20)

complete blood count（CBC）/ full blood count（FBC）全血细胞计数(1-2)

component /kəmˈpəonənt/ n. 组成部分,成分,组件,元件 (1-4)

compound light 复合光(2-9)

comprehensive metabolic panel（CMP）代谢功能全套试验 (1-4)

concavity /kɑːnˈkævəti/ n. 凹面(2-7)

concentration /ˌkɑːnsnˈtreɪʃn/ n. 浓度,浓缩(2-3)

condenser /kənˈdensər/ n. 冷凝器；［电］电容器；［光］聚光器(2-7)

condom /ˈkɑːndəm/ n. 避孕套(3-3)

configurable /kənˈfɪɡjərəbl/ adj. 可配置的,结构的(2-12)

confocal /kɑːnˈfəokl/ adj. ［数］共焦的,同焦点的(2-7)

confocal laser scanning microscopy 共聚焦激光扫描显微镜检查法(2-7)

conjecture /kənˈdʒektʃər/ vt. 推测,揣摩(5-2)

conjugated bilirubin 结合胆红素(3-12)

consist of... 由……组成(5-2)

consistency /kənˈsɪstənsi/ n. 浓度,稠度,一致性,相容性 (3-2)

consistently /kənˈsɪstəntli/ adv. 一贯地,坚持地(2-4)

constant /ˈkɑːnstənt/ adj. 不变的,恒定的 n. ［数］常数,恒量(3-9)

constituent /kənˈstɪtʃuənt/ n. 成分(2-3)

consumption /kənˈsʌmpʃn/ n. 消费,消耗(3-14)

contaminant /kənˈtæmɪnənt/ n. 污染物(2-3)

contaminate /kənˈtæmɪneɪt/ vt. 污染,弄脏(2-1)

contamination /kənˌtæmɪˈneɪʃn/ n. 污染,玷污,污染物(2-2)

contraction /kənˈtrækʃn/ n. 收缩,紧缩(3-8)

convalescent /ˌkɑːnvəˈlesnt/ n. 恢复中的病人,康复的人 adj. 康复的,恢复期的(2-6)

convert /kənˈvɜːrt/ vt. & vi. 转变,转换,变换(2-9)

coordination /kəoˌɔːrdɪˈneɪʃn/ n. 协调(3-11)

cord /kɔːrd/ n. 绳索,束缚(3-4)

corpuscular /kɔːrˈpʌskjulə/ adj. 血细胞的(3-1)

corresponding /ˌkɔːrəˈspɑːndɪŋ/ adj. 相当的,相应的,一致的 (3-7)

cottage cheese 白软干酪(3-3)

coulometry /kuːˈlɒmɪtri/ n. 电量分析,库仑分析法(2-10)

covalent /ˈkəoveɪlənt/ adj. 共价的(3-20)

cover slip / cover glass 盖玻片(2-7)

COVID-19 新型冠状病毒肺炎(3-17)

C-reactive protein（CRP） C 反应蛋白(5-3)

creatinine /kriˈætənin/ n. ［生化］肌氨酸酐,肌酸酐(1-4)

cross-matching blood 交叉配血(3-7)

crystal /ˈkrɪstl/ n. 晶体(1-2)

crystal violet 结晶紫(试剂)(1-6)

cues /kjuːz/ n. 线索(3-11)

curative /ˈkjʊrətɪv/ adj. 有疗效的(2-4)

custom-tailored /ˌkʌstəmˈteɪlərd/ adj. 定制的,量体裁衣的 (3-18)

cut off concentration 浓度界值(3-15)

cut-off /ˈkʌt ɔːf/ n. 截止,定点,界限(2-7)

cuvette /kjuˈvɛt/ n. [生化](分光光度计等仪器中盛样液用的)比色皿,比色杯(2-9)

cyanide-free SLS method 无氰血红蛋白测定方法(5-4)

cylindrical /səˈlɪndrɪkl/ adj. 圆柱形的(3-2)

cytogenetics /ˌsaɪtodʒəˈnɛtɪks/ n. 细胞遗传学(4-1)

cytokine /ˈsaɪtəkaɪn/ n. [细胞]细胞因子,细胞激素(3-5)

cytological smear 细胞涂片(4-2)

cytological /saiˈtɔlədʒɪkl/ adj. 细胞学的(3-5)

cytology /saiˈtɑːlədʒi/ n. 细胞学(1-1)

cytopathology /ˌsaitəupəˈθɒlədʒi/ n. [病理]细胞病理学 (1-1)

cytosine /ˈsaɪtoˌsin/ n. [生化]胞嘧啶(3-19)

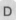

D

decantation /ˌdiːkænˈteiʃən/ n. [化工]倾析,倾注(2-8)

dedicated /ˈdedɪˌkeɪtɪd/ adj. 专用的,专注的(1-4)

dedifferentiate /diːˌdifəˈrenʃieit/ v. (细胞或组织)去分化 (3-13)

defecation /ˌdefəˈkeɪʃn/ n. 排便(3-2)

deformity /dɪˈfɔːrməti/ n. 畸形(5-3)

dehydration /ˌdiːhaɪˈdreɪʃn/ n. 脱水(3-8)

dehydrogenase /ˌdihaiˈdrɑdʒəˌnes/ n. [生化]脱氢酶(3-4)

Deming's cycle 戴明循环或 PDCA 循环(2-13)

demonstrate /ˈdemənstreɪt/ vt. 证明,展示,论证(2-13)

denaturation /diːˌnetʃəˈreʃən/ n. 变性(3-19)

denature /diˈneɪtʃə/ vt. 改变本性(使)变性,(使)改变 (3-14)

dengue /ˈdeŋgi/ n. 登革热(3-17)

deoxyribonuclease (DNase) /diˌoksiˌraiboˈnukliˌes/ n. [生化]脱氧核糖核酸酶(2-3)

deoxyribonucleic acid (DNA)脱氧核糖核酸(2-8)

derangement /dɪˈreɪndʒmənt/ n. 精神错乱(3-12)

derive from . . . 源出……,来自……(3-5)

designated /ˈdɛzɪɡˌnetɪd/ adj. 指定的,特定的(2-4)

designee /ˌdezɪɡˈniː/ n. 被指派者,被任命者(2-13)

detect /dɪˈtekt/ vt. 检测,探测,察觉,发现(1-5)

detection/dɪˈtekʃn/ n. 检查(3-15)

detection limit 检测范围(极限)(1-4)

detection of pathogen nucleic acids 病原体核酸检测(1-1)

detector /dɪˈtɛktər/ n. 探测器(3-1)

deviate /ˈdiːvieit/ vt. & vi. 偏离,脱离,越轨(2-9)

device /dɪˈvaɪs/ n. 设备,仪器(2-1)

diabetes /ˌdaɪəˈbiːtiːz/ n. 糖尿病(1-3)

diagnose /ˌdaɪəɡˈnoʊs/ vt. & vi. 诊断,断定,判断(4-2)

diagnoses /ˌdaɪəɡˈnəʊsiːz/ n. 诊断,调查分析,评价(diagnosis 的复数形式)(2-4)

diagnostic /ˌdaɪəɡˈnɑːstɪk/ adj. 诊断的,特征的 n. 诊断法,诊断结论(5-1)

diagnostics /ˌdaɪəɡˈnɑːstɪks/ n. 诊断学(用作单数)(1-1)

dialysis /daiˈæləsis/ n. [医][分化]透析,渗析(复数 dialyses)(2-5)

diaphragm /ˈdaɪəfræm/ n. 光圈(2-7)

diarrhea /ˌdaɪəˈriə/ n. 腹泻(3-2)

dideoxy /ˈdɪdiːɒksi/ n. 双脱氧法(1-7)

dietary fiber 膳食纤维(3-2)

differentiate /ˌdɪfəˈrenʃieit/ v. 分化,区分(3-5)

differentiation /ˌdɪfəˌrenʃiˈeiʃn/ n. [生物]变异,分化,区别 (2-1)

diffraction /diˈfrækʃn/ n. 衍射(2-7)

digestive /daiˈdʒestiv/ n. 助消化药 adj. 消化的,助消化的 (3-2)

digestive tract 消化道(3-2)

diluent /ˈdɪljuənt/ n. 稀释液(2-4)

dilute /daɪˈluːt/ v. 稀释(2-5)

dimension /daɪˈmenʃn/ n. 方面,维,尺寸(3-16)

diode laser 半导体激光器(5-4)

dipstick /ˈdɪpstɪk/ n. 试纸条(3-2)

direct bilirubin 直接胆红素(3-12)

discipline /ˈdɪsəplɪn/ n. 学科,纪律,训练,惩罚(2-12)

disease-causing microorganism 致病微生物(2-1)

disinfectant /ˌdɪsɪnˈfektənt/ n. 消毒剂 adj. 消毒的(2-2)

disinfection /ˌdɪsɪnˈfekʃn/ n. 消毒,杀菌(2-2)

disparate /ˈdɪspərət/ adj. 不同的,全异的(2-12)

dissociate /dɪˈsoʊʃieit/ v. 离解,分离(2-3)

dissolve /dɪˈzɑːlv/ v. 溶解,分解(2-3)

distinctive /dɪˈstɪŋktɪv/ adj. 独特的,有特色的,与众不同的 (3-3)

distribute /dɪˈstrɪbjuːt/ vt. 分配,散布,分开,把……分类(3-13)

disturbance /dɪˈstɜːrbəns/ n. 失调,紊乱(等于 disorder)(3-8)

diverse /daɪˈvɜːrs/ adj. 不同的(3-5)

domain /doʊˈmeɪn/ n. 结构域(3-20)

donor /ˈdoʊnər/ n. 捐赠者,供者(3-7)

double helix 双螺旋(3-19)

downdraft /ˈdaʊndræft/ n. 下坡,向下之气流或风(2-2)

draw blood 抽血(5-1)

drill /drɪl/ v. 钻孔(2-8)

dropper /ˈdrɑːpər/ n. 滴管(2-8)

drug resistance test 耐药性检测(1-7)

dry heat sterilization 干热灭菌(2-2)

dual wavelength method 双波长法(2-9)

due to . . . 由于……，因为……(2-3)

duplication /ˌduːplɪˈkeɪʃn/ n. 复制(3-19)

duration /duˈreɪʃn/ n. 持续，持续的时间，期间(3-13)

dye /daɪ/ n. 染色，染料(4-2)

dysfunction /disˈfʌŋkʃn/ n. 功能紊乱，功能障碍(3-12)

E

edema /iˈdimə/ n. ［病理］水肿，瘤腺体（等于 oedema）(3-4)

EDTA（Ethylene Diamine Tetraacetic Acid）乙二胺四乙酸(1-4)

efficiency /ɪˈfɪʃnsɪ/ n. 效率，效能(2-11)

electric charge 电荷(3-8)

electrical impedance 电阻抗(3-1)

electrical resistivity 电阻系数(2-4)

electroactive /ˌɪlektrəʊˈæktɪv/ adj. 电活性(2-10)

electrocardiogram /ˌɪlektroʊˈkɑːrdɪougræm/ n. ［内科］心电图(5-2)

electrochemical /ˌɪlektrəʊˈkemɪkəl/ adj. ［物化］电化学的，电气化学的(2-10)

electrode /ɪˈlektroʊd/ n. ［电］电极(2-8)

electrolyte /ɪˈlektrəlaɪt/ n. 电解液，电解质(1-1)

electromagnetic /ˌɪlektroʊmæɡˈnetɪk/ adj. 电磁的(2-7)

electromagnetic radiation 电磁辐射(2-7)

electron beam 电子束(2-7)

electrophoresis /ɪˌlektrofəˈrɪsɪs/ n. ［化学］电泳(1-4)

elevate /ˈelɪveɪt/ vt. 提升，举起(2-5)

elevation /ˌelɪˈveɪʃn/ n. 提升(2-5)

eliminate /ɪˈlɪmɪneɪt/ vt 消除，排除(2-9)

elimination /ɪˌlɪmɪˈneɪʃn/ n. 排除，除去(2-3)

embed /ɪmˈbed/ v. ［医］植入，埋藏(4-1)

embolism /ˈembəlɪzəm/ n. 栓塞，闰日(3-4)

emit /iˈmɪt/ vt. 发出，放射(2-9)

empirical /ɪmˈpɪrɪkl/ adj. 凭经验的(3-18)

endocrine /ˈendəkrɪn/ adj. 内分泌（腺）的 n. 内分泌，内分泌腺，内分泌物(1-4)

endocrine disorder 内分泌紊乱(3-11)

endocrinology /ˌendoʊkrɪˈnɑːlədʒi/ n. 内分泌学(3-11)

endoscope /ˈendəskoʊp/ n. ［临床］内镜(2-2)

enroll /ɪnˈroʊl/ v. 参加，登记(2-1)

enzyme /ˈenzaɪm/ n. ［生化］酶(3-14)

enzyme-linked immunosorbent assay（ELISA）酶联免疫吸附测定(1-5)

eosin /ˈiːəusin/ n. 曙红（鲜红色的染料）(4-3)

eosinophil /ˌiəˈsɪnəfɪl/ n. 嗜酸性粒细胞(1-2)

epidemiology /ˌepɪˌdiːmiˈɑːlədʒi/ n. 流行病学，传染病学(1-6)

epithelial /ˌɛpɪˈθilɪəl/ adj. ［生物］上皮的(1-2)

epithelium /ˌɛpəˈθilɪəm/ n. ［组织］上皮细胞(3-2)

equilibrium /ˌiːkwɪˈlɪbriəm/ n. 平衡，均衡(3-14)

erosion /ɪˈroʊʒn/ n. 侵蚀(5-3)

erythroblastosis /ɪˌrɪθroblæsˈtosɪs/ n. 骨髓成红血细胞增多症(3-7)

erythrocyte sedimentation rate（ESR, or sed rate）红细胞沉降率(5-3)

erythrocyte sedimentation rate 红细胞沉降率，红细胞沉降速度(2-6)

esterify /ɛsˈtɛrɪˌfai/ v. （使）酯化(3-10)

esters /ˈestəs/ n. 酯类(3-10)

etch /etʃ/ v. 蚀刻(2-7)

evaluate /ɪˈvæljʊeɪt/ vt. & vi. 评价，评估(3-13)

evaluation /ɪˌvæljuˈeɪʃn/ n. 评价；［审计］评估，估价，求值(2-4)

excrete /ɪkˈskriːt/ vt. 排泄，分泌(5-3)

expedite /ˈekspədaɪt/ v. 加快(3-1)

explosive /ɪkˈsploʊsɪv/ adj. 爆炸(性)的(2-1)

external quality assessment（EQA）室间质量评价(1-4)

external quality assessment programme（EQAP）室间质量评价计划(2-13)

extracellular /ˌekstrəˈsɛljʊlə/ adj. ［生物］(位于或发生于)细胞外的(2-6)

extraction /ɪkˈstrækʃn/ n. 取出，抽出，拔出，萃取(2-9)

extraction method 萃取法(2-9)

extra-laboratory testing 检验科外的检验(3-15)

extremity /ɪkˈstreməti/ n. 末端，极端，手足(3-6)

eyepiece /ˈaɪpiːs/ n. ［光］目镜，接目镜(2-7)

F

fall into the category 归为……（类别）(3-5)

fall into . . . 分成……(5-2)

fasting plasma glucose 空腹血糖(3-11)

fatigue /fəˈtiːg/ n. 疲劳，疲乏(2-12)

fecal /ˈfiːkl/ adj. 排泄物的(1-2)

fecal occult blood test 粪便隐血检查(1-2)

feces /ˈfiːsiːz/ n. 排泄物，粪便，渣滓(1-2)

femoral artery 股动脉，股骨动脉(3-9)

fermentation /fɜːmenˈteɪʃ(ə)n/ n. 发酵(1-6)

fertility /fərˈtɪləti/ n. 生育力(3-3)

fetalis /ˈfetəlɪs/ n. 胎儿(3-7)

fetus /ˈfiːtəs/ n. 胎儿(1-7)

fiber /ˈfaɪbə/ n. 纤维,光纤(等于 fibre)(4-3)

fingerstick /ˈfɪŋgəstik/ n. 手指穿刺,刺刺(2-5)

fishy /ˈfɪʃɪ/ adj. 鱼的(3-3)

fixation /fɪkˈseɪʃn/ n. 固定,定位,定影(4-1)

flammable /ˈflæməbl/ adj. 易燃的,可燃的(2-1)

flow cytometry 流式细胞术(1-3)

fluid /ˈfluɪd/ n. 液体(1-1)

fluidity /fluˈɪdəti/ n. [流] 流质,流动性(度),易变性(3-10)

fluorescein /ˌfluəˈresiɪn/ n. [试剂] 荧光素,荧光黄(1-5)

fluorescence /fləˈresns/ n. 荧光,荧光性(3-16)

fluorescent flow cytometry 荧光流式细胞术(5-4)

fluorescent tagging 荧光标记(4-3)

fluoride /ˈflɔːraɪd/ n. 氟化物(1-4)

fluoride-selective electrode 氟离子电极(2-10)

fluoroimmunoassay /ˈfluərəˌɪˈmjənoˌæse/ n. 荧光免疫技术(1-5)

fluorophore /ˈfluərəˌfɔː/ n. [化学] 荧光团(3-20)

foam /fuːm/ n. 泡沫(3-3)

focus wheel 调焦旋钮(2-7)

for instance 例如(2-4)

formalin /ˈfɔrməlɪn/ n. [药] 福尔马林(4-1)

formalin-fixed 福尔马林固定(4-1)

formation /fɔːˈmeɪʃn/ n. 形成,队形,编队,构造(3-14)

formula /ˈfɔrmjələ/ n. 公式,准则,配方(3-9)

forward scatter 前向散射(3-16)

fragmentation /ˌfrægmenˈteɪʃn/ n. 破碎,分裂(3-6)

fructose /ˈfrʌktoʊs/ n. [有化] 果糖(3-3)

fundamental /ˌfʌndəˈmentl/ adj. 基本的,根本的(3-19)

fungi /ˈfʌndʒaɪ/ n. 真菌(fungus 的复数)(1-6)

G

gallstone /ˈgɔːlstoʊn/ n. [病理] 胆石(3-12)

gamma glutamyl transpeptidase γ 谷氨酰转肽酶(3-12)

gardnerella /gɑːdnɪrələ/ n. 加德纳菌属(3-3)

gardnerella vaginalis 阴道加德纳菌(3-3)

gaseous /ˈgæsɪəs/ adj. 气体的,气体状态的(2-3)

gastritis /gæˈstraɪtɪs/ n. [内科] 胃炎(5-2)

gauze /gɔz/ n. 纱布(2-5)

genetic code 遗传密码(3-19)

genetic disease 遗传病(1-7)

genetics /dʒəˈnetɪks/ n. 遗传学(genetic 遗传的,基因的)(1-1)

genital /ˈdʒenɪtl/ n. 生殖器 adj. 外阴部,生殖的(3-3)

genital warts 生殖器疣(3-3)

genome /ˈdʒiːnoʊm/ n. 基因组,染色体组(1-7)

genotype /ˈdʒenətaɪp/ n. 基因型,遗传型(1-7)

gestational diabetes 妊娠糖尿病(3-11)

Giemsa stain 吉姆萨染色(4-3)

glass-membrane electrode 玻璃膜电极(2-10)

glean /gliːn/ v. 收集(2-5)

glomerular filtration rate 肾小球滤过率(3-12)

glucose /ˈgluːkoʊs/ n. 葡萄糖,葡糖(等于 dextrose)(3-14)

glutamic acid decarboxylase 谷氨酸脱羧酶(3-11)

gonorrhea /ˌgɒnəˈrɪə/ n. [性病] 淋病(3-3)

gradient /ˈgreɪdɪənt/ n. 梯度,坡度(3-8)

Gram-negative bacteria 革兰氏阴性菌(5-4)

Gram-positive bacteria 革兰氏阳性菌(5-4)

Gram staining 革兰氏染色(1-6)

granularity /ˌgrænjuˈlærɪti/ n. 间隔尺寸(3-16)

granule /ˈgrænjuːl/ n. 颗粒(3-5)

granulocyte /ˈgrænjələˌsaɪt/ n. [组织] 粒细胞,粒性白细胞(3-5)

graph /græf/ n. 图表(2-9)

Graphical User Interface 图形用户界面(5-4)

graticule /ˈgrætɪkjuːl/ n. 显微镜的计数线(2-7)

Graves' disease 毒性弥漫性甲状腺肿,格雷夫斯病(3-11)

gross lesion 肉眼损害(4-1)

guanine /ˈgwɑnin/ n. [生化] 鸟嘌呤(3-19)

gynecologic /ˌgaɪnɪkəˈlɒdʒɪk/ adj. 妇科的,妇产科医学的(3-3)

gynecological smear 妇科涂片(4-2)

haematein /ˌhɛməˈtiɪn/ n. 氧化苏木精(4-2)

haematological /ˌhiːmətəʊˈlɒdʒɪkəl/ adj. 血液学的(3-1)

haematoxylin /ˌhiːməˈtɒksilin/ n. 苏木精(4-3)

half-cell /ˈhɑːfsel/ n. [物化] 半电池(2-10)

half-life period 半衰期(3-12)

Hashimoto's disease 慢性甲状腺炎,桥本病(1-5)

heart failure 心力衰竭(3-13)

heel stick 足跟采血(5-1)

helical /ˈhelɪkl/ adj. 螺旋形的(3-17)

hematocrit /hɪˈmætəkrɪt/ n. 血细胞比容(3-1)

hematology /ˌhiməˈtɑlədʒi/ n. [基医] 血液学(1-1)

hematopoietic /ˌhɛmətopɔɪˈitɪk/ adj. 造血的,生血的(1-3)

hematopoietic tissue 造血组织(1-3)

hemoglobin /ˈhɛmoˈgloʊbɪn/ n. [生化] 血红蛋白(等于 haemoglobin)(1-2)

hemolytic /hiːˈmɒlitik/ adj. [生理] [免疫] 溶血的(3-7)

hemolyze /ˈhɛməlaɪz/ vt. 使(红细胞)溶解 vi. 发生溶血(等于 haemolyze)(2-6) hemophilia /ˌhɛməˈfɪlɪr/ n. ［内科］血友病(等于 haemophilia) (1-3)

hemoptysis /hɪˈmɑptəsɪs/ n. ［临床］咯血,咳血(3-4)

hemorrhage /ˈhɛmərɪdʒ/ n. ［病理］出血(等于 haemorrhage) (1-1)

hemostasis /ˌhiːməʊˈsteɪsɪs/ n. ［医］止血,止血法(3-6)

heparin /ˈhɛpərɪn/ n. ［生化］肝素(用于防治血栓形成等), 肝磷脂(2-6)

hepatitis /ˌhepəˈtaɪtɪs/ n. 肝炎(2-1)

hepatitis B virus (HBV)乙型肝炎病毒(2-1)

hepatocyte /hɪˈpætəsaɪt/ n. ［细胞］肝细胞(3-12)

heredity /həˈredəti/ n. 遗传,遗传性(3-19)

hereinafter /ˌhɪrɪnˈæftər/ adv. 以下,在下文中(2-4)

herpes /ˈhɔːpiz/ n. ［皮肤］疱疹(3-3)

herpes simplex 单纯疱疹(3-3)

heteroduplex /ˌhetərəʊˈdjuːpleks/ adj. 异源双链核酸分子的 (1-7)

hexokinase /ˌheksəʊˈkaineis/ n. ［生化］己糖激酶(3-14)

hidden blood 隐血(3-2)

high-pressure steam sterilization 高压蒸汽灭菌(2-2)

high-throughput screening 高通量筛选(2-12)

histogenesis /ˌhɪstoˈdʒɛnɪsɪs/ n. ［胚］组织发生(3-11)

histogram /ˈhɪstəgræm/ n. ［统计］直方图,柱状图(3-16)

histological /ˌhɪstəˈlɒdʒɪkəl/ adj. 组织学的(2-7)

histological section 组织切片(4-3)

histologist /hisˈtɔlədʒist/ n. ［解剖］组织学家,组织论学家 (4-3)

histopathology /ˌhɪstəʊpəˈθɒlədʒi/ n. 组织病理学(1-1)

histotechnologist /ˌhɪstəˌtekˈnɑːlədʒist/ n. 组织病理技术员 (5-1)

homeostasis /ˌhoʊmɪəˈsteɪsɪs/ n. ［生理］体内平衡(复数 homeostases)(3-8)

horizontal /ˌhɔːrɪˈzɑːntl/ adj. 水平的,地平线的(2-2)

human chorionic gonadotropin (HGG)人体绒毛膜促性腺激素 (3-13)

human immunodeficiency virus (HIV) 人类免疫缺陷病毒 (1-5)

humidity /hjuːˈmɪdəti/ n. ［气象］湿度,湿气(3-8)

humoral /ˈhjuːmərəl/ adj. 体液的(1-4)

hybridization /ˌhaɪbrɪdəˈzeɪʃn/ n. ［化学］杂交,杂化,反应 (1-3)

hybridize /ˈhaɪbrɪdaɪz/ v. 杂交(3-20)

hydration /haɪˈdreɪʃn/ n. ［化学］水合作用(3-8)

hydrogen /ˈhaɪdrədʒən/ n. ［化学］氢(3-8)

hydrogen bond 氢键(3-19)

hydrophilic /ˌhaɪdrəˈfɪlɪk/ adj. ［化学］亲水的(等于 hydrophilous)(2-3)

hydrophobic /ˌhaɪdrəˈfoʊbɪk/ adj. 疏水的(2-3)

hypersensitivity /ˌhaɪpərˌsensəˈtɪvəti/ n. 过敏症(1-5)

hypertrophy /haɪˈpɜːrtrəfi/ n. ［病理］肥大,肥厚,过度增大 (5-2)

hypoalbuminemia /ˌhaipəuælˌbjuːməˈniːmiə/ n. ［内科］低白蛋白血症(3-12)

hypochlorite /ˌhaɪpəˈklɔːraɪt/ n. ［无化］次氯酸盐,低氧化氯 (2-5)

hypothetical /ˌhaɪpəˈθetɪkl/ adj. 假设的(2-12)

hypoxemic /ˌhaipɔkˈsiːmik/ adj. 血氧过低的(3-9)

I

icosahedral /ˌaikəusəˈhedrəl/ adj. ［数］二十面体的(3-17)

icteric /ɪkˈterɪk/ n. 治黄疸之药 adj. 黄疸的(2-6)

identification /aɪˌdentɪfɪˈkeʃn/ n. 鉴别,识别(2-4)

identifier /aɪˈdentɪfaɪər/ n. 标识符,认同者(2-12)

IgG antibody 免疫球蛋白 G 抗体(5-3)

Illumina /ɪˈljuːmɪnə/ n. 依诺米那(公司名)(3-20)

immerse /ɪˈmɜːrs/ vt. 沉浸,使陷入(4-3)

immersion /ɪˈmɜːrʒn/ n. 沉浸,陷入,专心(2-2)

immersion oil 镜油(1-6)

immune system 免疫系统(3-5)

immunoagglutination test 免疫凝集试验(1-5)

immunoassay /ˌɪmjənəˈæˌseɪ/ n. 免疫分析,免疫测定(1-5)

immunoblot /ˈɪmjʊnoʊblɒt/ n. 免疫印迹(1-5)

immunodeficiency /ɪˌmjuːnoʊdɪˈfɪʃnsi/ n. ［免疫］免疫缺陷 (2-1)

immunofluorescence /ˈɪmjunəʊˌfluəˈresns/ n. ［免疫］免疫荧光,免疫荧光法(1-5)

immunoglobulin /ˌɪmjənoʊˈglɑbjələn/ n. ［免疫］［生化］免疫球蛋白,免疫血球素(1-5)

immunohematology /ˌɪmjənoʊˌhiməˈtɑːlədʒi/ n. 免疫血液学 (1-1)

immunohistochemistry /ˈɪmjʊnəʊˌhɪstəʊˈkemɪstrɪ/ n. 免疫组织化学(4-1)

immunolabeling techniques 免疫标记技术(1-5)

immunology /ˌɪmjuˈnɑːlədʒi/ n. ［免疫］免疫学(1-1)

immunopathology /ˌɪmjʊnəʊpəˈθɒlədʒɪ/ n. 免疫病理学(1-5)

immunosorbent /ˌɪmjunəʊˈsɔːbənt/ adj. ［生化］免疫吸附的 n. 免疫吸附剂(1-5)

immunotherapy /ɪˈmjənoʊˈθerəpi/ n. 免疫疗法(2-6)

immunoturbidimetry /ˌɪmjənoʊtəˌbiˈdimitri/ n. 免疫比浊(1-5)

impaired /imˈperd/ adj. 受损的(3-12)

impedance /imˈpiːdns/ n. ［电］阻抗(3-1)

impregnate /imˈpregneɪt/ v. 浸透(2-7)

impregnation /ˌɪmpregˈneɪʃən/ n. 注入,受精,怀孕,受胎 (4-1)

impurities /ɪmˈpjʊrətiz/ n. 杂质(impurity 的复数)(2-3)

in accordance to . . . 根据……(5-2)

in addition to . . . 除……之外(还有,也)(5-2)

incompatibility /ˌɪnkəmˌpætəˈbɪləti/ n. 不相容,不一致(3-7)

incorporate /ɪnˈkɔːrpəreɪt/ vt. 包含(5-4)

incubation /ˌɪŋkjuˈbeɪʃn/ n. [病毒][医] 潜伏,孵化(3-17)

incubation period 潜伏期(5-3)

indication /ˌɪndɪˈkeɪʃn/ n. 指示,指出(3-18)

indicator /ˈɪndɪkeɪtər/ n. 指标,标志,迹象,指示器;[试剂] 指示剂(3-2)

indicator electrode 指示电极(2-10)

indices /ˈɪndɪsiːz/ n. 指标(index 的复数)(3-1)

indigestible /ˌɪndɪˈdʒestəbl/ adj. 难消化的(3-2)

inert separator gel 惰性分离胶(2-6)

infection /ɪnˈfekʃn/ n. 感染(3-1)

infectious /ɪnˈfekʃəs/ adj. 传染的,传染性的(1-1)

infectious agent 传染性试剂,传染因子(2-1)

infiltrate /ˈɪnfɪltreɪt/ v. 使浸润(2-7)

infiltrative /ɪnˈfɪltreɪtɪv/ adj. 渗透性的(3-12)

inflammation /ˌɪnfləˈmeɪʃn/ n. [病理] 炎症;[医] 发炎,燃烧,发火(3-3)

inflammatory /ɪnˈflæmətɔːri/ adj. 炎症性的(1-1)

influenza /ˌɪnfluˈenzə/ n. [内科] 流行性感冒(简写 flu),家畜流行性感冒(1-7)

influenza virus 流感病毒(3-17)

inhale /ɪnˈheɪl/ vt. 吸入(3-17)

initial test 初筛试验(3-17)

inorganic /ˌɪnɔːrˈɡænɪk/ adj. [无化] 无机的(3-2)

inorganic phosphorus 无机磷(2-12)

insight into . . . 深刻理解……,洞察……(2-13)

in-situ hybridization 原位杂交(1-7)

insulin /ˈɪnsəlɪn/ n. [生化][药] 胰岛素(3-11)

integrate /ˈɪntɪɡreɪt/ v. 使……成整体(2-12)

integrated /ˈɪntɪɡreɪtɪd/ adj. 集成的(5-4)

integrated program 综合课程(5-1)

integration /ˌɪntɪˈɡreɪʃn/ n. 集成(3-11)

intended /ɪnˈtendɪd/ adj. 有意的,打算中的(3-7)

intercourse /ˈɪntərkɔːrs/ n. 性交(3-3)

interface /ˈɪntərfeɪs/ v. 相互作用,交流(2-12)

interior /ɪnˈtɪriər/ n. 内部(3-10)

internal quality control (IQC) 室内质量控制(1-4)

International Standardization Organization (ISO) 国际标准化组织(2-3)

international society of blood transfusion (ISBT) 国际输血学会(3-7)

interpret /ɪnˈtɜːrprət/ v. 解释,理解(3-18)

intestine /ɪnˈtestɪn/ n. 肠(3-2)

intrahepatic /ˌɪntrəhiˈpætɪk/ adj. [解剖] 肝内的(3-12)

intraperitoneal /ˈɪntrəˌperɪtəuˈniːəl/ adj. 腹膜内的(3-13)

intravenous /ˌɪntrəˈviːnəs/ adj. 静脉内的(3-8)

intubation /ˌɪntjuːˈbeɪʃən/ n. [临床] 插管,插管法(2-2)

invalidate /ɪnˈvælɪdeɪt/ vt. 使无效,使无价值(2-6)

invasive procedures 创伤性操作,侵入性医疗作业(2-5)

inverted /ɪnˈvɜːtɪd/ adj. 倒转的,反向的(3-18)

in vitro 在(活)体外,在试管内(2-4)

in vivo 在活的有机体内(3-18)

ion /ˈaɪən/ n. 离子(2-4)

ion channel 离子通道(3-8)

ion selective electrode 离子选择性电极(3-8)

ionic /aɪˈɑːnɪk/ adj. 离子的(2-3)

ionizing radiation 电离辐射灭菌(2-2)

ion-selective electrode 离子选择电极(2-10)

irradiate /ɪˈreɪdieɪt/ vt. 辐射,辐照,照射,放射(2-9)

irradiation /ɪˌreɪdiˈeɪʃn/ n. 照射(2-7)

isoform /ˈaɪsəufɔːm/ n. 亚型,同种型(3-10)

isotype /ˈaɪsəutaɪp/ n. 同型抗原(1-5)

isozyme /ˈaɪsəuzaim/ n. [生化] 同工酶(等于 isoenzyme)(3-13)

it goes without saying that 不用说,不言而喻(2-5)

itch /ɪtʃ/ n. 痒,疥疮 vt. & vi. (使)发痒(3-3)

K

Karl Landsteiner 卡尔·兰德斯坦纳(人名)(3-7)

karyotype /ˈkærɪəˌtaɪp/ n. 核型(1-7)

kell system 凯尔系统(3-7)

ketone body 酮体(3-2)

kinase /ˈkɪnneɪz/ n. [生化] 激酶,致活酶(3-20)

Kirby-Bauer antibiotic testing K-B 药物敏感性试验(3-18)

kit /kɪt/ n. 试剂盒,成套用品(2-4)

krypton /ˈkrɪptɑːn/ n. [化学] 氪(3-16)

L

laboratory information system (LIS) 实验室信息系统(2-5)

laboratory management system 实验室管理系统(2-5)

lactate /ˈlækteɪt/ n. 乳酸,乳酸盐(3-4)

lactate dehydrogenase 乳酸脱氢酶(3-4)

Beer-Lambert law 比尔-朗伯定律(2-9)

laminar /ˈlæmɪnər/ adj. 层状的,薄片状的,板状的(2-2)

lancet /ˈlænsɪt/ n. [外科] 柳叶刀(2-5)

larvae /ˈlɑrvi/ n. 幼虫,幼体(larva 的复数)(1-2)

laryngitis /ˌlærɪnˈdʒaɪtɪs/ n. [耳鼻喉] 喉炎(3-4)

laser /ˈleɪzər/ n. 激光(3-16)

lavender /ˈlævəndər/ n. 薰衣草,淡紫色 adj. 淡紫色的(2-6)

leach /liːtʃ/ v. 浸出(2-3)

lecithin /ˈlesɪθɪn/ n. [生化] 卵磷脂,蛋黄素(3-10)

lengthwise /ˈlɛŋθˌwaɪz/ adv. 纵长地(3-19)

lesion /ˈliːʒn/ n. 功能障碍(4-2)

leukemia /luˈkimɪə/ n. ［内科］［肿瘤］白血病(1-3)

leukocyte /ˈlʊkəˌsaɪt/ n. 白细胞(等于 leucocyte)(1-3)

leukotriene /ˌljuːkəuˈtraiən/ n. ［生化］白三烯(3-5)

Lewis system 路易斯系统(3-7)

lifespan /ˈlaɪfspæn/ n. 寿命,预期生命期限(3-6)

linearity /ˌlɪnɪˈærəti/ n. 线性,直线性(2-11)

lining /ˈlaɪnɪŋ/ n. (身体器官内壁的)膜(5-3)

lipoprotein /ˌlɪpəˈprəutiːn/ n. ［生化］脂蛋白(3-10)

liquid immersion 液浸灭菌(2-2)

lithium ion battery 锂离子电池(3-8)

logarithm /ˈlɔːgərɪðəm/ n. ［数］对数(2-10)

logarithmic /ˌlɔːgəˈrɪðmɪk/ adj. 对数的(3-16)

low-density lipoprotein（LDL）低密度脂蛋白(3-10)

lubricant /ˈluːbrɪkənt/ n. 润滑剂,润滑油(3-3)

lymphatic /lɪmˈfætɪk/ adj. 淋巴的(3-10)

lymphocyte /ˈlɪmfəsaɪt/ n. ［免疫］淋巴细胞,淋巴球(1-2)

lymphocytopenia /ˌlɪmfəsaɪtəˈpiːnɪə/ n. ［内科］淋巴球减少,
　淋巴细胞(球)减少症(3-5)

lymphocytosis /ˌlɪmfosaɪˈtosɪs/ n. ［内科］淋巴球增多,淋巴细
　胞(球)过多症(3-5)

lymphoma /lɪmˈfoumə/ n. ［肿瘤］淋巴瘤(3-16)

lysate /ˈlaiseit/ n. 溶菌产物,溶解产物(3-20)

lysis /ˈlaɪsɪs/ n. (生物)溶胞,溶菌,溶解,分解(1-6)

lysosome /ˈlaɪsəˌsom/ n. ［细胞］(细胞中的)溶酶体(3-5)

M

macromolecular /ˌmækrəuməuˈlekjulə/ adj. ［化学］大分子的
　(3-14)

magnesium /mægˈniːzɪəm/ n. ［化学］镁,镁离子(3-8)

major cross-match 主侧配血(3-7)

make up 组成,构成,占据(2-3)

malaria /məˈleərɪə/ n. ［内科］疟疾,瘴气(4-3)

Mallory body 酒精小体,马洛里小体(4-3)

mammal /ˈmæml/ n. ［脊椎］哺乳动物(3-5)

manually /ˈmænjuəli/ adv. 手动地(3-1)

marine /məˈriːn/ n. 海运业(3-16)

marrow /ˈmærou/ n. 髓,骨髓,精华,活力(1-2)

masturbate /ˈmæstərbeɪt/ vi. 手淫 vt. 对……行手淫(3-3)

matrix /ˈmeɪtrɪks/ n. ［生物］基质,母体,子宫(2-6)

maturation /ˌmætʃuˈreɪʃn/ n. 成熟,化脓(3-17)

MCHC 平均红细胞血红蛋白浓度(3-1)

mean corpuscular volume（MCV）平均红细胞体积(3-1)

measurement /ˈmeʒərmənt/ n. 测量,度量,尺寸(3-18)

measurement range 测量范围(1-4)

mechanism /ˈmekənɪzəm/ n. 原理,机制(3-8)

meconium /məˈkonɪəm/ n. 胎便(3-2)

median cubital vein 肘正中静脉(2-5)

medication /ˌmedɪˈkeɪʃn/ n. 药物治疗,药物(2-1)

medium /ˈmiːdɪəm/ n. 介质(2-8)

megakaryocyte /ˌmegəˈkærɪəusait/ n. ［组织］巨核细胞(3-6)

melt off 熔化掉(4-1)

membrane /ˈmembreɪn/ n. 膜,薄膜(2-1)

menstrual /ˈmenstruəl/ adj. 月经的(3-3)

menstrual cycle 月经周期(3-3)

mercury /ˈmɜːrkjəri/ n. ［化学］汞,水银(3-16)

messenger RNA 信使 RNA(3-19)

metabolic /ˌmetəˈbɑːlɪk/ adj. 变化的,新陈代谢的(1-3)

metabolite /mɛˈtæbəlaɪt/ n. ［生化］代谢物(3-15)

metabolome /metæbouˈlɒm/ n. 代谢组(1-7)

metal mould 金属铸模(4-1)

metastases /məˈtæstəsiːs/ n. 转移(metastasis 的复数)(3-13)

meter /ˈmiːtər/ n. 仪表,计量器(2-10)

methylation /ˌmeθɪˈleɪʃən/ n. ［有化］甲基化,甲基化作用
　(1-7)

methylene blue 亚甲蓝(4-3)

microalbuminuria /ˌmaɪkrəuælˈbjuminˈnʊrɪə/ n. 微白蛋白尿,
　微量白蛋白尿(3-12)

microarray /ˌmaɪkrəuəˈrei/ n. 微阵列,微阵列芯片(3-20)

microarray profiling 微阵列谱(3-20)

microbiology /ˌmaɪkroubaɪˈɑːlədʒi/ n. 微生物学(1-1)

microelectrode /ˌmaɪkrəuiˈlektrəud/ n. 微电极(2-10)

micronized silica 二氧化硅微粒(2-6)

micronutrient /ˌmaɪkroˈnjutrɪənt/ n. ［生化］微量营养素
　(1-3)

microorganism /ˌmaɪkrouˈɔːrgənɪzəm/ n. ［微］微生物(1-1)

microscope /ˈmaɪkrəskoup/ n. 显微镜(4-2)

microscope slide 显微镜载物片(2-7)

microscopic /ˌmaɪkrəˈskɑːpɪk/ adj. 微观的(3-20)

microscopy /maɪˈkrɑːskəpi/ n. 显微镜学(1-1)

microtome /ˈmaɪkrəˌtom/ n. 显微镜用薄片切片机(2-7)

migrate /ˈmaɪgreɪt/ v. 迁移,移居(3-5)

milky /ˈmɪlkɪ/ adj. 乳状的,乳白色的(3-3)

minimum inhibitory concentration（MIC）最小抑菌浓度,最低
　抑菌浓度(1-6)

minor cross-match 次侧配血(3-7)

misleading /ˌmɪsˈliːdɪŋ/ adj. 令人误解的,引入歧途的(3-14)

mitigate /ˈmɪtɪgeɪt/ v. 使缓和,使减轻(2-4)

mitochondria /ˌmaɪtoˈkɑndrɪr/ n. 线粒体(mitochondrion 的复
　数)(3-13)

molar /ˈmoulər/ adj. 磨碎的,臼齿的;［物理］质量上的;［化
　学］摩尔的(3-14)

molar absorptivity 摩尔吸光系数(2-9)

molarity /moʊˈlærɪti/ n. ［化学］摩尔浓度(2-3)

molecular /məˈlekjələr/ *adj.* 分子的,由分子组成的(1-1)

molecular pathology 分子病理学(4-1)

molecule /ˈmɑːlɪkjuːl/ *n.* ［化学］分子,微粒(3-14)

monitor /ˈmɑːnɪtər/ *n.* 监视器,监听器,班长 *vt.* 监控(3-13)

monochromatic light 单色光(2-9)

monochromator /ˌmɔnəuˈkrəumeitə/ *n.* ［光］单色仪,单色器,单色光镜(2-9)

monoclonal /ˌmɑnoˈklonəl/ *adj.* 单细胞繁殖的(3-15)

monocyte /ˈmɑːnəsaɪt/ *n.* ［基医］单核细胞(1-2)

morpheme /ˈmɔːrfiːm/ *n.* ［语］词素(5-2)

morphological /ˌmɔːrfəˈlɑːdʒɪkl/ *adj.* 形态学的(1-1)

mosquito /məˈskiːtoʊ/ *n.* 蚊子(3-17)

motility /məʊˈtɪlətɪ/ *n.* 运动性(1-6)

mucopurulent /ˌmjuːkəʊˈpjuərulənt/ *adj.* 黏脓性的(3-4)

mucous /ˈmjuːkəs/ *adj.* 黏液的(2-1)

mucus /ˈmjuːkəs/ *n.* 黏液(3-2)

Mueller-Hinton agar plates 水解酪蛋白培养基琼脂平板(3-18)

multidisciplinary /ˌmʌltiˈdɪsəpləneri/ *adj.* 有关各种学问的(4-1)

multipotent /mʌlˈtipətənt/ *adj.* 多能的(3-5)

mutation /mjuˈteʃn/ *n.* 突变(1-7)

myasthenia gravis 重症肌无力(1-5)

mycobacteria /ˌmaikəubækˈtiəriə/ *n.* ［微］分枝杆菌(1-6)

myelogenous /ˌmaiəˈlɔdʒənəs/ *adj.* 骨髓性的(3-16)

myeloperoxidase /ˌmaiələupəˈrɔksideis/ *n.* 髓过氧化物酶(3-4)

myocardial /ˌmaɪəˈkardɪəl/ *n.* 心肌衰弱(1-4)

myocardial infarction（MI）心肌梗死(3-6)

myocyte /ˈmaɪəsaɪt/ *n.* 肌细胞,肌丝层(3-13)

myoglobin /ˈmaɪoˌglobɪn/ *n.* ［生化］肌红蛋白(等于 myohemoglobin)(3-13)

N

naked eye（unaided eye）肉眼(1-2)

National Committee for Clinical Laboratory Standards（NCCLS）美国临床实验室标准化委员会(2-3)

negative /ˈnegətɪv/ *adj.* ［医］［化学］阴性的(2-8)

neoplasm /ˈnioplæzm/ *n.* ［医］赘生物,瘤,新生物(3-6)

nephrotic syndrome 肾病综合征(3-12)

nephrotoxic /ˌnefrəˈtɔksɪk/ *adj.* ［医］对肾脏有害处的(3-12)

Nernst Equation 能斯特方程(2-10)

nervous /ˈnɜːrvəs/ *adj.* 神经的(3-4)

neurological /ˌnʊrəˈlɑːdʒɪkl/ *adj.* 神经病学的,神经学上的(3-8)

neurologist /nʊˈrɑːlədʒɪst/ *n.* 神经学家,神经科专业医师(5-2)

neurology /nʊˈrɑːlədʒi/ *n.* 神经病学,神经学(5-2)

neuron-specific enolase（NSE）神经特异性烯醇(3-13)

neutral /ˈnuːtrəl/ *adj.* 中性的,中立的(3-5)

neutrophil /ˈnjuːtrəfil/ *n.* 中性粒细胞(1-2)

nicotinamide adenine dinucleotide phosphate 烟酰胺腺嘌呤二核苷酸磷酸,辅酶Ⅱ(3-14)

nicotinamide adenine dinucleotide 烟酰胺腺嘌呤二核苷酸,辅酶Ⅰ(3-14)

NIDA（the national institute on drug abuse）国家药物滥用研究所(3-15)

noncondensing /ˈnɔnkənˈdensɪŋ/ *adj.* 不凝固的,不凝结的(3-8)

nonelectrolyte /ˌnɔnɪˈlektrəlaɪt/ *n.* 非电解质(2-3)

non-invasive prenatal screening 无创产前筛查(1-7)

norovirus /ˈnɔːrouvaɪrəs/ *n.* 诺瓦克病毒(3-17)

nuclear magnetic resonance spectroscopy 磁共振光谱法(2-9)

nucleate /ˈnjʊklɪɪt/ *v.* (使)成核 *adj.* 有核的(3-5)

nuclei /ˈnjʊklɪˌai/ *n.* 核心,核子(4-2)

nucleic acid 核酸(2-8)

O

objective turret 物镜转换器(2-7)

observed value 观测值(2-11)

obstruction /əbˈstrʌkʃn/ *n.* 阻塞,障碍(3-4)

occult /əˈkʌlt/ *adj.* 被掩蔽的(3-2)

occult blood 潜血(3-2)

occupational exposure 职业暴露(2-1)

Occupational Safety and Health Administration（OSHA）职业安全与健康管理局(2-1)

ocular /ˈɑːkjələr/ *adj.* 眼睛的,视觉的,目击的 *n.* ［光］目镜(2-7)

odor /ˈoʊdər/ *n.* 气味(1-2)

odorless /ˈodərlɪs/ *adj.* 无气味的,无臭的(2-3)

oil-soluble 油溶的(3-10)

oligonucleotide /ˌɔligəuˈnjuːklɪəutaid/ *n.* ［生化］寡核苷酸(3-20)

on the basis of … 根据……(5-1)

oncofetal antigens 癌胎抗原(3-13)

oncogene /ˈɑŋkəˌdʒin/ *n.* ［遗］［肿瘤］致癌基因(1-7)

oncology /ɑːnˈkɑːlədʒi/ *n.* ［肿瘤］肿瘤学(3-13)

opaque /oʊˈpeɪk/ *adj.* 不透明的(3-4)

optical /ˈɑːptɪkl/ *adj.* 光学的(2-7)

optical microscope 光学显微镜(4-1)

optimize /ˈɑːptɪmaɪz/ *v.* 使最优化,使完善(2-5)

optimum /ˈɑːptɪməm/ *adj.* 最佳的,最适宜的(3-14)

oral glucose tolerance test（OGTT）口服葡萄糖耐量试验

（3-11）

order of draw 采血顺序（2-5）

organic compound 有机化合物（4-3）

organism /ˈɔːrgənɪzəm/ n. 有机体，生物体，微生物（3-14）

organogenesis /ˌɔːgænoˈdʒʒsɪsɪs/ n. ［胚］器官发生，器官形成（3-11）

orientation /ˌɔːriənˈteɪʃn/ n. 方向，定向，适应，情况介绍（4-1）

osmotic /ɑːzˈmɑːtɪk/ adj. 渗透性的（3-8）

osology /oʊˈsɑlədʒɪ/ n. 体液学（1-1）

osteoarthritis /ˌɑːstiʊɑːrˈθraɪtɪs/ n. ［外科］骨关节炎（5-3）

outline /ˈaʊtlaɪn/ n. 轮廓，大纲，概要，略图 vt. 概述，略述，描画……轮廓（3-19）

ovarian /oʊˈveriən/ adj. ［解剖］卵巢的，子房的（3-13）

ovary /ˈoʊvəri/ n. ［解剖］卵巢（复数 ovaries）（3-11）

over-secretion /ˈəʊvə siˈkriːʃn/ n. 分泌过多（3-11）

ovum /ˈoʊvəm/ n. ［细胞］［组织］卵子（复数 ova）（3-2）

oxygenate /ˈɑːksɪdʒəneɪt/ vt. 氧化，充氧，以氧处理（3-9）

packed cells 浓集细胞（3-7）

packed-cell volume 血细胞比容（3-1）

palpable /ˈpælpəbl/ adj. 明显的，可感知的，易觉察的

pancreas /ˈpæŋkrɪəs/ n. ［解剖］胰腺（1-4）

panel /ˈpænl/ n. 仪表板，嵌板（3-1）

Pap smear 帕普涂片，巴氏涂片，宫颈涂片（4-2）

Papanicolaou stain 巴氏染色法（4-2）

parabasal cell 副底层细胞（4-2）

paracetamol /ˌpærəˈsiːtəmɑːl/ n. 对乙酰氨基酚（3-12）

paraffin section 石蜡切片（4-1）

paraffin wax 固体石蜡（4-1）

parameter /pəˈræmɪtər/ n. 参数，系数，参量（2-4）

parasitic /ˌpærəˈsɪtɪk/ adj. 寄生的（等于 parasitical）（1-2）

parasitology /ˌpærəsaɪˈtɑlədʒi/ n. 寄生虫学（1-1）

parathyroid /ˌpærəˈθaɪrɔɪd/ n. 甲状旁腺（3-8）

parathyroid hormone 甲状旁腺素（3-8）

parenchymal /pərənˈkəməl/ adj. 薄壁组织的（3-12）

parenteral /pəˈrɛntərəl/ adj. 肠胃外的（2-1）

Pasteur pipette 巴斯德吸管（2-8）

pathogen /ˈpæθədʒən/ n. ［基医］病原体，病原菌，致病菌（1-1）

pathogenic /ˌpæθəˈdʒenɪk/ adj. 致病的，病原的，发病的（等于 pathogenetic）（1-1）

pathological /ˌpæθəˈlɑːdʒɪkl/ adj. 病理（学）的（等于 pathologic）（3-2）

pathological diagnosis 病理学诊断（4-1）

pathologist /pəˈθɑːlədʒɪst/ n. 病理学家（5-1）

pathology /pəˈθɑːlədʒi/ n. 病理（学）（1-1）

pathophysiology /ˌpæθoˌfɪziˈɑlədʒi/ n. 病理生理学（1-1）

pediatric /ˌpiːdiˈætrɪk/ adj. 小儿科的（5-2）

pediatrician /ˌpiːdiəˈtrɪʃən/ n. 儿科医生（等于 paediatrician）（5-2）

penetrate /ˈpenətreɪt/ vt. & vi. 渗透，穿透，刺入（2-9）

penetration /ˌpenəˈtreɪʃn/ n. 穿入，侵入，渗透（3-17）

pepsin /ˈpepsɪn/ n. 胃蛋白酶，助消化药（3-14）

perception /pərˈsepʃn/ n. 知觉（3-11）

percutaneous /ˌpɜːrkjuːˈteɪniəs/ adj. 通过皮肤的（2-1）

perform /pərˈfɔːrm/ v. 执行（3-19）

performance /pərˈfɔːrməns/ n. 性能，绩效，表演，执行，表现（1-4）

performance characteristics 运行特性（2-4）

perinuclear /ˌperəˈnjuklɪə/ adj. 细胞核周围的（3-5）

periodic /ˌpɪriˈɑːdɪk/ adj. 周期的，定期的（3-9）

periodically /ˌpɪriˈɑːdɪkli/ adv. 定期地，周期性地（2-13）

peripheral blood 外周血（3-1）

peripheral blood smear 外周血涂片（3-5）

permanent /ˈpɜːrmənənt/ adj. 永久的，永恒的，不变的（4-3）

permeability /ˌpɜːrmiəˈbɪləti/ n. 渗透性（3-10）

perpendicular /ˌpɜːrpənˈdɪkjələr/ adj. 垂直的（2-5）

personnel /ˌpɜːrsəˈnel/ n. 人员（5-1）

perspective /pərˈspektɪv/ n. 观点，远景（2-12）

pertain to 关于（5-2）

petri plate 培养皿（3-18）

pharmacogenetics /ˌfɑrməkodʒəˈnɛtɪks/ n. 遗传药理学（1-7）

pharmacopeia /ˈfɑrməkəˈpiə/ n. 药典，处方汇编（2-4）

phlebotomist /fliˈbɑtəmist/ n. 采血员，抽血者（5-1）

phlegm /flem/ n. 痰，黏液（3-4）

phosphate /ˈfɑːsfeɪt/ n. 磷酸盐，磷肥（3-14）

phosphatidic acid 磷脂酸（3-10）

phosphatidylcholine /ˈfɔsfəˌtaidilˈkɔuliːn/ n. ［生化］卵磷脂，磷脂酰胆碱（3-10）

phosphatidylethanolamine /ˌfɔsfəˈtaidilˌeθəˈnɔləmiːn/ n. ［生化］磷脂酰乙醇胺（3-10）

phosphatidylglycerol /ˌfɔsfəˈtaidilˈglisərɔl/ n. ［生化］磷脂酰甘油（3-10）

phosphatidylinositol /ˌfɔsfəˈtaidiliˈnəusitɔl/ n. ［生化］磷脂酰肌醇（3-10）

phosphatidylserine /fɔsfəˈtaidilsəriːn/ n. ［生化］磷脂酰丝氨酸（3-10）

phosphotungstic acid 磷钨酸（4-2）

photometric /ˌfəʊtəʊˈmetrik/ adj. 测光的（5-4）

phthalate /ˈ(f)θæleɪt/ n. 邻苯二甲酸酯（2-10）

physically /ˈfɪzɪkli/ adv. 身体上地（5-2）

physician /fɪˈzɪʃn/ n. 医师，内科医师（1-6）

physiology /ˌfɪziˈɑːlədʒi/ n. 生理学（1-1）

picomole /ˈpaikəuməul/ n. 皮摩尔,微微摩尔(3-20)

pigment /ˈpɪgmənt/ n. [物][生化] 色素,颜料(3-13)

pipette /paɪˈpet/ n. 移液管,吸移管(2-11)

pituitary /pɪˈtuːəteri/ n. 脑垂体(3-11)

placental /pləˈsentl/ adj. 胎盘的(3-12)

plasma /ˈplæzmə/ n. [生理] 血浆(1-3)

plasticizer /ˈplæstəˌsaɪzə/ n. 塑化剂(2-10)

platelet /ˈpleɪtlət/ n. [组织] 血小板,薄片(3-6)

play a key role in ... 在……中起关键作用(3-5)

pneumococcus /ˌnjuːməˈkɑkəs/ n. [微][基医] 肺炎球菌(3-4)

pneumonia /nuːˈmounɪə/ n. 肺炎(3-4)

polarity /pəˈlærəti/ n. [物] 极性,两极,对立(2-3)

polyacrylamide /ˈpɔliˌækriˈlæmaɪd/ n. [高分子] 聚丙烯酰胺(2-8)

Polymerase chain reaction 聚合酶链式反应(1-3)

polymorphonuclear neutrophils 多形核中性粒白细胞(3-2)

polyvinyl chloride 聚氯乙烯(2-10)

poor nutrient 营养不良(3-2)

portmanteau /pɔːrtˈmæntou/ n. 混成词(3-2)

positive /ˈpɑːzətɪv/ adj. [医][化学] 阳性的(2-8)

post baccalaureate degree 硕士学位(5-1)

post-analytical stage 分析后阶段(2-13)

potassium /pəˈtæsiəm/ n. [化学] 钾,钾离子(3-8)

potentiometry /pəˌtenʃiˈɔmitri/ n. [电] 电势测定法,电位测定法(2-10)

pre-analytical stage 分析前阶段(2-13)

precaution /prɪˈkɔːʃn/ n. 预防(措施),警惕(2-1)

precipitate /prɪˈsɪpɪteɪt/ n. 沉淀物(2-3)

precipitation reaction 沉淀反应(1-5)

precise /prɪˈsaɪs/ adj. 精确的(3-1)

precursor /priˈkɜːrsər/ n. 前体,前体物(3-6)

predetermine /ˌpriːdɪˈtɜːrmɪn/ vt. 预先确定,预先决定,预先查明(2-6)

prediabetes /ˌpriːdaɪəˈbitɪs/ n. [内科] 前驱糖尿病(3-11)

pregnancy /ˈpregnənsi/ n. 怀孕(3-15)

primary standard 基准物质(2-4)

primer /ˈpraɪmər/ n. 引物(3-19)

probe /proub/ n. 探针,调查(2-11)

professional/prəˈfeʃənl/ adj. 专业的,职业的 n. 专业人员(5-1)

proficiency /prəˈfɪʃnsi/ n. 精通,熟练(2-13)

proficiency testing (PT)能力比对验证,能力验证(2-13)

progenitor /prouˈdʒenɪtər/ n. 祖先,起源(3-5)

prognosis /prɑːgˈnousɪs/ n. [医] 预后,预知(复数 prognoses)(1-1)

prognostic /prɑːgˈnɑːstɪk/ n. 预兆,预后症状 adj. 预后的,医学预测的(3-12)

programmable /ˈprougræməbl/ adj. [计] 可编程的,可设计的(3-19)

proliferation /prəˌlɪfəˈreɪʃn/ n. 增殖,扩散(3-11)

property/ˈprɑːpərti/ n. 性质,性能,财产,所有权(复数 properties)(3-14)

prostate /ˈprɑːsteɪt/ adj. 前列腺的 n. 前列腺(3-13)

prostate specific antigen (PSA)前列腺特异抗原(3-13)

prostatic /ˈprɔsteitik/ adj. 前列腺的(1-2)

protein /ˈproutiːn/ n. 蛋白质,朊(1-1)

protein engineering 蛋白质工程(3-16)

proteinaceous /proutiːˈneɪʃəs/ adj. 蛋白质的(3-2)

protein-protein interaction 蛋白质-蛋白质相互作用(3-20)

proteinuria /ˌprotiːnˈjuəriə/ n. [泌尿] 蛋白尿(症)(3-12)

proteolytic /ˌprəutiəˈlɪtɪk/ adj. [生化] 蛋白水解的,解蛋白的(3-3)

proteolytic enzyme 蛋白水解酶(3-3)

proteome /ˈprəutɪəum/ n. 蛋白质组(1-7)

prothrombin /proˈθrɑmbin/ n. 凝血素,凝血酶原(3-6)

protocol /ˈproutəkɑːl/ n. 草案(5-4)

provision /prəˈvɪʒn/ n. 供应,规定(2-13)

pulmonary abscess 肺脓肿(3-4)

pulmonary embolism 肺栓塞,肺血管阻塞症(3-6)

puncture /ˈpʌŋktʃər/ v. 刺穿,戳破,揭穿 n. 穿刺,刺痕(2-2)

purify /ˈpjʊrɪfaɪ/ v. 净化(3-19)

purine /ˈpjuriːn/ n. [有化] 嘌呤(3-19)

purulent /ˈpjʊrələnt/ adj. 化脓的,脓的(3-4)

pus /pʌs/ n. 脓,脓汁(3-5)

putative /ˈpjuːtətɪv/ adj. 推定的,假定的(5-1)

pyrimidine /paɪˈrɪməˌdin/ n. [生化] 嘧啶(3-19)

Q

qualitative /ˈkwɑːlɪteɪtɪv/ adj. 定性的(3-15)

quality assurance (QA)质量保证,质量评价(2-13)

quality assurance programme (QAP)质量保证计划(2-13)

quantitatively/ˈkwɒntəteɪtɪvli/ adv. 数量上,分量上(2-11)

R

rack /ræk/ n. 架子,样本架,行李架(2-12)

radial artery 桡动脉,桡骨动脉(3-9)

radial artery puncture 桡动脉穿刺(2-5)

radiation /ˌreɪdiˈeɪʃn/ n. 辐射,放射物(2-2)

radioactive /ˌreɪdiouˈæktɪv/ adj. [核] 放射性的(2-1)

radioimmunoassay /ˈrediˌoɪmjənoˈæse/ n. 放射免疫检定法(1-5)

radionuclide /ˈredioˈnjuˌklaɪd/ n. [核] 放射性核素(1-5)

random plasma glucose 随机血糖(3-11)

rash /ræʃ/ n. (皮肤)皮疹(3-3)

reabsorption /ˌriːəbˈsɔːpʃən/ n. 再吸收(1-4)

reactant /rɪˈæktənt/ n. 〔化学〕反应物,反应剂(2-4)

reaction /rɪˈækʃn/ n. 反应(3-15)

readout /ˈriːdˌaut/ n. 显示器,读出器,示值读数(2-9)

reagent /riˈeɪdʒənt/ n. 〔试剂〕试剂,反应物(2-4)

reagent-quality 试剂质量(2-4)

reassurance /ˌriːəˈʃurəns/ n. 使安心,再保证,放心(2-11)

recalibrate /riˈkælɪbreɪt/ v. 重新校准(2-11)

receptor /rɪˈseptər/ n. 〔生化〕受体,接受器,感觉器官(3-20)

recipient /rɪˈsɪpiənt/ n. 接受者,容纳者(3-7)

recognize /ˈrekəgnaɪz/ v. 承认,认可,识别(3-7)

recombinant immunoblot assay (RIBA)重组免疫印迹试验(3-17)

rectal /ˈrektəl/ adj. 直肠的(3-13)

rectum /ˈrektəm/ n. 直肠(复数 rectums 或 recta)(3-2)

redox /ridˈɑks/ n. 〔化学〕氧化还原反应(3-14)

reducing substances 还原物质(3-2)

refer to ... 指的是……(5-2)

refer to ... as ... 把……称作……(2-3)

reference electrode 参比电极(2-10)

reference range 参考范围(3-6)

reference value 参考值(3-4)

reflection /riˈflekʃn/ n. 反射(2-7)

refraction /riˈfrækʃn/ n. 折射(2-7)

rehabilitation /ˌriːəˌbɪlɪˈteɪʃn/ n. 复原,康复(1-1)

relate to ... 与……有关(5-2)

release /rɪˈliːs/ v. 释放,发射 n. 释放,发布(2-3)

relevant /ˈreləvənt/ adj. 相关的(5-2)

renal /ˈriːnl/ adj. 〔解剖〕肾脏的(3-12)

renal function 肾功能(3-8)

repeatability/riˈpiːtəˌbiliti/ n. 重复性;〔计〕可重复性,再现性(2-11)

repetitive /rɪˈpetətɪv/ adj. 重复的(2-12)

replicate /ˈreplɪkeɪt/ v. 复制,折叠(3-17)

reproducibility/riprəˌdjuːsəˈbiliti/ n. 〔自〕再现性(2-11)

reproducible /ˌriːprəˈduːsəbl/ adj. 可再生的(2-10)

reservoir /ˈrezərvwɑːr/ n. 储液槽(2-7)

residual /rɪˈzɪdʒuəl/ n. 剩余,残渣 adj. 剩余的,残留的(2-2)

resistance /rɪˈzɪstəns/ n. 耐药性(3-18)

respiratory /ˈrespərətɔːri/ adj. 呼吸的(1-3)

respiratory therapist 呼吸治疗师(3-9)

respiratory acidosis 呼吸性酸中毒(3-9)

retention /rɪˈtenʃn/ n. 保留,扣留,滞留,记忆力(3-9)

retrospectively /ˌretrəˈspektɪvli/ adv. 回顾地(2-13)

revolutionize /ˌrevəˈluːʃənaɪz/ vt. 发动革命(2-7)

revolver /rɪˈvɑːlvər/ n. 旋转器(2-7)

rhesus antigens 恒河猴抗原(3-7)

rheumatoid arthritis 类风湿性关节炎(5-3)

rheumatoid factor 类风湿因子(5-3)

rheumatology /ˌruːməˈtɒlədʒɪ/ n. 风湿病学(3-15)

ribonuclease (RNase) /ˌraɪboˈnjʊklɪez/ n. 〔生化〕核糖核酸酶(2-3)

ribonucleic acid (RNA)核糖核酸(2-8)

robustness /roʊˈbʌstnəs/ n. 〔计〕稳健性(2-4)

rotation /roʊˈteɪʃn/ n. 旋转(2-8)

rotavirus /ˌrotəˈvaɪrəs/ n. 轮状病毒(1-2)

routine and microscopy (R&M)常规与显微镜检验(3-2)

rung /rʌŋ/ n. 阶梯(3-19)

S

safranin /ˈsæfrənɪn/ n. 盐基性红色染料(1-6)

saliva /səˈlaɪvə/ n. 唾液(2-1)

salt bridge 盐桥(2-10)

sample /ˈsæmpl/ n. 样本(3-15)

SARS (severe acute respiratory syndromes)严重急性呼吸综合征(3-17)

saturated /ˈsætʃəreɪtɪd/ adj. 饱和的,渗透的(3-10)

scattered /ˈskætərd/ adj. 散射的(2-7)

secrete /sɪˈkriːt/ vt. 藏匿,私下侵吞,分泌(3-13)

secretion /sɪˈkriːʃn/ n. 分泌(物)(1-4)

section /ˈsekʃn/ n. 截面,节段,型材 v. 把……切成片,把……作成截面(4-1)

sediment /ˈsedɪmənt/ n. 沉淀物,沉积物,沉渣(3-5)

sedimentation /ˌsedɪmenˈteɪʃn/ n. 沉淀(2-8)

selenium /səˈliːniəm/ n. 〔化学〕硒(1-5)

semen /ˈsiːmən/ n. 〔生理〕精液,精子(1-1)

semisolid /ˌsemiˈsɒlɪd/ n. 半固体(3-2)

sensitive /ˈsensətɪv/ adj. 敏感的,灵敏的(3-16)

sensitivity /ˌsensəˈtɪvəti/ n. 敏感,敏感度,敏感性(1-1)

sensor /ˈsensər/ n. 传感器(3-1)

sensory /ˈsensəri/ adj. 感觉的(3-11)

sensory perception 感官知觉(3-11)

sequelae /sɪˈkwili/ n. 后遗症(sequela 的复数)(2-4)

sequence /ˈsiːkwəns/ n. 〔数〕〔计〕序列,顺序,续发事件(3-19)

sequencing /ˈsiːkwənsɪŋ/ n. 〔计〕排序,测序(1-7)

serologically /siˈrɒlədʒikli/ adv. 血清学地(3-7)

serum /ˈsɪrəm/ n. (免疫)血清,浆液(3-13)

serum glutamic oxaloacetic transaminase (SGOT)血清谷氨酰草酰乙酸转氨酶(3-12)

serum glutamic pyruvate transaminase (SGPT)血清谷氨酰丙

酮酸转氨酶(3-12)

sexually /ˈsekʃəli/ adv. 两性之间地(4-2)

sheath fluid 鞘液(3-16)

shield /ʃiːld/ vi. 防御,起保护作用(3-16)

sickle cell anemia 镰状细胞贫血(1-7)

side scatter 侧向散射(3-16)

silica /ˈsɪlɪkə/ n. 二氧化硅;[材] 硅土(2-3)

silicate /ˈsɪlɪkeɪt/ n. [矿物] 硅酸盐(2-10)

silicon /ˈsɪlɪkən/ n. [化学] 硅,硅元素(3-20)

silver /ˈsɪlvər/ n. 银(3-20)

simultaneous /ˌsaɪmlˈteɪniəs/ adj. 同时的,联立的,同时发生的(1-7)

skeletal /ˈskelətl/ adj. 骨骼的(3-10)

slide /slaɪd/ n. 载玻片(2-7)

sliding calipers 游标卡尺(3-18)

slip /slɪp/ n. 片(2-7)

slot /slɑːt/ n. 位置(2-8)

smear tests 涂片检查,子宫抹片检查(4-2)

soluble /ˈsɑːljəbl/ adj. [化学] 可溶解的(2-3)

solvent /ˈsɑːlvənt/ n. 溶剂(2-3)

sophisticated /səˈfɪstɪkeɪtɪd/ adj. 精密的(2-5)

sore /sɔːr/ n. 疡,褥疮(3-17)

specific /spəˈsɪfɪk/ adj. 特定的,具有特效的(3-15)

specific gravity 比重(2-6)

specificity /ˌspesɪˈfɪsəti/ n. [免疫] 特异性,特征,专一性(1-4)

specimen /ˈspesɪmən/ n. 样品,样本,标本(1-1)

specimen holder 标本夹,样品夹,试样架(4-1)

spectrophotometer /ˌspektrofoˈtɑːmətər/ n. [光] 分光光度计(2-9)

spectrophotometric /ˌspektrəufəuˈtɔmitrik/ adj. 分光光度计的,光谱仪的(3-14)

spectrophotometry /ˌspektrəuˈfəuˈtɔmitri/ n. [分化] [光] 分光光度(测定)法(2-9)

spectroscopy /spekˈtrɑːskəpi/ n. [光] 光谱学(2-9)

spectrum /ˈspektrəm/ n. 光谱,频谱(1-4)

sperm /spɜːrm/ n. 精子,精液(3-3)

spinal /ˈspaɪnl/ adj. 脊髓的,脊柱的(3-4)

spinal cord 脊髓,脊椎神经(3-4)

split /splɪt/ v. 分离(3-19)

sputum /ˈspjuːtəm/ n. [生理] 痰,唾液(1-2)

squamous /ˈskweməs/ adj. 鳞状的(等于 squamosa 或 squamose)(3-2)

stabilize /ˈsteɪbəlaɪz/ vt. 使安定,使坚固(3-14)

stain /steɪn/ vt. 给……着色(2-7)

standard operating procedure (SOP)标准操作程序(2-11)

starch /stɑːrtʃ/ n. 淀粉(2-8)

STAT analyzer 急诊分析仪(5-4)

state of the art 当前发展状况(2-13)

stem cell 干细胞(3-5)

stem from ... 来自……(3-11)

stepwise /ˈstepwaɪz/ adv. 逐步地,阶梯式地(2-11)

sterile /ˈsterəl/ adj. 无菌的,不生育的(2-3)

sterilization /ˌsterələˈzeɪʃn/ n. [医] [食品] 杀菌,使不孕,无用状态(2-2)

steroid /ˈsterɔɪd/ n. [有化] 类固醇,甾族化合物(3-10)

steroid hormones 类固醇激素,甾体激素(3-10)

stippled /ˈstɪpld/ adj. 带有小圆点的,布满斑点的(3-3)

stool /stuːl/ n. 粪便(1-2)

streak /striːk/ n. 条纹,线条(3-2)

streptococcus pneumoniae 肺炎链球菌(3-18)

stringency /ˈstrɪndʒənsi/ n. 严格(3-20)

strip /strɪp/ n. 条,长条(1-2)

stroke /stroʊk/ n. 中风(3-6)

subarachnoid /ˌsʌbəˈræknɔɪd/ adj. 蛛网膜下的(3-4)

subsequently /ˈsʌbsɪkwəntli/ adv. 随后,其后,后来(2-11)

substrate /ˈsʌbstreɪ/ n. [生化] 基质,基片,酶作用物(等于 substratum)(3-14)

sufficient /səˈfɪʃnt/ adj. 足够的,充足的(2-4)

superficial cell 表层细胞(4-2)

supernatant liquid 上层液体(2-8)

supernate /ˈsjuːpəneɪt/ n. [免疫] 上清液(2-8)

supplemental /ˌsʌpləˈmentl/ adj. 补充的,追加的(3-9)

supplies /səpˈlaɪz/ n. (复数) 物资,医疗设备和用品(2-5)

surface antigen 表面抗原(5-3)

surface engineering 表面工程(3-20)

surfactant /sɜːrˈfæktənt/ n. 表面活性剂(3-17)

surgeon /ˈsɜːrdʒən/ n. 外科医生(5-2)

surgical /ˈsɜːrdʒɪkl/ adj. 外科的(1-3)

susceptible /səˈseptəbl/ adj. 易受影响的,易受感染的(2-5)

suspend /səˈspend/ vt. & vi. 延缓,使暂停,悬浮(3-16)

suspension /səˈspenʃn/ n. 悬浮,暂停,停职(2-6)

swell /swel/ v. 肿胀(5-3)

symptom /ˈsɪmptəm/ n. [临床] 症状,征兆(3-17)

synthesize /ˈsɪnθəsaɪz/ vt. 合成(3-20)

syphilis /ˈsɪfɪlɪs/ n. [性病] 梅毒(3-4)

syphilis serology 梅毒血清学(3-4)

syringe /sɪˈrɪndʒ/ vt. 注射,冲洗 n. 注射器,洗涤器(3-9)

systematic error 系统误差(2-11)

T

tailor /ˈteɪlər/ v. 量身定制,使合适,使适应(2-1)

take ... for example 以……为例(5-2)

tap water 自来水(4-3)

tapered /ˈtepərd/ adj. 锥形的(2-8)

Taq DNA polymerase Taq DNA 聚合酶(3-19)

template /ˈtemplət/ *n.* 模板(3-19)

terminology /ˌtɜːrmɪˈnɑːlədʒi/ *n.* 术语,术语学,用辞(5-1)

test kit 试剂盒(3-17)

testis /ˈtestɪs/ *n.* ［解剖］睾丸(3-11)

tetrazolium /ˌtetrəˈzəuliəm/ *n.* ［化学］四唑(3-14)

texture /ˈtekstʃər/ *n.* 质地,质感(3-3)

the first-generation sequencing technique 第一代测序技术
(1-7)

therapeutic /ˌθerəˈpjuːtɪk/ *adj.* 治疗的,治疗学的(1-1)

thermal /ˈθəːrml/ *adj.* 热的(2-5)

thermal cycler 热循环仪(3-19)

thermal printer 热敏印刷机(3-8)

thermophilic /ˌθəːməuˈfilik/ *adj.* 嗜热的(3-14)

thrombocyte /ˈθrɑmbəˌsaɪt/ *n.* ［组织］血小板,凝血细胞
(1-2)

thrombocytopathy /θrɑmbəˈsitəpəθi/ *n.* ［内科］血小板病
(3-6)

thrombocytopenia /ˌθrɑmbəˌsaɪtəˈpiniə/ *n.* ［内科］血小板减
少(症)(3-6)

thrombocytosis /ˌθrɔmbəusaiˈtəusis/ *n.* ［内科］血小板增多
(症)(3-6)

thromboembolism /ˌθrɒmbəuˈembəlɪzəm/ *n.* ［病理］血栓栓
塞(3-6)

thromboplastin /ˌθrɑmbəˈplæstɪn/ *n.* ［生化］促凝血酶原激
酶,血栓形成质(3-6)

thrombosis /θrɑːmˈbousɪs/ *n.* ［病理］血栓形成,血栓症(复
数 thromboses)(1-1)

throughput /ˈθruːpʊt/ *n.* 生产量,生产能力,通量,吞吐量
(1-7)

thymine /ˈθaɪmɪn/ *n.* ［生化］胸腺嘧啶(3-19)

thyroid /ˈθaɪrɔɪd/ *n.* 甲状腺(1-1)

thyrotoxicosis /ˌθaɪroˌtɑksəˈkosɪs/ *n.* ［内科］甲状腺功能亢
进,甲状腺毒症(3-11)

titration /tɪˈtreɪʃn/ *n.* ［分化］滴定,滴定法(2-4)

tourniquet /ˈtəːrnəkət/ *n.* ［外科］止血带,压脉器,压血带
(2-5)

toxic /ˈtɑːksɪk/ *adj.* 有毒的,中毒的(5-3)

toxicity /tɑːkˈsɪsəti/ *n.* ［毒物］毒效(3-12)

trachea /ˈtreɪkiə/ *n.* ［脊椎］［解剖］气管;［植］导管(3-4)

transaminase /trænsˈæmɪnez/ *n.* ［生化］转氨酶,氨基转移酶
(3-13)

transcription /trænˈskrɪpʃn/ *n.* 转录(3-20)

transcriptome /trænskˈrɪptɒm/ *n.* 转录组(1-7)

transducer /trænzˈduːsər/ *n.* ［自］传感器;［电子］变换器,
换能器(2-10)

transfusion /trænsˈfjuːʒn/ *n.* ［临床］输血,输液(1-1)

transitional cell 移行细胞(3-2)

transmission electron microscopy 透射电子显微镜检查法
(2-7)

transparent /trænsˈpærənt/ *adj.* 透明的,显然的,坦率的,易
懂的(2-7)

tray /treɪ/ *n.* 电泳槽(2-8)

triacylglycerol /traiˈæsilglisərəul/ *n.* ［生化］三酰甘油,甘油
三酯(3-10)

triage/ˈtriɑːʒ/ *n.* 伤员验伤分类,分类(3-15)

trichomoniasis /ˌtrɪkəuməˈnaɪəsɪs/ *n.* 滴虫病(3-3)

trimming /ˈtrɪmɪŋ/ *n.* 整理,装饰品,配料,修剪下来的东西
(4-1)

Trisomy 21 syndrome (Down's syndrome) 21 三体综合征(唐
氏综合征)(1-7)

troponin /ˈtroupənɪn/ *n.* ［生化］肌钙蛋白(1-4)

tuberculosis /tuːbɜːrkjəˈlousɪs/ *n.* 肺结核(1-7)

tubular /ˈtuːbjələr/ *adj.* 管状的(3-2)

tumorigenesis /ˌtʊmərəˈdʒɛnɪsɪs/ *n.* 肿瘤发生(1-7)

tumour /ˈtuːmər/ *n.* ［肿瘤］瘤,肿瘤,肿块(3-13)

turret /ˈtɜːrət/ *n.* 转台(2-7)

U

ubiquitous /juˈbɪkwɪtəs/ *adj.* 普遍存在的(2-3)

ultra /ˈʌltrə/ *adj.* 过激的(2-3)

ultrafiltrate /ˌʌltrəˈfiltreit/ *n.* ［化学］超滤液(3-4)

ultra-pure water 超纯净水(2-3)

ultraviolet-visible spectroscopy 紫外可见光光谱法(2-9)

unbranched /ˈʌnˈbrɑːntʃt/ *adj.* 无支链的(3-10)

uncoating /ˌʌnˈkəutiŋ/ *n.* 病毒脱壳(3-17)

unconjugated bilirubin 未结合胆红素(3-12)

under-secretion /ˌʌndə siˈkriːʃn/ *n.* 分泌低下(3-11)

United States Patent(USP) 美国专利(2-4)

unresponsive /ˌʌnrɪˈspɑːnsɪv/ *adj.* 反应迟钝的(3-11)

urea /jʊˈriːə/ *n.* ［肥料］尿素(1-4)

urea nitrogen 尿素氮(2-12)

urinalysis /ˌjʊrəˈnæləsɪs/ *n.* 尿液分析(1-2)

urinary casts 尿管型(1-2)

urine /ˈjʊrɪn/ *n.* 尿,小便(3-15)

urothelial /jʊˈrɑːˈθiliəl/ *adj.* 泌尿道上皮的(3-2)

V

vacutainer /ˈvækjʊteɪnə/ *n.* 真空采血管(2-5)

vacuum /ˈvækjuːm/ *n.* 真空,空间 *adj.* 真空的,利用真空的,
产生真空的(2-6)

vaginal /vəˈdʒaɪnl/ *adj.* ［解剖］阴道的(1-2)

vaginal discharge 阴道分泌物(2-7)

vaginal smear 阴道涂片(3-3)

validate /ˈvælɪdeɪt/ v. 证实,验证(2-4)

validation /ˌvælɪˈdeɪʃn/ n. 确认,批准,生效(2-11)

vasodilation /ˌveɪzoʊdaɪˈleɪʃn/ n. 血管舒张(3-9)

vendor /ˈvendər/ n. 供应商,销售商(2-12)

venipuncture /ˈveniˌpʌŋktʃə/ n. 静脉穿刺(等于 venepuncture)(5-1)

venous /ˈviːnəs/ adj. 静脉的(2-1)

ventilation /ˌventɪˈleɪʃn/ n. 通风设备,空气流通(3-9)

vertebrate /ˈvɜːrtɪbrət/ adj. 脊椎动物的 n. 脊椎动物(3-5)

vertical /ˈvɜːtɪkl/ adj. 垂直的,直立的 [解剖] 头顶的,顶点的(2-2)

very low-density lipoprotein (VLDL)极低密度脂蛋白(3-10)

via /ˈvaɪə/ prep. 通过(3-20)

vinyl /ˈvaɪnl/ n. 乙烯基(化学)(2-10)

viral nucleic acid quantification of infectious diseases 感染性疾病病毒核酸定量(1-1)

virion /ˈvaɪərɪˌɑn/ n. [病毒] 病毒粒子,病毒体(3-17)

virulence /ˈvɪrələns/ n. 毒力,毒性,恶意(等于 virulency)(3-17)

virulent /ˈvɪrələnt/ adj. 剧毒的(1-6)

virus /ˈvaɪrəs/ n. 病毒(1-6)

viscosity /vɪˈskɑːsəti/ n. 黏性,黏度(2-8)

volt /voʊlt/ n. 伏特(电压单位)(2-10)

voltage /ˈvoʊltɪdʒ/ n. [电] 电压(2-11)

voltammetry /voʊlˈtæmitri/ n. [分化] 伏安法(2-10)

voltmeter /ˈvoʊltmiːtər/ n. 伏特计,电压表(2-10)

wafer /ˈweɪfər/ n. 圆片,晶片,薄片(3-18)

warfarin /ˈwɔːrfərɪn/ n. 华法林(1-7)

wart /wɔːrt/ n. [皮肤] 疣(等于 verruca)(3-3)

wavelength limits 波长范围(2-9)

waxy /ˈwæksi/ adj. 像蜡的(3-10)

western blot 免疫印迹(法)(3-17)

white cell differential 白细胞分类(5-3)

WHO Model List of Essential Medicines WHO 基本药物示范目录(2-6)

Widal test 肥达试验(1-5)

winged infusion needle 有翼输液针(2-5)

work flow 工作流程(2-5)

workup /ˈwɜːrkʌp/ n. 病情检查(2-5)

xenon /ˈzenɑːn/ n. [化学] 氙(3-16)

yeast /jiːst/ n. 泡沫,酵母,酵母片(3-3)

zone of inhibition 抑菌圈(3-18)